Opioid Use, Overuse, and Abuse in Otolaryngology

Opioid Use, Overuse, and Abuse in Otolaryngology

Edited by

Ryan J. Li, MD FACS

Associate Professor
Oregon Health & Science University
Otolaryngology-Head and Neck Surgery

ELSEVIER

Publisher: Sarah Barth
Acquisitions Editor: Jessica L. McCool
Editorial Project Manager: Tracy Tufaga
Project Manager: Sreejith Viswanathan
Cover Designer: Matthew Limbert

3251 Riverport Lane
St. Louis, Missouri 63043

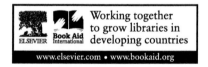

Working together to grow libraries in developing countries

www.elsevier.com • www.bookaid.org

Contents

CHAPTER 8   Nonopioid pain management in otolaryngology—head and neck surgery: the pharmacist's perspective 151

Rebecca Britton, PharmD, BCPS, Kylee Kastelic,
PharmD, Robert Osten, PharmD, BCPS, BCGP
and Renita Patel, PharmD, BCPS

CHAPTER 9   Addiction management in the outpatient setting .. 169

Julia M. Shi, MD, FACP, Benjamin J. Slocum, DO,
Jeanette M. Tetrault, MD, FACP, FASAM and
Ken Yanagisawa, MD, FACS

CHAPTER 10   International perioperative pain management approaches... 189

*Catherine P.L. Chan, MRCSEd (ENT), MRes, MB ChB
and Jason Y.K. Chan, MBBS*

Contributors

Brittany Abud, MD
Department of Otolaryngology, University of Illinois Chicago, Chicago, IL, United States

Virginie Achim, MD, FACS
Head and Neck Surgeon, ENT, Columbia Surgical Specialists, Spokane, WA, United States

Rebecca Britton, PharmD, BCPS
Department of Pharmacy, Oregon Health and Science University, Portland, OR, United States

Catherine P.L. Chan, MRCSEd (ENT), MRes, MB ChB
Department of Ear, Nose and Throat, Prince of Wales Hospital, Shatin, Hong Kong SAR, China

Jason Y.K. Chan, MBBS
Department of Otorhinolaryngology, Head and Neck Surgery, The Chinese University of Hong Kong, Shatin, Hong Kong SAR, China

Ravi A. Chandra, MD, PhD
Oregon Health & Science University, Department of Radiation Medicine, Portland, OR, United States

Ruth J. Davis, MD
Department of Otolaryngology—Head and Neck Surgery, Johns Hopkins University School of Medicine, Baltimore, MD, United States

Nyssa Fox Farrell, MD
Washington University in St. Louis School of Medicine, Department of Otolaryngology-Head and Neck Surgery, St. Louis, MO, United States

Jay K. Ferrell, MD
Division of Head and Neck Surgery, Department of Otolaryngology-Head and Neck Surgery, UT Health San Antonio Long School of Medicine, San Antonio, TX, United States

Abhishek Gami, BS
Johns Hopkins University, School of Medicine, Baltimore, MD, United States

Andrew W. Joseph, MD, MPH
Department of Otolaryngology—Head and Neck Surgery, University of Michigan Medical School, Ann Arbor, MI, United States

Kylee Kastelic, PharmD
Department of Pharmacy, Oregon Health and Science University, Portland, OR, United States

Cymon Kersch, MD, PhD
Providence Portland Medical Center, Department of Internal Medicine, Medical Education, Portland, OR, United States

Ryan Li, MD
Oregon Health & Science University, Department of Otolaryngology-Head and Neck Surgery, Portland, OR, United States

Choopong Luansritisakul, MD, FRCAT
Department of Anesthesiology, Faculty of Medicine Siriraj Hospital, Mahidol University, Bangkok, Thailand

Christopher Mularczyk, MD
Department of Otolaryngology, University of Illinois Chicago, Chicago, IL, United States

Robert Osten, PharmD, BCPS, BCGP
Department of Pharmacy, Oregon Health and Science University, Portland, OR, United States

Adlai Pappy, MD, MBA
Department of Anesthesiology, Perioperative, and Pain Medicine, Brigham and Women's Hospital, Harvard Medical School, Boston, MA, United States

Renita Patel, PharmD, BCPS
Department of Pharmacy, Oregon Health and Science University, Portland, OR, United States

Julia M. Shi, MD, FACP
Medical Director, Primary Care Services, APT Foundation, New Haven, CT, United States; Associate Clinical Professor of Medicine, Yale University School of Medicine, New Haven, CT, United States

Maisie L. Shindo, MD
Head & Neck Endocrine Surgery, Thyroid and Parathyroid Center, Department of Otolaryngology-Head and Neck Surgery, Oregon Health and Science University, Portland, OR, United States

Benjamin J. Slocum, DO
Family Medicine, Central Maine Healthcare, Gray, ME, United States

Timothy Smith, MD, MPH
Oregon Health & Science University, Department of Otolaryngology-Head and Neck Surgery, Portland, OR, United States

Daniel Q. Sun, MD
Johns Hopkins University, Department of Otolaryngology-Head and Neck Surgery, Baltimore, MD, United States

Jeanette M. Tetrault, MD, FACP, FASAM
Professor of Medicine and Public Health, Vice Chief for Education, Section of
General Internal Medicine, Program Director, Addiction Medicine Fellowship,
Associate Director for Education and Training, Program in Addiction Medicine,
Yale University School of Medicine, New Haven, CT, United States

David E. Tunkel, MD
Department of Otolaryngology—Head and Neck Surgery, Johns Hopkins
University School of Medicine, Baltimore, MD, United States

Yanjun Xie, MD
Department of Otolaryngology—Head and Neck Surgery, University of Michigan
Medical School, Ann Arbor, MI, United States

Ken Yanagisawa, MD, FACS
Managing Partner, Southern New England Ear Nose Throat & Facial Plastic
Surgery Group, LLP, New Haven, CT, United States; Section Chief of
Otolaryngology, Yale New Haven Hospital, New Haven, CT, United States;
Associate Clinical Professor of Surgery, Yale University School of Medicine, New
Haven, CT, United States; Assistant Clinical Professor of Surgery, Frank H. Netter
MD School of Medicine, Quinnipiac University, Hamden, CT, United States

Nantthasorn Zinboonyahgoon, MD
Department of Anesthesiology, Faculty of Medicine Siriraj Hospital, Mahidol
University, Bangkok, Thailand

Introduction

The experience of pain and the management thereof can be exhausting and frustrating for both patients and healthcare providers. There is a science and an art in the care of patients suffering from pain. There is a heightened awareness of opioid misuse in recent years. However, the pendulum can swing so far in the direction of opioid avoidance as to create an unnecessarily restrictive analgesia pathway. A few years ago an experienced head and neck surgeon reminded me that the presence of pain indicates a real problem. This may have seemed obvious, but it highlighted the need to earnestly investigate pain symptoms, and put aside cynicism.

Throughout this book, authors from otolaryngology-head and neck surgery subspecialties, addiction medicine specialists, pharmacists, radiation oncologists, and anesthesiologists have contributed perspective from their clinical experience in the management of pain. They also provide a thorough review of salient pain management literature across multiple disciplines. These good works have informed logical approaches to preoperative, intraoperative, and postoperative analgesia in otolaryngology-head and neck surgery, and head and neck cancer treatment. The discussion continues with a contemporary update on the monitoring of opioid utilization, and the humane treatment of patients with opioid use disorder. Perspective from a head and neck surgery program in Hong Kong provides insight into analgesic approaches internationally. This book can be read from beginning to end, or as chapters with value on their own. We appreciate the opportunity to share our experience and lessons learned from our colleagues in responsible opioid utilization and compassionate pain management.

Ryan J. Li, MD FACS

The evolution of perioperative pain management in otolaryngology—head and neck surgery

Virginie Achim, MD, FACS [1], **Christopher Mularczyk, MD** [2], **Brittany Abud, MD** [2]

[1]*Head and Neck Surgeon, ENT, Columbia Surgical Specialists, Spokane, WA, United States;*
[2]*Department of Otolaryngology, University of Illinois Chicago, Chicago, IL, United States*

Overview and historical pain management

Perioperative pain management is an essential component of surgical care. In the United States, an estimated 360,000—420,000 head and neck surgeries are performed annually.[10] Pain severity tends to differ depending upon the type of otolaryngological procedure performed as well as with the anatomic location of the procedure.[11] Opioid pain medications have been a mainstay in the treatment of acute perioperative pain in head and neck surgery. Early publications from the 1930s demonstrate that pain control was primarily achieved with opioids and salicylates for tonsillectomy and adenoidectomy. In the 1950s, the addition of adjunctive local anesthetics, such as effocaine, to tonsillectomy procedures provided further pain control.[12–14]

Oncology patients make up a significant proportion of patients requiring pain control, with nearly 50% of cancer patients undergoing treatment reporting pain.[15] In the United States, an estimated 54,000 new oral cavity and pharyngeal cancers, 12,600 new laryngeal cancers, and 44,200 new thyroid cancers will be diagnosed in 2021.[16] Additionally, an estimated 586,000 thyroid, 377,000 lip/oral cavity, 184,000 larynx, 133,000 nasopharynx, 98,000 oropharynx, 84,000 hypopharynx, and 53,000 salivary gland malignancies will be diagnosed in 2020 worldwide.[17] Surgical resection is a mainstay for the treatment of many head and neck cancers, and therefore, a strong understanding of perioperative pain management is essential for the care of head and neck oncology patients.[18]

Pain management continues to evolve in the otolaryngology practice, and several shifts in prescribing patterns have occurred over the past several decades. Notably, an increase in the prevalence of opioid prescription began in the 1990s, which coincided with an increase in opioid dependence, and opioid-related deaths within the United States have brought attention to prescribing practices among physicians.[19] These consequences have been a major driving force in the evolution of pain management within otolaryngology and include the introduction and implementation of multimodal analgesic strategies and enhanced recovery protocols that aim to limit the use of opioid analgesics. Another notable shift in perioperative pain management includes the cessation of codeine-containing analgesia for pediatric patients undergoing adenotonsillectomy as a result of deaths among patients who hypermetabolize the drug into its active opioid.[20]

The first enhanced recovery after surgery (ERAS) protocol specific to otolaryngology was published by Coyle et al. in 2016. Their ERAS protocol was developed specifically for patients undergoing head and neck oncology procedures. Further ERAS protocols have been subsequently tailored to more specific procedures such as head and neck cancer resection with free-flap reconstruction and thyroid/parathyroid surgery. ERAS protocols are multifaceted with an overall goal of improving the perioperative experience for the patient and improving outcomes of major surgeries by decreasing length of hospitalization and reducing postoperative complication rates. Pain control is a key component of all ERAS protocols, and a majority of these protocols involve a multimodal pain management strategy in an effort to decrease the number of opioid analgesics utilized during recovery. These strategies will be further discussed within this chapter.[4,21,22]

Typical pain management regimens

A strong understanding of perioperative pain management provides a basis for safe perioperative care in patients undergoing head and neck surgery. Perioperative pain regimens often include a combination of opioid and/or nonopioid medications that are oriented toward decreasing each medication's side effects and limiting the overall use of opioids. The exact pain management regimen selected is often based on provider preference and patient factors such as medication allergies, renal and liver function, enteral status, the type of procedure performed, and expected pain levels. Care should also be taken for patients who undergo procedures requiring airway manipulation and in patients with obstructive sleep apnea, as opioids pose a risk of sedation and respiratory depression.[19] Several nonopioid analgesics including nonsteroidal anti-inflammatory drugs, acetaminophen, anticonvulsants such as gabapentin, corticosteroids, and locoregional anesthetics may be utilized in an effort to decrease the risks associated with opioid use in patients undergoing head and neck surgery. Medications commonly utilized within the perioperative period are included in Table 1.1.

Table 1.1 Various commonly used medications in the treatment of perioperative pain.

Route of administration	Class	Medication	Dose	Mechanism of action	Special considerations	Side effects	History
Oral/ Nasogastic tube/ Gastrostomy tube	Analgesic/ Antipyretic	Acetaminophen	650 mg Q6h-950 mg Q8h	Activation of descending serotonergic inhibitory pathways in CNS	Hepatic dosing	Hearing loss, skin rash	First used clinically in 1893, did not appear commercially until 1950s in the US[33]
	NSAID	Ibuprofen	200–400 mg Q4-6h	Reversibly inhibits COX-1 and 2 resulting in decreased prostaglandin production	Renal dosing or omit in patients with CKD or decreased GFR Cardiovascular considerations	Decreased hemoglobin, increased serum ALT and AST, edema, dyspepsia, nausea, vomiting, prolonged bleeding time, rash	COX genes were characterized in the 1980s and NSAIDs were developed shortly after.[25]
		Celecoxib	Preop: 200 mg once Postop: 200 mg BID and continue for 5 days postop[1]	Decreases prostaglandin synthesis by selectively inhibiting the activity of COX-2		Acute myocardial infarction, angina, palpitations, alopecia, dermatitis, GI symptoms, GERD, anemia, thrombocytopenia, increased liver enzymes, bronchospasm	
	Anticonvulsants	Gabapentin	300–1200 mg TID	Not well known. Proposed	Renal dosing or omit in patients	Somnolence, dizziness, ataxia,	Gabapentin was originally approved

Continued

Table 1.1 Various commonly used medications in the treatment of perioperative pain.—*cont'd*

Route of administration	Class	Medication	Dose	Mechanism of action	Special considerations	Side effects	History
		Pregabalin	50–300 mg BID	mechanisms include the class being structurally related to GABA, antagonism of calcium channels in CNS, and antagonism of NMDA receptors	with CKD or decreased GFR, need for up-titration based on side effects	asthenia, hypertension, hyperglycemia, weight gain, skin rash, constipation, nausea, impotence, infection, emotional lability	in the United Kingdom in 1993. Pregabalin was approved in Europe in 2014[26]
	Opioid	Tramadol	50 mg Q4-6h PRN	Partial mu agonist, in addition to central GABA, catecholamine, and serotonergic activities.	Renal dosing may interfere with serotonin and norepinephrine	Constipation, nausea, drowsiness, orthostatic hypotension, pruritus, hyperglycemia	It was first synthesized in 1962 and has been available for pain treatment since 1977[27]
		Acetaminophen-hydrocodone Oxycodone	325–5 mg Q6h PRN 5–10 mg Q4-6h PRN	Mu opioid receptor agonist	Hepatic dosing	Sedation, tolerance respiratory depression, constipation, nausea/vomiting, urinary retention, hearing loss, skin rash	Oxycodone has been in clinical use since 1917[28]
Intravenous (IV)	Opioid	Morphine Hydromorphone	1–4 mg IV Q1-4h PRN 0.2–1 mg IV Q2-3h PRN	Mu opioid receptor agonists	Renal dosing	Sedation, tolerance respiratory depression, constipation, nausea/vomiting, urinary retention	Morphine was isolated in 1804 by a German pharmacist[29]

Class	Drug	Dose	Mechanism	Dosing Considerations	Side Effects	Notes
Analgesic/Antipyretic	Acetaminophen	650 mg IV Q6H	Activation of descending serotonergic inhibitory pathways in CNS	Hepatic dosing	Nausea, vomiting	
Corticosteroid	Dexamethasone	8–10 mg IV Q8h	Suppresses neutrophil migration, decreases the production of inflammatory mediators, and reverses increased capillary permeability; suppresses normal immune response	Dose reduction in diabetic patients	Cardiac arrhythmias, bradycardia, depression, euphoria, insomnia, psychosis, acne vulgaris, adrenal suppression, decreased glucose tolerance, growth suppression, hirsutism, weight gain, infection, fractures, osteoporosis, impaired wound healing	Dexamethasone was introduced in the 1950s[30]
NSAIDs	Ketorolac	15–30 mg IV Q6h PRN	Decreases prostaglandin synthesis by weakly inhibiting both COX-1 and COX-2	Should be limited to 72 h of use maximum. Consider renal dosing	Dyspepsia, increased liver enzymes, headache, hypertension, pruritus, gastrointestinal ulcer, heartburn, prolonged bleeding time, anemia	

Continued

Table 1.1 Various commonly used medications in the treatment of perioperative pain.—*cont'd*

Route of administration	Medication	Class	Dose	Mechanism of action	Special considerations	Side effects	History
Patient-controlled analgesia (PCA)	Morphine	Opioid	Demand dose: 0.5–2 mg Lockout (min): 6–10 Continuous basal: 0–2 mg/h (not recommended)	Mu opioid receptor agonists	Renal dosing	Sedation, tolerance respiratory depression, constipation, nausea/vomiting, urinary retention	Morphine was isolated in 1804 by a German pharmacist.
	Hydromorphone		Demand dose: 0.1–0.4 mg Lockout (min): 6–10 Continuous basal: 0.0.4 mg/h (not recommended)		Renal dosing		
	Fentanyl		Demand dose: 5–50 µg Lockout (min): 5–10 Continuous basal: 0–2 mg/h (not recommended)		Preferred opioid for patients with renal or hepatic dysfunction		

			Dosing	Mechanism	Pharmacokinetics	Adverse effects
Transdermal	Opioid	Fentanyl	Apply 1 device (40 mcg dose delivered over 10 min; maximum 6 doses per hour). 1 device operates for 24 h or 80 doses. Reapply Q24h for a maximum duration of up to 72 h	Mu opioid receptor agonist	Has a lag time of 6–12 h to onset of action, and typically reaches a steady state in 3–6 days. After removal, a subcutaneous reservoir remains, and drug clearance may take up to 24 h	Peripheral edema, hyperhidrosis, dehydration, hypokalemia, abdominal pain, nausea, vomiting, constipation, anemia, confusion, drowsiness, dyspnea, pneumonia
	Local anesthetics (amides and esters)	Lidocaine	3.5%–4% patch: apply to the affected area for up to 12 h in a 24-h period	Blocks initiation and conduction of nerve impulses by decreasing the neuronal membrane's permeability to sodium ions, which results in inhibition of depolarization with resultant blockade of conduction		Erythema, petechia, edema, pruritus, nausea, flushing, metallic taste, dermatitis, burning

BID, *twice daily*; CKD, *chronic kidney disease*; COX, *cyclooxygenase*; GFR, *glomerular filtration rate*; NMDA, *N-methyl-ᴅ-aspartate*; NSAID, *nonsteroidal antiinflammatory drug*; PRN, *pro re nata*; Q, *every*; TID, *3 times a day.*

Doses are a range compiled from different published articles and are provided as a guideline. The doses should be adjusted and titrated when appropriate. Additionally, dosing adjustments or medication alternatives must be implemented for patients with hepatic or renal dysfunction when appropriate, or other contraindications to the medications listed.[1,2,23–32]

Opioids and changes in prescribing habits within otolaryngology

The opioid epidemic remains an important health crisis that continues to shape how prescribers manage perioperative pain. Between 1991 and 2010, the number of opioid prescriptions in the United States nearly tripled as a result of several contributing factors.[34] Routine documentation of patients' pain levels as a vital sign was recommended in a consensus statement introduced in 1995 by the American Pain Society. The consensus statement also advised frequent pain assessments, prompt pain control, and assessment of pain response to analgesics provided.[35] In the late 1990s, state medical boards reduced restrictions on opioid prescriptions for non-cancer patients, and in 2000 the Joint Commission on the Accreditation of Health Care Organizations introduced new inpatient and outpatient pain management standards. Other factors that may have compounded the increase in opioid utilization included an increase in patient awareness of pain control via opioid medication, claims of undertreatment of pain, physician promotion, and marketing by the pharmaceutical industry.[36,37] Several misconceptions regarding opioids exist including the belief that they are a uniquely powerful pain reliever, that they are particularly effective for acute pain, and that short-term courses do not pose a risk of long-term use or opioid use disorders. These misconceptions also likely contributed to their overuse.[38] Risks of opioid prescription have long been established and include respiratory depression, constipation, nausea, vomiting, sedation, tolerance, opioid dependence, overdose, and opioid-related death. Additionally, more recent studies suggest that opioids modulate immune function and contribute to delayed wound healing that may further negatively impact postoperative recovery, however, these findings require further investigation.[19,39,40]

The increase in opioid prescribing has been correlated with an increase in opioid-related deaths and hospital admissions.[41,42] The most recently published cause of mortality data by the Centers for Disease Control and Prevention (CDC) ranges from 1999 to 2019. The age-adjusted death rate in the United States involving all opioids increased from 2.9 per 100,000 population in 1999 to 15.5 per 100,000 population in 2019.[43] Between 2013 and 2019, death from drug overdose increased by 56.5%, with a total of 70,360 opioid-related deaths reported in 2019. Of these opioid-related deaths within the United States, the age-adjusted death rate from synthetic opioids increased from 1.0 (2013) to 11.4 (2019) per 100,000 population, and the prescription opioid-related death rate decreased from 4.4 (2013) to 4.2 (2019) per 100,000 population.[44]

The CDC Annual Surveillance Report of Drug-Related Health Risks was most recently updated for 2019. This report demonstrated that the total volume of opioid prescriptions in the United States peaked in 2012 with an annual dispense rate of 81.3 per 100 persons, accounting for 255 million prescriptions. Additionally, in 2012, surgeons accounted for 9.8% of the total annual opioid prescriptions made and prescribed opioids at a rate of 36.5% of their total prescriptions.[45] A steady decline in prescription dispense rate has occurred between 2012 and 2019, with a dispense rate of 46.7 per 100 persons and 153 million prescriptions written in 2019.[46]

The risk of developing long-term opioid use has been correlated with the duration of the initial prescription. Alam et al. performed a retrospective cohort study to assess long-term opioid use in patients who underwent short stay surgery between 1999 and 2008 and demonstrated patients who received an opioid pain medication within 7 days of an outpatient procedure were 44% more likely to become long term users than those who did not receive an opioid. Long-term use was defined as having filled an opioid prescription greater than 10 months from the initial procedure date.[47] Characteristics that have been proposed to increase the likelihood of long-term opioid use include the duration of the prescription, number of refills provided, and providing second opioid prescriptions. Likelihood of long-term opioid use begins to rise in patients who receive postoperative opioid prescriptions longer than 3 days duration, with the sharpest increase in likelihood at the 10th day and 30th day of a prescription. An estimated one in seven patients who receive opioid refills, or a second opioid prescriptions, remain on opioids 1 year later.[48] Additionally, an estimated 33% of patients who undergo a resection for head and neck cancer continue opioid use >90 days after the procedure, with an increased likelihood in patients with preoperative opioid use.[49]

Otolaryngologists continue to make efforts to transition away from opioid utilization. Nonopioid strategies and strategies that decrease the number of opioids prescribed for postoperative pain management have demonstrated success in many studies and often involve a multimodal approach. These multimodal strategies include the use of local and regional anesthesia, acetaminophen and nonsteroidal antiinflammatory drugs (NSAIDs), γ-aminobutyric acid agonists (i.e., Gabapentin, pregabalin), tramadol, as well as the implementation of advanced recovery after surgery protocols.[19] While many studies demonstrate a reduced opioid requirement with multimodal approaches to analgesia, the true analgesia requirements for various procedures remain poorly understood due to the heterogeneity of the procedures performed by the otolaryngologist.[50] Subsets of procedures have been explored to include head and neck oncologic surgeries, neck dissection, and endocrine surgeries.[4−6,21]

Additional factors that have facilitated a decrease in opioid prescription by physicians include governmental legislation. While the 2016 opioid prescribing guidelines for chronic pain by the CDC does not specifically address perioperative pain management, the guideline does discuss treatment of acute pain. It states when using opioids for acute pain, the lowest effective dose of immediate-release opioids should be used, and the quantity should be no greater than the expected duration of pain severe enough to require opioids. They conclude that 3 days or less of opioids is often sufficient for acute pain, and rarely is more than 7 days of opioids required.[51] Since its publication in 2016, 49 states have implemented a prescription drug monitoring program (PDMP) and have demonstrated success in the reduction of opioid prescription within otolaryngology. Rubin et al. assessed the effectiveness of Massachusetts' prescription awareness tool specifically on otolaryngologic procedures and demonstrated a statistically significant reduction in opioid prescriptions for thyroidectomy, tonsillectomy, and parotidectomy since their states program initiation in 2016.[52] Legislation that limits the duration of opioid prescription have also been shown to significantly decrease the duration of opioids prescribed, decrease the proportion of patients receiving an opioid, and decrease the total opioid dose prescribed postoperatively specifically within otolaryngology.[53]

In 2021, the American Academy of Otolaryngology—Head and Neck Surgery published their first clinical practice guidelines addressing opioid prescribing for analgesia after common otolaryngology operations. The guidelines outlined 10 key action statements can be found in Table 1.2.[9]

Table 1.2 A brief overview of key action statements as outline by the American Academy of Otolaryngology—Head and Neck Surgery in 2021.

Statement	Action: clinicians should...	Strength
Statement 1: Expected pain	Preoperatively advise patients and those involved in the postoperative care about expected severity and duration of pain	Recommendation
Statement 2: Modifying factors	Preoperatively gather information about specific patient factors that may modulate the severity or duration of pain	Recommendation
Statement 3A: Risk factors for opioid use disorder	Preoperatively identify patient-specific risk factors for opioid use disorder when analgesia with opioids is anticipated	Strong recommendation
Statement 3B: Patients at risk for opioid use disorder	Preoperative evaluate the need for modification of postoperative pain management plan in patients at risk for opioid use disorder	Recommendation
Statement 4: Shared decision making	Encourage shared decision making by informing patients of the benefits and risks of postoperative pain treatments that include nonopioid analgesics, opioid analgesics, and nonpharmacologic interventions	Recommendation
Statement 5: Multimodal therapy	Develop a multimodal treatment strategy for the management of postoperative pain	Recommendation
Statement 6: Nonopioid analgesia	Advocate for the use of nonopioid medications as the first line for postoperative pain management	Strong recommendation
Statement 7: Opioid prescribing	Limit therapy to the lowest effective dose and shortest duration when treating pain with opioids	Recommendation

Table 1.2 A brief overview of key action statements as outline by the American Academy of Otolaryngology—Head and Neck Surgery in 2021.—*cont'd*

Statement	Action: clinicians should…	Strength
Statement 8A: Patient feedback	Educate patients and caregivers on how to communicate if pain is not controlled, or if side effects are experienced from pain medications	Recommendation
Statement 8B: Stopping pain medications	Recommend patients discontinue opioids when pain is controlled with nonopioids, and discontinue all analgesics when pain has resolved.	Recommendation
Statement 9: Storage and disposal of opioids	Recommend patients or caregivers securely store opioids, and dispose of unused opioids through take-back programs or other accepted means	Strong recommendation
Statement 10: Assessment of pain control with opioids	Inquire within 30 days postoperatively whether a patient has stopped use of opioids, has properly disposed of unused opioids, and was satisfied with their postoperative pain management plan	Recommendation

Table adapted from Anne S, Mims J, Tunkel DE, et al. Clinical practice guideline: opioid prescribing for analgesia after common otolaryngology operations. *Otolaryngol Head Neck Surg. 2021;164(2_suppl): S1—S42.*

Perioperative considerations for patients on long-term opioid therapy

Perioperative pain management is commonly performed by the anesthesiologist in addition to the surgeon. Perioperative regimens typically combine opioid and non-opioid adjuvants to enhance analgesia in a synergistic fashion via central and peripheral pathways.[54] Roughly 80% of head and neck cancer patients experience pain before treatment, and greater than 40% of these patients receive opioid pain medications before treatment.[55] Otolaryngologists must be aware of tolerance as a result of chronic opioid use, which may require an increased dose of opioid medication to achieve a desired therapeutic effect.[3,56]

Patients receiving long-term opioid medications such as methadone and buprenorphine for substance use disorder or chronic pain require special considerations. Methadone should be continued postoperatively, and the appropriate dose should be confirmed through PDMPs or by calling the patient's methadone clinic, as these clinics do not typically report to PDMPs. Surgeons should also establish a discharge plan, which may include resuming these medications, however, the patient should not be discharged with a prescription or refill as methadone and buprenorphine require a DEA-X license to prescribe, and therefore appropriate follow-up with the patient's outpatient provider is essential.[3]

Buprenorphine may create particular difficulty in the management of acute perioperative pain, as its properties as a partial agonist, its long half-life, and high receptor binding affinity interfere with the effectiveness of other opioids. No current consensus exists for the optimal management strategy for patients receiving buprenorphine. Therefore, a pain management strategy involving input from the perioperative team of surgeons, anesthesiologists, addiction specialists, nurses, and the patient should be developed when possible. Preoperative and postoperative medication transitions should be managed by addiction and/or pain specialists, as abrupt discontinuation of buprenorphine in the stressful perioperative period risks relapse of opioid use disorder. The risks and benefits of continuing or discontinuing buprenorphine perioperatively and the risks of using alternative opioids should be explicitly discussed with patients. Additionally, the surgeon should inquire about the patient's beliefs regarding pain and the planned procedure, and their coping strategies when under stress. If additional opioids are necessary for postoperative pain control after discharge, a safety plan should be developed that may involve limiting the number of pills prescribed, using a locked medication box, or having a family member hold the medication.[57]

Evolution in pain management for pediatric tonsillectomy

Pain control in children represents a challenge as some children may not be able to accurately communicate their pain. Many pediatric pain management regimens may include acetaminophen, NSAIDs such as ibuprofen or ketorolac, opioids including morphine or oxycodone, nerve blockade with local anesthetics, and use of adjuncts such as dexamethasone.[58]

Approximately 530,000 children in the United States undergo tonsillectomy alone or adenotonsillectomy per year.[59] Codeine had previously been a mainstay for management of posttonsillectomy pain in the pediatric population; however, the use of opioids for postoperative analgesia in children has fallen out of favor due to the severe side effects of opioids that includes respiratory depression and associated deaths.[60] Notably, there is a small percentage of children that rapidly metabolize codeine into morphine, causing elevated and potentially fatal blood opioid levels despite prescription of standard doses of codeine. This phenotype was associated with a functional duplication of the CYP2D6 allele that encodes cytochrome p450 2D6.[20,61] In 2013, the United States Food and Drug Administration issued a black box warning and contraindication for codeine use in children after tonsillectomy and/or adenoidectomy after deaths in children with obstructive sleep apnea occurred with evidence of ultrarapid metabolization.[62] While codeine has demonstrated adverse events in hypermetabolizers, providers must also be aware that postoperative opioid use, even in normal metabolizers, has been linked to oxygen desaturations in pediatric patients with obstructive sleep apnea when used in the immediate postoperative period.[63] Currently, the American Academy of Otolaryngology Clinical Practice Guideline for tonsillectomy makes a strong recommendation against prescribing any medication containing codeine in children under 12 years of age.[64]

Post-tonsillectomy bleeding has been reported to occur at a mean of 4.5% based on a meta-analysis.[65] There has been controversy surrounding whether NSAIDs are associated with an increased risk of postoperative bleeding in children after tonsillectomy. D'Souza et al. conducted a retrospective chart review of children who received acetaminophen and ibuprofen following intracapsular tonsillectomy with or without adenoidectomy. They found that the incidence of posttonsillectomy hemorrhage (PTH) requiring a return to the operating room was higher in the NSAID group when compared to the narcotic group.[66] A 2003 systemic review by Moiniche et al. concluded that NSAIDS use and an associated increased bleeding risk after tonsillectomy remains ambiguous. They also demonstrated a lack of evidence for whether a single-dose versus multiple-dose NSAID regimen impacted the rates of PTH. Additionally, their study suggested that NSAIDs are equianalgesic to opioid therapy. Another review by Lewis et al. assessing NSAIDs in children undergoing elective tonsillectomy or adenotonsillectomy concluded there is insufficient evidence to exclude an increased risk of bleeding when NSAIDs are used in pediatric tonsillectomy.[67] It has also been speculated that there may be a difference in the risk of postoperative bleeding between adult and pediatric populations. A 2014 systematic review and meta-analysis evaluating posttonsillectomy hemorrhage rates in subjects receiving perioperative ketorolac found that adults are at five times increased risk for posttonsillectomy hemorrhage with ketorolac use while children are not at a statistically significantly increased risk.[68]

On the other hand, a 2013 meta-analysis demonstrated no evidence of an increase in postoperative bleeding risk, more severe bleeding, or an increased need for operative control of posttonsillectomy bleeding among pediatric or adult patients receiving NSAIDs postoperatively. Subgroups analyzed for the specific NSAID used (ibuprofen, diclofenac, ketorolac, ketoprofen, and Lornoxicam) also demonstrated no significant increased bleeding risk.[69] A double-blind, multicentric clinical trial by Diercks et al. compared posttonsillectomy bleeding rates between acetaminophen and ibuprofen. A group of 688 pediatric patients were assessed and monitored for type 3 posttonsillectomy bleeding (bleeding requiring a return to the operating room for control of hemorrhage). Their results could not conclude that there is no difference between ibuprofen and acetaminophen and posttonsillectomy bleeding rates.[70] The American Academy of Otolaryngology clinical practice guidelines for tonsillectomy, updated in 2019, currently makes a strong recommendation for the use of postoperative NSAIDs, acetaminophen, or both. The use of ketorolac remains controversial and provider dependent, and no formal recommendation was made in the guidelines.[64]

Multimodal approaches to analgesia

Awareness of the risks of opioids and an increasing shift away from opioid utilization has placed importance on multimodal approaches to analgesia. Several pain management strategies have been developed over several decades that treat pain in a multimodal fashion. These strategies may allow for the reduction in perioperative opioid requirements, and often include the use of NSAIDs, acetaminophen, and gabapentin. In 2021, The American Academy of Otolaryngology—Head and Neck Surgery Clinical Practice Guideline, "Opioid Prescribing for Analgesia After Common Otolaryngology Operations," recommended nonopioid multimodal analgesia as a first-line approach to perioperative pain, representing a paradigm shift in perioperative pain management within the field of otolaryngology.[9]

NSAIDs play an important role in multimodal analgesia (MMA), and NSAID-based regimens should be considered the first-line analgesia after head and neck surgery. In 2018, Nguyen et al. performed the first prospective single-blind trial to assess the efficacy of ibuprofen versus opioids (acetaminophen-hydrocodone) as a primary analgesic after outpatient otolaryngological procedures. Procedures assessed in the study included thyroidectomy, parathyroidectomy, functional endoscopic sinus surgery, septoplasty, endolaryngeal surgery, and otologic procedures. They demonstrated no significant difference in patient-reported pain scores and a statistically significantly lower opioid consumption in the group who received ibuprofen as a primary analgesic. Additionally, no adverse postoperative bleeding or hematomas were experienced in their ibuprofen group.[71] Gabapentin is another important medication utilized for MMA, often given as a single dose 1—2 h before a procedure at a dose range of 300—1,200 mg. Preoperative gabapentin has been associated with a reduction in postoperative pain scores in various procedures for various specialties including otolaryngology.[72,73]

Thuener et al.[74] assessed the effect of implementing a pain management protocol on patients undergoing head and neck procedures with an expected mild postoperative pain level. The procedures stratified into the "mild postoperative pain" category included parotidectomy, thyroidectomy, parathyroidectomy, open lymph node biopsy, neck dissection without mucosal resection, and cutaneous wide local excisions. Their protocol included the use of postoperative tramadol as a first-line analgesic, and ibuprofen and/or acetaminophen as an adjuvant, resulting in a reduction in the number of patients receiving oxycodone, and reduction of both quantity of pills and refills prescribed.[74] Banik et al. demonstrated a statistically significant reduction in opioid utilization specifically for patients undergoing unilateral neck dissection with or without concomitant thyroidectomy, parotidectomy, glossectomy, or tonsillectomy through preoperative patient education, multimodal analgesia, and multidisciplinary collaboration to accurately assess and manage pain. Their multimodal regimen included scheduled preoperative acetaminophen (1000 mg) once within 2 h of surgery, intraoperative local anesthesia at the incision with 10 mL of 1% lidocaine with 1:100,000 epinephrine and bilateral cervical nerve blocks with 10 mL of 0.25% bupivacaine before incision and after closure, and postoperative acetaminophen (1000 mg) every 6 h, ibuprofen (600 mg) every 6 h, use of menthol throat lozenges, chloramphenicol throat spray, ice packs, and other adjuncts in the postanesthesia care unit.[50] A reduction in opioid utilization through multimodal analgesia in more complex head and neck procedures including free-flap reconstruction has also been explored. A recent retrospective study by Eggerstedt et al.[75]

demonstrated a reduction in opioid prescription and improvement in postoperative pain score with a regimen consisting of preoperative oral acetaminophen (975 mg orally) and gabapentin (900 mg orally) and intraoperative intravenous acetaminophen (1000 mg intravenously). Their postoperative regimen included scheduled acetaminophen (950 mg every 8 h), gabapentin (300 mg every 8 h), celecoxib (200 mg every 12 h), and ketorolac (15 mg every 6 h intravenously as needed, limited to three consecutive days to reduce risk of renal injury), and intravenous fentanyl pushes if pain remained uncontrolled. Of note, ketorolac and celecoxib use was not associated with an increased risk of perioperative bleeding or free flap failure in their MMA cohort.[75]

In 2021, Cramer et al. performed a review further highlighting recommendations regarding NSAID use. They reiterated that a combination of ibuprofen and acetaminophen is equal to or more effective than standard dosing of oxycodone and that opioids are most useful when other therapies are contraindicated. Additionally, NSAID-based multimodal regimens have not been found to increase the risk of postoperative hemorrhage. However, if a concern of bleeding still exists for a specific patient, selective COX-2 inhibitors (Celecoxib) can be used instead which may reduce the theoretical bleeding risk. While a concern regarding cardiac risks exists with the specific selective COX-2 inhibitor rofecoxib, the PRECISION Trial assessed the safety of celecoxib among 24,081 randomized participants and found no significantly increased risk of cardiac events when compared to ibuprofen or naproxen.[23] Furthermore, a retrospective cohort study by Carpenter et al. assessed 51 patients undergoing free flap surgery and found no increased risk of free flap complications in patients receiving celecoxib compared with retrospective controls, and also found patients receiving celecoxib required less opioids.[24] Therefore, celecoxib should be considered an acceptable alternative to other NSAIDs for head and neck surgeries.

Preoperative evaluation

Preoperative evaluation of patients is important for optimization of postoperative pain management and includes obtaining a thorough pain history, screening for substance abuse, discussion of perioperative and postoperative expectations, and development of a postoperative analgesia plan in conjunction with the patient. Care must be taken to identify patients with cardiopulmonary risk factors that may increase postoperative opioid induced respiratory depression.[76] Additionally, special considerations must be made for patients on long-term opioid medications such as methadone or buprenorphine as discussed earlier in this chapter.[3] Other important considerations exist with the utilization of NSAIDs in a multimodal regimen. For example, NSAIDs may be of limited use in patients with renal dysfunction (use with caution in patients with stage 2 chronic kidney disease, and avoid in patients with stage 3–5 chronic kidney disease) or in sinonasal surgery due to high rates of concomitant aspirin-exacerbated respiratory disease, and therefore alternative medications may be advised.[23,77]

Preemptive analgesia

Preemptive analgesia is a treatment strategy that is thought to improve postsurgical pain by preventing the development of altered central and/or peripheral processing of pain. Woolf first introduced the concept of a central component to postinjury pain in 1983. It was understood that a noxious stimulus sufficient to produce tissue injury, such as a skin incision, may be capable of generating prolonged poststimulus sensory disturbances such as continued pain, increased sensitivity to noxious stimuli, and pain triggered by innocuous stimulation. Woolf demonstrated his hypothesis using an animal model and found that increases in the excitability of flexion neurons due to injury arise partly from changes in activity within the spinal cord, suggestive of central processing changes in addition to peripheral changes as a result of a noxious injury.[78] Preemptive analgesia takes this concept into account with a goal of reducing the development of pathological pain, as opposed to physiological pain. Pathological pain is considered pain that is excessive in intensity and localization and can be triggered by low-intensity stimuli.[79]

Preemptive analgesia can take place preoperatively, intraoperatively, and immediately postoperatively. One definition suggests that preemptive analgesia involves the initiation of therapy before the introduction of a noxious stimulus to reduce the sensitization of the peripheral and/or central pathways; however, several definitions exist and have not been uniform. Emphasis must be placed on preventing altered sensory pathways and does not simply imply initiation of therapy before incision.[80] Preemptive analgesia must be robust enough to prevent the formation of pathologic pain, and therefore regimens that do not produce sufficient analgesia cannot be considered preemptive.[79,80] Two requirements for ensuring the adequacy of preemptive analgesia include verification of the effectiveness of the pharmacological treatment, such as verification of sufficient neural blockade, and extension of the antinociceptive treatment 12–48 h into the postoperative period for more significant inflammatory nociceptive stimuli. Therapeutic regimens and medications studied for preemptive analgesia include NSAIDs, opioids, N-methyl-D-aspartate-receptor antagonists, epidural analgesia, peripheral local anesthetic and nerve blockade, and wound infiltration.[81,82]

The efficacy of preemptive treatment remains controversial.[83] A large systematic review performed in 2002 by Møiniche et al. demonstrated limited evidence supporting preemptive analgesia when focused solely on the timing of analgesia, comparing preincisional and postincisional initiation of analgesics. Definitions of preemptive analgesia have not been uniform, which may contribute to the controversial views and inconclusive studies of the strategy.[82] A more recent 2005 meta-analysis by Ong et al. concluded that there was an overall benefit to preemptive analgesia that was most apparent in studies utilizing systemic NSAIDs, local wound infiltration, and epidural analgesia. This was concluded using surrogate outcome measures including time to first rescue analgesic, total analgesic consumption, and postoperative pain scores. While NSAIDs and local wound infiltration demonstrated a reduced total analgesic consumption and increased time to first analgesic, only epidural analgesia demonstrated consistent improvement in all three of these outcome measures.[80]

Few studies have been performed to assess preemptive analgesia efficacy within otolaryngology. Select studies of preoperative gabapentin and/or pregabalin have shown potential benefit in tonsillectomy, thyroidectomy, tympanoplasty, and nasal surgeries by reducing postoperative analgesic consumption or postoperative pain score.[84–86] Additionally, a single-institution study assessing preemptive analgesia in pediatric tonsillectomy found that ropivacaine with or without clonidine may improve postoperative tonsillectomy pain through a reduction in visual analog scale pain scores, medication use, and sooner return to normal activity.[87] Further studies are warranted given the current paucity of studies and evidence for preemptive analgesia in head and neck surgery.

Enhanced recovery after surgery

ERAS is a protocol that was first developed in Europe by a group of academic surgeons in 2001 and first described for colonic resection in 2005 by Fearon et al. The ERAS clinical care protocol describes a multimodal approach to perioperative care developed from evidence-based and consensus methodology.[12] ERAS addresses preadmission, preoperative, intraoperative, and postoperative elements that are carried out by various medical professionals including surgeons, anesthesiologists, and nursing staff to optimize postoperative outcomes. ERAS protocols typically have several elements, which may differ depending on the procedure for which it is implemented, but these elements have one similar emphasis: minimization of physiological stress and improvement of the stress response. This is typically done through introducing and standardizing perioperative care such as preoperative counseling, nutrition optimization, preoperative medical optimization, smoking cessation, minimizing drain use and early removal of drains, appropriate fluid balance intraoperatively and postoperatively, early postoperative mobilization, early resumption of an oral diet, and incorporation of multimodal opioid-sparing pain regimens. Evaluation of ERAS implementation has revealed improved outcomes that include decreased complication rates, decreased length of hospitalization, and decreased number of readmissions. Additionally, a higher compliance to a proposed protocol has been associated with improved results.[13]

An important component of an ERAS protocol includes a reduction in pain by various strategies including multimodal analgesia with opioid-sparing agents, early mobilization, early removal of urinary catheters and lines, and restrictive use of drains to decrease pain and improve mobility.[13] Guidelines for patients undergoing head and neck cancer surgery were first described for Otolaryngology in 2016 by Coyle et al. Formation of this protocol involved recommendations involved input from otolaryngologists, oral and maxillofacial surgeons, nursing, speech and language therapists, anesthetists, dieticians, and physical therapists.[14] The implementation of ERAS in head and neck surgery has been shown to reduce opioid use.

Postoperative pain management guidelines for major head and neck oncology procedures include intravenous opioid infusion for ventilated patients. If unventilated in the intensive care unit or ward, recommendations are determined by PO status. Patients who can take oral medications are recommended to begin scheduled acetaminophen, scheduled NSAIDs, scheduled tramadol (with a 50 mg test dose first

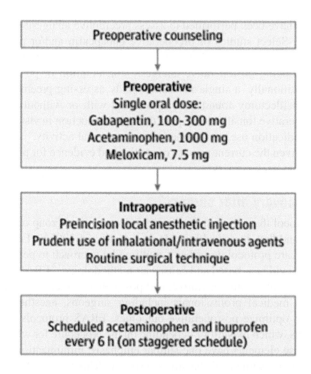

FIGURE 1.1

Outline of institutional multimodal analgesia protocol.

Militsakh O, Lydiatt W, Lydiatt D, et al. Development of multimodal analgesia pathways in outpatient thyroid and parathyroid surgery and association with postoperative opioid prescription patterns. JAMA Otolaryngol Head Neck Surg. *2018;144(11):1023–1029. Requires permissions.*

to assess side effects), oral morphine as needed or patient-controlled analgesia (PCA) as indicated, and naloxone. Patients unable to take PO medications, but with a gastrostomy/nasogastric tube were recommended to have scheduled intravenous acetaminophen, scheduled tramadol (with a 50 mg test dose), oral morphine as needed or PCA as indicated, and naloxone. These medications should be continued on postoperative day 1. If a patient requires a PCA, the requirement should be reviewed on postoperative day 2 and discontinued if able. On postoperative day 3, NSAIDs should be discontinued if they were utilized (Fig. 1.1).

ERAS protocols have been applied to multiple aspects of head and neck surgery including free-flap reconstruction and thyroid/parathyroid surgery. Dort el al first described an ERAS protocol for head and neck cancer surgery with free-flap reconstruction. Pain recommendations included preoperative medications with short-term anxiolytics and avoidance of long-term anxiolytics or opioids. Postoperative pain recommendations include the use of NSAIDs, COX inhibitors, and acetaminophen to avoid opioid use. Patient-controlled analgesia was considered if multimodal analgesia approaches were insufficient. No additional recommendation regarding postoperative nerve blockade was made in the setting of head and neck free flap reconstruction.[15] Furthermore, Jandali et al. demonstrated their ERAS protocol reduced total narcotic use during the course of major head and neck surgery, a statistically significant reduction in pain score at 72 h postoperatively, and a lower number of patients discharged with opioid pain medication (21.7% ERAS group vs. 90.3% control group).[6]

Lide et al. implemented an ERAS protocol in 2018 for ambulatory thyroid and parathyroid surgery with a focus on reducing opioid prescriptions. They implemented their ERAS protocol at a single institution that consisted of preoperative ibuprofen, acetaminophen, gabapentin, scopolamine, and a superficial cervical plexus block with bupivacaine 0.25% bilaterally, and postoperative ibuprofen and acetaminophen. Intraoperatively, patients received ketamine, dexamethasone, and ondansetron. They demonstrated a statistically significant reduction in postoperative prescription morphine milligram equivalents (MME) from 163 MME per prescription to 72 MME, and fewer patients were prescribed opioids (68.7% from 97.1%). 96% of the post-ERAS protocol received tramadol as their prescribed opioid, and 4% received an opioid-acetaminophen combination. This contrasted to their pre-ERAS opioid prescribing patterns that consisted of hydrocodone-containing medications (40%), oxycodone-containing medications (32%), and tramadol (26%). Opioid administration, determined by average MME, was not significantly different intraoperatively or in the postanesthesia care unit (PACU) between pre-ERAS and post-ERAS groups, pain scores in the PACU were not significantly different, and mean PACU time was not different.[5]

Narcotic free regimens in thyroid and parathyroid surgery

The recent transition toward an opioid-free postoperative pain regimen has been successfully demonstrated through various studies in patients who have undergone parathyroidectomy and thyroidectomy. Several groups have developed multimodal analgesia strategies that have demonstrated a decrease in postoperative opioid prescribing patterns. Strategies often involve preoperative counseling regarding the postoperative pain management plan, preoperative risks stratification of pain based on procedure type, standardized prescription regimens, and postoperative assessment.[74]

Militsakh et al. developed a multimodal analgesia strategy that was applied at a single institution in 2015 that consisted of acetaminophen, NSAIDS, and gabapentin. 528 patients who underwent thyroid and parathryoid surgery between 2015 and 2017 were retrospectively reviewed. Patients were preoperatively counseled regarding the management strategy and also made aware of the option for opioid analgesics as an option in case of unexpected severe, intolerable pain. Patients who qualified (those without significant renal dysfunction, liver dysfunction, or other contraindications to the aforementioned medications) received this strategy if agreeable. The described protocol consisted of preoperative oral gabapentin 100–300 mg, acetaminophen 1000 mg, and meloxicam 7.5 mg. Intraoperatively, preincisional local anesthesia was used, and postoperatively patients received a staggered dose of acetaminophen and ibuprofen every 6 h (Fig. 1.2). Their study demonstrated significant patient adherence to an opioid-free protocol for thyroid and parathyroid surgery. Adherence to their 3-medication protocol increased over the course of its implementation from 0% to 87%, and opioid prescription decreased from 13% to 1% upon discharge from 2015 to 2017.[7,88]

University Hospitals Bristol **NHS**
NHS Foundation Trust

Clinical Professional Standard
Head and Neck Major Surgery Postop Pain Management

SETTING   Clinical inpatient areas within Division of Surgery Head & Neck

FOR STAFF   All clinical staff involved in caring for patients

PATIENTS   Major surgery for Head and Neck Oncology

Patients returning to ICU ventilated:

• Intravenous opioid infusion

Patients returning to the ward or unventilated on ICU:

• Ensure the patient is prescribed the following unless contraindicated:

• Able to take oral medication
  ◦ Regular paracetamol
  ◦ Regular non steroidal anti-inflammatory†
  ◦ Regular tramadol – stop after test dose of 50 mg if unwanted side effects
  ◦ Oramorph prn or PCA as indicated
  ◦ Naloxone

• Unable to take oral medication but has ng/gastrostomy
  ◦ Regular i.v. paracetamol
  ◦ Regular tramadol – stop after test dose of 50 mg if unwanted side effects
  ◦ Oramorph prn or PCA as indicated
  ◦ Naloxone

Postop Day 1

• Continue medication as above

Postop Day 2

• Review requirement for PCA
• Continue other medication as above

Postop Day 3

• Stop non steroidal anti-inflammatories if prescribed.

†NSAID prescribed only if the patient is <70 years old, urine output > 30 mls/hr for 4 hours, no evidence of renal failure, no peptic ulcer disease and no excess alcohol intake

FIGURE 1.2

Appendix 2: Pain protocol for head and neck oncology patients.

From: Coyle MJ, Main B, Hughes C, et al. Enhanced recovery after surgery (ERAS) for head and neck oncology patients. Clin Otolaryngol. *2016;41(2):118–126.*

Shindo et al. performed a retrospective study demonstrating a significant reduction in postoperative opioid need in parathyroid and thyroid surgeries after initiation of preoperative patient education and increasing use of nonopioid pain medications.

Additionally, they found a statistically significant reduction in the number of postoperative phone calls for refills in the groups prescribed lower dose or no opioids. They found the greatest variability in postoperative opioid use was in the immediate postoperative anesthesia care unit.[8]

While perioperative NSAID use raises the concern for postoperative hematoma and intraoperative bleeding, studies applying a strategy utilizing perioperative NSAIDS have not yet demonstrated a significant increase in postoperative bleeding events.[7]

Regional differences in postoperative pain management in otolaryngology

Pain management strategies vary across different populations. While a profound opioid epidemic exists within the United States, no clear data from Asia and Europe exist to indicate an opioid epidemic within those regions.[89] A comparative study by Li et al. carried out between 820 patients at the Chinese University of Hong Kong (CUHK) and Oregon Health and Science University (OHSU) regarding opioid prescribing habits after major head and neck procedures demonstrated a significantly lower rate of opioid use in Hong Kong compared to the United States. No significant difference in the number of acetaminophen, NSAIDs, or anxiolytic medications used existed between the two institutions. CUHK utilized significantly more tramadol than OHSU postoperatively. Factors hypothesized to influence these differences include cultural and patient expectations, industry drivers of opioid use, alternatives to opioid pain regimens, and the metrics by which pain is assessed.[89] Further studies about global prescribing trends are warranted as publications addressing global prescribing habits within otolaryngology are scarce.

References

1. Bobian M, Gupta A, Graboyes EM. Acute pain management following head and neck surgery. *Otolaryngol Clin North Am.* 2020;53(5):753.
2. Schwartz MA, Naples JG, Kuo C, Falcone TE. Opioid prescribing patterns among otolaryngologists. *Otolaryngol Head Neck Surg.* 2018;158(5):854−859.
3. Matar N, Pashkova AA. Preoperative optimization for perioperative analgesia. *Otolaryngol Clin North Am.* 2020;53(5):729.
4. Dort JC, Farwell DG, Findlay M, et al. Optimal perioperative care in major head and neck cancer surgery with free flap reconstruction: a consensus review and recommendations from the enhanced recovery after surgery society. *JAMA Otolaryngol Head Neck Surg.* 2017;143(3):292−303.
5. Lide RC, Creighton EW, Yeh J, et al. Opioid reduction in ambulatory thyroid and parathyroid surgery after implementing enhanced recovery after surgery protocol. *Head Neck.* 2021.

6. Jandali DB, Vaughan D, Eggerstedt M, et al. Enhanced recovery after surgery in head and neck surgery: reduced opioid use and length of stay. *Laryngoscope*. 2020;130(5):1227−1232.

7. Militsakh O, Lydiatt W, Lydiatt D, et al. Development of multimodal analgesia pathways in outpatient thyroid and parathyroid surgery and association with postoperative opioid prescription patterns. *JAMA Otolaryngol Head Neck Surg*. 2018;144(11):1023−1029.

8. Shindo M, Lim J, Leon E, Moneta L, Li R, Quintanilla-Dieck L. Opioid prescribing practice and needs in thyroid and parathyroid surgery. *JAMA Otolaryngol Head Neck Surg*. 2018;144(12):1098−1103.

9. Anne S, Mims J, Tunkel DE, et al. Clinical practice guideline: opioid prescribing for analgesia after common otolaryngology operations. *Otolaryngol Head Neck Surg*. 2021;164(2_suppl):S1−S42.

10. Bhattacharyya N. The increasing workload in head and neck surgery: an epidemiologic analysis. *Laryngoscope*. 2011;121(1):111−115.

11. Sommer M, Geurts JW, Stessel B, et al. Prevalence and predictors of postoperative pain after ear, nose, and throat surgery. *Arch Otolaryngol Head Neck Surg*. 2009;135(2):124−130.

12. Hamblen-Thomas C. Factors in painless tonsillectomy. *Postgrad Med J*. 1938;14(151):147.

13. Penn SE. Control of post-tonsillectomy pain. *AMA Arch Otolaryngol*. 1952;56(1):59−60.

14. Allen RT. New method for relieving postoperative pain following tonsillectomy. *AMA Arch Otolaryngol*. 1953;57(1):86.

15. Money S, Garber B. Management of cancer pain. *Curr Emerg Hospital Med Rep*. 2018;6(4):141−146.

16. Siegel RL, Miller KD, Fuchs HE, Jemal A. Cancer statistics, 2021. *CA Cancer J Clin*. 2021;71(1):7−33. https://doi.org/10.3322/caac.21654. Accessed April 18, 2021.

17. Sung H, Ferlay J, Siegel RL, et al. Global cancer statistics 2020: GLOBOCAN estimates of incidence and mortality worldwide for 36 cancers in 185 countries. *CA Cancer J Clin*; 2021. https://doi.org/10.3322/caac.21660. Accessed April 18, 2021.

18. *National Comprehensive Cancer Network. Clinical Practice Guidelines in Oncology*; 2021. https://www.nccn.org/professionals/physician_gls/pdf/head-and-neck.pdf. Accessed April 18, 2021.

19. Cramer JD, Wisler B, Gouveia CJ. Opioid stewardship in otolaryngology: state of the art review. *Otolaryngol Head Neck Surg*. 2018;158(5):817−827.

20. Ciszkowski C, Madadi P, Phillips MS, Lauwers AE, Koren G. Codeine, ultrarapid-metabolism genotype, and postoperative death. *N Engl J Med*. 2009;361(8):827−828.

21. Coyle MJ, Main B, Hughes C, et al. Enhanced recovery after surgery (ERAS) for head and neck oncology patients. *Clin Otolaryngol*. 2016;41(2):118−126.

22. Ljungqvist O, Scott M, Fearon KC. Enhanced recovery after surgery: a review. *JAMA Surg*. 2017;152(3):292−298.

23. Cramer JD, Barnett ML, Anne S, et al. Nonopioid, multimodal analgesia as first-line therapy after otolaryngology operations: primer on nonsteroidal anti-inflammatory drugs (NSAIDs). *Otolaryngol Head Neck Surg*. 2021;164(4):712−719.

24. Carpenter PS, Shepherd HM, McCrary H, et al. Association of celecoxib use with decreased opioid requirements after head and neck cancer surgery with free tissue reconstruction. *JAMA Otolaryngol Head Neck Surg*. 2018;144(11):988−994.

25. Bacchi S, Palumbo P, Sponta A, Coppolino MF. Clinical pharmacology of non-steroidal anti-inflammatory drugs: a review. *Anti-Inflamm Anti-Aller Agents Med Chem*. 2012; 11(1):52−64.

26. Kong V, Irwin MG. Gabapentin: a multimodal perioperative drug? *Br J Anaesth*. 2007; 99(6):775−786.

27. Grond S, Sablotzki A. Clinical pharmacology of tramadol. *Clin Pharmacokinet*. 2004; 43(13):879−923.

28. Kalso E. Oxycodone. *J Pain Symptom Manage*. 2005;29(5):47−56.

29. Trescot AM, Datta S, Lee M, Hansen H. Opioid pharmacology. *Pain Phys*. 2008;11(2 Suppl):133.

30. Hench PS, Kendall EC, Slocumb CH, Polley HF. Effects of cortisone acetate and pituitary ACTH on rheumatoid arthritis, rheumatic fever and certain other conditions: a study in clinical physiology. *Arch Intern Med*. 1950;85(4):545−666.

31. Tiippana EM, Hamunen K, Kontinen VK, Kalso E. Do surgical patients benefit from perioperative gabapentin/pregabalin? A systematic review of efficacy and safety. *Anesthes Analges*. 2007;104(6):1545−1556.

32. Grass JA. Patient-controlled analgesia. *Anesthes Analges*. 2005;101(5S):S44−S61.

33. Prescott LF. Paracetamol: past, present, and future. *Am J Ther*. 2000;7(2):143−147.

34. Brady JE, Wunsch H, DiMaggio C, Lang BH, Giglio J, Li G. Prescription drug monitoring and dispensing of prescription opioids. *Publ Health Rep*. 2014;129(2):139−147.

35. Max MB, Donovan M, Miaskowski CA, et al. Quality improvement guidelines for the treatment of acute pain and cancer pain. *J Am Med Assoc*. 1995;274(23):1874−1880.

36. Van Zee A. The promotion and marketing of oxycontin: commercial triumph, public health tragedy. *Am J Public Health*. 2009;99(2):221−227.

37. Manchikanti L, Helm 2nd S, Fellows B, et al. Opioid epidemic in the United States. *Pain Phys*. 2012;15(3 Suppl):ES9−ES38.

38. Barnett ML. Opioid prescribing in the midst of crisis-myths and realities. *N Engl J Med*. 2020;382(12):1086−1088.

39. Roy S, Wang J, Kelschenbach J, Koodie L, Martin J. Modulation of immune function by morphine: implications for susceptibility to infection. *J Neuroimmu Pharmacol*. 2006; 1(1):77−89.

40. Shanmugam VK, Couch KS, McNish S, Amdur RL. Relationship between opioid treatment and rate of healing in chronic wounds. *Wound Rep Regen*. 2017;25(1): 120−130.

41. Compton WM, Boyle M, Wargo E. Prescription opioid abuse: problems and responses. *Prev Med*. 2015;80:5−9.

42. Modarai F, Mack K, Hicks P, et al. Relationship of opioid prescription sales and overdoses, North Carolina. *Drug Alcohol Depend*. 2013;132(1−2):81−86.

43. *Multiple Cause of Death 1999-2019 on CDC Wonder Online Database*. Centers for Disease Control, National Center for Health Statistics; 2020.

44. Mattson CL, Tanz LJ, Quinn K, Kariisa M, Patel P, Davis NL. Trends and geographic patterns in drug and synthetic opioid overdose Deaths—United States, 2013−2019. *Morb Mortal Weekly Rep*. 2021;70(6):202.

45. Levy B, Paulozzi L, Mack KA, Jones CM. Trends in opioid analgesic−prescribing rates by specialty, US, 2007−2012. *Am J Prev Med*. 2015;49(3):409−413.

46. *U.S. Opioid Dispensing Rate Maps|Drug Overdose|CDC Injury Center*; 2020. https://www.cdc.gov/drugoverdose/maps/rxrate-maps.html. Accessed April 18, 2021.

47. Alam A, Gomes T, Zheng H, Mamdani MM, Juurlink DN, Bell CM. Long-term analgesic use after low-risk surgery: a retrospective cohort study. *Arch Intern Med.* 2012;172(5): 425–430.

48. Shah A, Hayes CJ, Martin BC. Characteristics of initial prescription episodes and likelihood of long-term opioid use—United States, 2006–2015. *Morb Mortal Weekly Rep.* 2017;66(10):265.

49. Saraswathula A, Chen MM, Mudumbai SC, Whittemore AS, Divi V. Persistent postoperative opioid use in older head and neck cancer patients. *Otolaryngol Head Neck Surg.* 2019;160(3):380–387.

50. Banik GL, Kraimer KL, Shindo ML. Opioid prescribing in patients undergoing neck dissections with short hospitalizations. *Otolaryngol Head Neck Surg.* 2021;164(4): 792–798.

51. Dowell D, Haegerich TM, Chou R. CDC guideline for prescribing opioids for chronic pain—United States, 2016. *J Am Med Assoc.* 2016;315(15):1624–1645.

52. Rubin S, Wulu JA, Edwards HA, Dolan RW, Brams DM, Yarlagadda BB. The impact of MassPAT on opioid prescribing patterns for otolaryngology surgeries. *Otolaryngol Head Neck Surg.* 2021, 0194599820987454.

53. Katz AP, Misztal C, Ghiam MK, Hoffer ME. Changes in single-specialty postoperative opioid prescribing patterns in response to legislation: single-institution analysis over time. *Otolaryngol Head Neck Surg.* 2021, 0194599820986577.

54. Kumar K, Kirksey MA, Duong S, Wu CL. A review of opioid-sparing modalities in perioperative pain management: methods to decrease opioid use postoperatively. *Anesthes Analges.* 2017;125(5):1749–1760.

55. McDermott JD, Eguchi M, Stokes WA, et al. Short-and long-term opioid use in patients with oral and oropharynx cancer. *Otolaryngol Head Neck Surg.* 2019;160(3):409–419.

56. Mitra S, Sinatra RS, Warltier DC. Perioperative management of acute pain in the opioid-dependent patient. *Journal Am Soc Anesthesiol.* 2004;101(1):212–227.

57. Anderson TA, Quaye AN, Ward EN, Wilens TE, Hilliard PE, Brummett CM. To stop or not, that is the question: acute pain management for the patient on chronic buprenorphine. *Anesthesiology.* 2017;126(6):1180–1186.

58. Rodríguez MC, Villamor P, Castillo T. Assessment and management of pain in pediatric otolaryngology. *Int J Pediatr Otorhinolaryngol.* 2016;90:138–149.

59. Erickson BK, Larson DR, St Sauver JL, Meverden RA, Orvidas LJ. Changes in incidence and indications of tonsillectomy and adenotonsillectomy, 1970-2005. *Otolaryngol Head Neck Surg.* 2009;140(6):894–901.

60. Goldman JL, Ziegler C, Burckardt EM. Otolaryngology practice patterns in pediatric tonsillectomy: the impact of the codeine boxed warning. *Laryngoscope.* 2018;128(1): 264–268.

61. Kelly LE, Rieder M, van den Anker J, et al. More codeine fatalities after tonsillectomy in north american children. *Pediatrics.* 2012;129(5):e1343–e1347.

62. *Safety Review Update of Codeine Use in Children; New Boxed Warning and Contraindication on Use after Tonsillectomy and/or Adenoidectomy*; 2013. https://www.fda.gov/media/85072/download. Accessed March 25, 2021.

63. Kelly LE, Sommer DD, Ramakrishna J, et al. Morphine or ibuprofen for posttonsillectomy analgesia: a randomized trial. *Pediatrics.* 2015;135(2):307–313.

64. Mitchell RB, Archer SM, Ishman SL, et al. Clinical practice guideline: tonsillectomy in children (update). *Otolaryngol Head Neck Surg.* 2019;160(1_suppl):S1–S42.

65. Blakley BW. Post-tonsillectomy bleeding: how much is too much? *Otolaryngol Head Neck Surg.* 2009;140(3):288−290.

66. D'Souza JN, Schmidt RJ, Xie L, Adelman JP, Nardone HC. Postoperative nonsteroidal anti-inflammatory drugs and risk of bleeding in pediatric intracapsular tonsillectomy. *Int J Pediatr Otorhinolaryngol.* 2015;79(9):1472−1476.

67. Lewis SR, Nicholson A, Cardwell ME, Siviter G, Smith AF. Nonsteroidal anti-inflammatory drugs and perioperative bleeding in paediatric tonsillectomy. *Cochrane Database Syst Rev.* 2013;(7).

68. Chan DK, Parikh SR. Perioperative ketorolac increases post-tonsillectomy hemorrhage in adults but not children. *Laryngoscope.* 2014;124(8):1789−1793.

69. Riggin L, Ramakrishna J, Sommer DD, Koren GA. Updated systematic review & meta-analysis of 36 randomized controlled trials; no apparent effects of non steroidal anti-inflammatory agents on the risk of bleeding after tonsillectomy. *Clinical otolaryngology.* 2013;38(2):115−129.

70. Diercks GR, Comins J, Bennett K, et al. Comparison of ibuprofen vs acetaminophen and severe bleeding risk after pediatric tonsillectomy: a noninferiority randomized clinical trial. *JAMA Otolaryngol Head Neck Surg.* 2019;145(6):494−500.

71. Nguyen KK, Liu YF, Chang C, et al. A randomized single-blinded trial of ibuprofen-versus opioid-based primary analgesic therapy in outpatient otolaryngology surgery. *Otolaryngol Head Neck Surg.* 2019;160(5):839−846.

72. Hurley RW, Cohen SP, Williams KA, Rowlingson AJ, Wu CL. The analgesic effects of perioperative gabapentin on postoperative pain: a meta-analysis. *Reg Anesth Pain Med.* 2006;31(3):237−247.

73. Turan A, Memis D, Karamanlioglu B, Yagiz R, Pamukçu Z, Yavuz E. The analgesic effects of gabapentin in monitored anesthesia care for ear-nose-throat surgery. *Anesthes Analges.* 2004;99(2):375−378.

74. Thuener JE, Clancy K, Scher M, et al. Impact of perioperative pain management protocol on opioid prescribing patterns. *Laryngoscope.* 2020;130(5):1180−1185.

75. Eggerstedt M, Stenson KM, Ramirez EA, et al. Association of perioperative opioid-sparing multimodal analgesia with narcotic use and pain control after head and neck free flap reconstruction. *JAMA Facial Pastic Surg.* 2019;21(5):446−451.

76. Dahan A, Aarts L, Smith TW. Incidence, reversal, and prevention of opioid-induced respiratory depression. *J Am Soc Anesthesiol.* 2010;112(1):226−238.

77. Gill AS, Virani FR, Hwang JC, et al. Preoperative gabapentin administration and its impact on postoperative opioid requirement and pain in sinonasal surgery. *Otolaryngol Head Neck Surg.* 2021;164(4):889−894.

78. Woolf CJ. Evidence for a central component of post-injury pain hypersensitivity. *Nature.* 1983;306(5944):686−688.

79. Kissin I, Weiskopf RB. Preemptive analgesia. *J Am Soc Anesthesiol.* 2000;93(4):1138−1143.

80. Ong CK, Lirk P, Seymour RA, Jenkins BJ. The efficacy of preemptive analgesia for acute postoperative pain management: a meta-analysis. *Anesthes Analges.* 2005;100(3):757−773.

81. Dahl JB, Møiniche S. Pre-emptive analgesia. *Br Med Bull.* 2005;71(1):13−27.

82. Møiniche S, Kehlet H, Dahl JB. A qualitative and quantitative systematic review of pre-emptive analgesia for postoperative pain relief: the role of timing of analgesia. *J Am Soc Anesthesiol.* 2002;96(3):725−741.

83. Kissin I. Preemptive analgesia: why its effect is not always obvious. *J Am Soc Anesthesiol.* 1996;84(5):1015−1019.

84. Teharia RK, Rathore VS. Use of pregabalin as preemptive analgesia for decreasing postoperative pain in tympanoplasty. *Indian J Otolaryngol Head Neck Surg.* 2020:1−4.

85. Kim JH, Seo MY, Hong SD, et al. The efficacy of preemptive analgesia with pregabalin in septoplasty. *Clin Exp Otorhinolaryngol.* 2014;7(2):102.

86. Sanders JG, Dawes PJ. Gabapentin for perioperative analgesia in otorhinolaryngology—head and neck surgery: systematic review. *Otolaryngol Head Neck Surg.* 2016;155(6):893−903.

87. Giannoni C, White S, Enneking FK, Morey T. Ropivacaine with or without clonidine improves pediatric tonsillectomy pain. *Arch Otolaryngol Head Neck Surg.* 2001;127(10):1265−1270.

88. Oltman J, Militsakh O, D'Agostino M, et al. Multimodal analgesia in outpatient head and neck surgery: a feasibility and safety study. *JAMA Otolaryngol Head Neck Surg.* 2017;143(12):1207−1212.

89. Li RJ, Li ML, Leon E, et al. Comparison of opioid utilization patterns after major head and neck procedures between Hong Kong and the United States. *JAMA Otolaryngol Head Neck Surg.* 2018;144(11):1060−1065.

Pain management in the care of otolaryngology patients: an anesthesiologist and pain physician's perspective

Nantthasorn Zinboonyahgoon, MD [1], **Adlai Pappy, MD, MBA** [2], **Choopong Luansritisakul, MD, FRCAT** [1]

[1]Department of Anesthesiology, Faculty of Medicine Siriraj Hospital, Mahidol University, Bangkok, Thailand; [2]Department of Anesthesiology, Perioperative, and Pain Medicine, Brigham and Women's Hospital, Harvard Medical School, Boston, MA, United States

Introduction

Pain has recently been redefined as "an unpleasant sensory and emotional experience associated with, or resembling that associated with, actual or potential tissue damage."[1] Pain is not only an undesirable experience, but also is associated with many consequences, including lower patient satisfaction, delayed recovery from surgery, and increased perioperative mortality and morbidity.[2] Moreover, a prolonged period of pain can lead to long-term detrimental effects on quality of life, psychological and social function, and the economy.[3]

Even though pain can cause the aforementioned consequences, improper pain management can lead to even more harmful complications such as an overdose or death from opioids as evidenced by the opioid crisis in some countries.[4,5] Pain is the most common reason that patients seek medical care,[6] and the surgeon will encounter various types, both in the outpatient and inpatient setting. Thus, a fundamental understanding of pain management is an essential part of education for all surgeons, including otolaryngologists.

This chapter will describe the pain conditions that can be commonly found in the otolaryngologist's practice from acute perioperative pain, chronic noncancer pain, and chronic cancer pain.

Acute perioperative pain in otolaryngology

In the United States, more than 50 million inpatient operations are performed annually;[7] however, less than half of these patients report adequate postoperative pain relief.[8]

Inadequate pain control causes physiological changes in multiple systems and can lead to delayed recovery, morbidity, and mortality as follows:[2]

- Cardiovascular system: increased sympathetic output, increased blood pressure, heart rate and myocardial oxygen demand, and cardiac arrhythmias
- Respiratory system: increased risk for atelectasis, pneumonia, and respiratory failure secondary to splinting
- Gastrointestinal system: increased postoperative ileus
- Nervous system: increased risk of postoperative delirium, increased risk of chronic postsurgical pain
- Endocrine system: increased cortisol levels, elevated blood glucose, sodium and water retention, and protein catabolism
- Immune system: immunosuppression and increased risk of postoperative infection, increased potential for cancer recurrence
- Hematological system: increased risk for deep vein thrombosis due to immobilization

Magnitude of pain in otolaryngology surgery

Otolaryngology surgery can be associated with a variable degree of postoperative pain.[4] A study showed groups of patients who underwent otolaryngology surgery have a 48%−58% incidence of moderate-to-severe pain after surgery in the oral region, pharynx, larynx, neck, and salivary glands, 4−10 times higher than when compared to ear surgery.[9] Moreover, contrary to the general understanding that endoscopic procedures are quite painless, they have been associated with a 30%−35% incidence of moderate to severe pain on postoperative day zero.[9]

The type of surgery is not the only predicting factor for the degree of acute postoperative pain. Besides the operative site, preoperative pain and pain catastrophizing (an exaggerated negative mental set brought to bear during an actual or anticipated painful experience) are independent risk factors of moderate-to-severe pain after surgery.[9]

Management of perioperative pain

Pain assessment and measurement

The first step of successful pain management is the recognition and assessment of pain (RAT model; recognition, assess, and treat).[10] The recognition starts from understanding the high incidence of pain and asking or noticing if the patient has pain, especially during the perioperative period (recognition). Recording pain intensity as "the fifth vital sign"—originally intended to improve recognition and acute pain management—contributed to unrealistic goals, such as being pain-free and excessive opioid use leading to overdoses, deaths from opioids, and the opioid crisis in North America. In 2018, the USA Joint Commission on Accreditation of Healthcare Organizations (JCAHO) implemented new and revised pain assessment and management standards, by focusing more on the impact of pain on patients' physical function, rather than pain intensity.[11]

Pain assessment should be obtained from a thorough medical history and physical examination, pain history, functional impact, and adverse effects of treatment. Pain history can be obtained by the acronym PAIN: place (site of pain), amplitude (intensity), intensifier, and nullifier. At the end of taking the history, physicians should have a clear understanding of the type of pain, pain intensity, and individual physical and psychological factors contributing to the pain to determine a treatment plan.[10]

Types of pain

There are many ways to classify pain (acute/chronic, cancer/noncancer, nociceptive/neuropathic). However, classifying by pathophysiology into nociceptive and neuropathic will help the clinician choose from the correct group of medications for treatment. The differences between nociceptive and neuropathic pain are shown in Table 2.1.

Contrary to a general understanding that nociceptive pain is the exclusive type of pain in acute postoperative pain, acute postoperative pain can be a mixed component of nociceptive and neuropathic pain.[12] Additionally, the concept of mixed pain has been studied in many chronic pain conditions, which were previously recognized as purely nociceptive pain. The prevalence of neuropathic pain in chronic low back pain is 20%–55% and 19%–39% in cancer pain.[13]

As acute postoperative pain is mixed pain by nature, neuropathic pain medications such as gabapentinoids also have roles in acute postoperative pain. However, the high dose of gabapentinoids can be associated with sedation, and specific studies of gabapentinoids for otolaryngologic surgery are still limited. Finally, because opioids can alleviate both acute nociceptive and neuropathic pain, opioids have been popular analgesics in the acute pain setting (but not recommended as the first line for chronic noncancer pain).

Table 2.1 The differences between nociceptive and neuropathic pain.

	Nociceptive pain	Neuropathic pain
Definition	Pain that arises from nonneural tissue and is due to the activation of nociceptors	Pain caused by a lesion or disease of the somatosensory nervous system
Example	Acute: fracture, incisional pain Chronic: bone metastasis	Acute: nerve injuries, stump pain Chronic: chronic postsurgical pain
Characteristic	Dull aching pain	Sharp shooting pain Numbness, hyperalgesia, allodynia
Treatment	Acetaminophen Nonsteroidal anti-inflammatory drugs (NSAIDs) Opioids	Gabapentinoids Tricyclic antidepressants Serotonin and norepinephrine reuptake inhibitors (SNRIs) Opioids

Pain intensity

The pain intensity or severity will determine the strength of treatment, according to the analgesic ladder. Many pain measurement tools have been applied in clinical practice. However, self-reporting tools such as the Visual Analog Scale or Verbal Numerical Rating Scale (0—10 or 0—100) are the gold standard measurement of pain intensity and are most commonly used. Typically, the pain scale from 0 to 10 is classified into mild (0—3), moderate (4—6), or severe (7—10) pain.

There is little evidence that one pain assessment tool is superior to others. However, for certain patient populations where self-report is difficult or impossible, adapted scales or behavioral tools may be used instead. Examples of pain measurement tools for these specific populations include[11]

- *Face, Legs, Activity, Cry, Consolability Scale* for children ages between 1 and 6 years old (However, Face Pain Scale, which provides images from smiling to crying faces for the children to choose, is a self-reporting tool and is suitable for children ages more than 6 years old.)[11]
- *Critical Care Pain Observation Tool* for critically ill patients who are incapable of reporting their pain
- *Pain Assessment in Advanced Dementia Scale* for cognitively impaired patient

Factors contributing to pain management

There are a number of factors that have been shown to have significant effects on pain management. These include

- *Physical factors* such as allergies and comorbidities, especially any conditions that might affect pharmacological choice, such as a history of gastrointestinal (GI) bleeding, history of cardiovascular disease, kidney and liver function
- *Psychological factors* such as depression, anxiety, and catastrophizing

Treatment of acute postoperative pain

The options for pain treatment include both nonpharmacological and pharmacological treatment.

Nonpharmacological treatment

Nonpharmacologic treatment can commence preoperatively with good education about the surgery and continue postoperatively with good communication and reassurance. There are many additional techniques to attenuate pain, such as distraction for children, application of cold, transcutaneous electrical nerve stimulation (TENS), relaxation therapy, music therapy, meditation, and acupuncture.

Pharmacological treatment

The World Health Organization's (WHO's) analgesic ladder originally intended to provide a stepped approach to the management of cancer pain (Fig. 2.1A); however, clinicians also apply it for acute pain.[14] The model starts with nonopioids (acetaminophen, NSAIDs) for mild pain, then escalates to weak opioids (codeine, tramadol) for moderate pain, and strong opioids (morphine, fentanyl) for severe pain.[15]

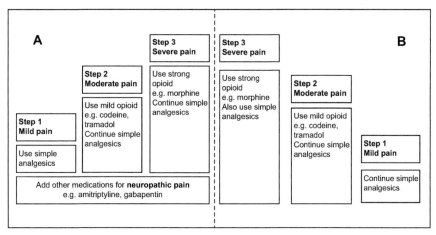

FIGURE 2.1

(A) The analgesic ladder for cancer pain, (B) The reverse analgesic ladder for acute pain.[10]

Used with permission from Dr. Roger Goucke, Essential pain management, workshop manual, second edition.

Remembering that it is appropriate to start at the top of the ladder for acute severe nociceptive pain. As postoperative pain is usually acute and severe and tends to improve over time, the reverse ladder approach, which starts with strong opioids and steps down subsequently, has been applied for acute pain (Fig. 2.1B).[10]

Nonopioid analgesics Nonopioid analgesics including nonsteroidal anti-inflammatory drugs (NSAIDs), acetaminophen, ketamine, local anesthetics (systemic, local infiltration, and regional block), clonidine, and gabapentin. Commonly used nonopioid analgesics, mechanism of action, route, and precaution are listed in Table 2.2.[2] The combination of two or more medications or techniques (such as combination with local anesthetic infiltration or regional anesthesia) that act by different mechanisms for providing analgesia is termed multimodal analgesia.[16]

Multimodal analgesia improves pain control, reduces opioid requirements, reduces opioid-related side effects, and has the potential to reduce costs in patients undergoing surgery.[17] Strong evidence shows that NSAIDs, gabapentin, pregabalin, systemic lidocaine, and ketamine are opioid-sparing medications and reduce opioid-related adverse effects.[11]

Opioid analgesics Opioids are strong analgesics, acting at μ-opioid receptors in the brain and spinal cord, which inhibits transmission of the nociceptive signal. Opioids can be administered by many routes, including oral and intravenous, intramuscular, subcutaneous, buccal, transdermal, or neuraxial (spinal, epidural). Commonly used opioids in the perioperative period and comments are shown in Table 2.3.

Even if opioids are effective in managing postoperative pain, they are often associated with adverse events, including nausea, vomiting, itching, ileus and constipation,

Table 2.2 Commonly used nonopioid analgesics, mechanism of action, and precaution.[2]

Agents	Mechanism of actions	Route	Precautions	Side effects
Acetaminophen	Unknown, may involve cyclooxygenase, endocannabinoid, TRPV1, and serotonin	PO, PR, IV	Liver failure	Minimal, unless overdose (recommended dose less than 3–4 g/day)
Traditional NSAIDs (e.g., ibuprofen, naproxen, ketorolac)	Central and peripheral COX inhibitors	PO, IV	Allergy to NSAIDs. Decrease dose in renal impairment, elderly or bodyweight <50 kg	GI bleeding, renal failure and surgical bleeding, possible risk of anastomotic leakage after colorectal surgery
COX-2 inhibitors (e.g., celecoxib)	COX-2 inhibitors	PO	Cross allergy with sulfonamides	Fewer GI side effects. Minimal effect on platelets. Similar renal risk but increased cardiovascular events with long-term use
Local anesthetics	Sodium channel blockers	IV (lidocaine), local infiltration nerve block	Allergy to local anesthetic	Local anesthetic systemic toxicity
Ketamine	NMDA receptor antagonist	IV, IM, PO	Patient with psychosis	Hallucination, delirium, hypertension, tachycardia
Gabapentin, Pregabalin	Calcium channel blockers	PO	Adjust dose for renal function (CrCl <60 mL/min), elderly	Somnolence, dizziness

COX, cyclooxygenase; CrCl, creatinine clearance; GI, gastrointestinal; IM, intramuscular; IV, intravenous; NMDA, N-methyl-D-aspartate; NSAIDs, nonsteroidal anti-inflammatory drugs; PO, per os; PR, per rectum; TRPV1, transient receptor potential cation channel subfamily V member 1.
Adapted with permission from Nantthasorn Z. Acute pain: Operative and postoperative pain, trauma, obstetric pain. In: Hogans B, Barreveld A, eds. Pain Care Essentials, Oxford University Press:2020.

Table 2.3 Commonly used opioids in perioperative period.[2]

Agents	Mechanism	Comment
Codeine	Weak μ agonist	Need CYP2D6 enzyme that converts codeine to morphine; poor metabolizers (8%–10%) do not respond, whereas ultrarapid metabolizers (3%–5%) are at risk of toxicity
Fentanyl	μ agonist	Transdermal route (fentanyl patch) results in 12 h of onset and offset delay, not recommended for acute pain, but useful for basal delivery in opioid-tolerant patients
Meperidine	μ agonist	Associated with an increased risk of delirium in the postoperative period compared to other opioids
Morphine	μ agonist	Contraindicated in end-stage renal disease
Hydromorphone	μ agonist	May produce less nausea and vomiting than morphine in some patients
Methadone	μ agonist (L-isomer), NMDA antagonist (D-isomer)	Long half-life, analgesic dose is twice or thrice a day and once daily as methadone maintenance therapy for the management of opioid addiction. May also have NMDA antagonist effect, thus decreasing opioid tolerance
Oxycodone	μ agonist	Often coformulated with acetaminophen (Percocet), requiring caution in patients where there is a potential to take a larger than recommended dose, and patients should be warned about not also taking tylenol (acetaminophen) simultaneously when these coformulations are used.
Hydrocodone	μ agonist	Often coformulated with acetaminophen (Vicodin), see caution above.
Nalbuphine (Nubain)	μ antagonist, κ agonist	Contraindicated in chronic opioid users (precipitating withdrawal). Used in labor and delivery due to lower risk of neonatal respiratory depression. Low dose (5 mg IV) used for the treatment of pruritus (side effect) from other narcotics.
Buprenorphine (Subutex)	Partial μ agonist, κ antagonist	Lower risk of respiratory depression. Use in patients with previous problems with opioid addiction. High affinity to mu receptor, preventing euphoric/analgesic effect from other opioids, should stop 3–5 days before a major operation and monitor for withdrawal symptoms.

Adapted with permission from Nantthasorn Z. Acute pain: Operative and postoperative pain, trauma, obstetric pain. In: Hogans B, Barreveld A, eds. Pain care essentials. *Oxford University Press:2020.*

sedation, dizziness, confusion, urinary retention, respiratory depression and tolerance, and dependence. Nausea is dose related and the most common side effect (32%).[11]

Postsurgical patients who experienced an opioid-related adverse event had a 55% longer length of hospital stay, 47% higher costs, 36% increased risk of readmission, and 3.4 times higher risk of inpatient mortality.[11] As discussed, nonopioid analgesics have been administrated as part of multimodal analgesia to reduce opioid use and the aforementioned side effects.

Benefits of early pain control

Intense nociceptive stimulation leads to peripheral and central sensitization, which affects pain in the short and long term. Early and adequate pain control may decrease central sensitization, thus allowing better pain control and preventing persistent pain.

The strategy of early pain control by the administration of an analgesic before an acute nociceptive stimulus is called preemptive analgesia. Even though the laboratory studies found preemptive analgesia effectively minimized dorsal horn changes, which are associated with central sensitization more than if the same analgesic is given after the pain state was established, clinical studies have shown conflicting results.[11]

Preventive analgesia is a subsequent strategy that focuses on preventing central sensitization, rather than time. As postoperative pain relates not only to the skin incision but also to intraoperative tissue and nerve injuries and postoperative effects; preventive analgesia initiates analgesics or interventions not only before a nociceptive stimulus but also continues until the majority of nociceptive stimuli have abated.[18] Preventive analgesia provides the persistence of analgesic efficacy beyond its pharmacological duration, including long-term outcomes such as any effect on chronic postsurgical pain. Local anesthetics (systemic, local, or regional block) and ketamine demonstrate a preventive analgesic effect in the perioperative period, whereas studies on gabapentinoids have shown conflicting results.[11]

Perioperative management for chronic opioid users

Perioperative management of patients receiving opioid therapy is quite challenging. Several studies have suggested that these patients have an increased risk of poor surgical outcome, inadequate pain control, and perioperative opioid-related adverse events, which require particular attention and multidisciplinary treatment. Evidence shows that preoperative opioid misuse is associated with considerable postoperative morbidity and mortality, such as surgical site infection, respiratory failure, and pneumonia.[19]

Before the operation, patients should be assessed for the likelihood of opioid-related adverse events. This depends on the dosage and the duration of preoperative opioid use combined with other factors, such as uncontrolled psychiatric comorbidities, a history of a substance use disorder, and surgery likely to give a high incidence of severe postoperative pain. Generally, patients receiving more than 60 oral morphine milligram equivalents (MME) per day in the 7-day period before surgery are considered high risk.[20] For elective surgery, it is recommended to wean down opioids preoperatively to the minimum effective dose, where possible, as there is a correlation between preoperative opioid dose and poor surgical outcomes.[11] In addition, these patients should be educated to promote shared pain management expectations, and a perioperative pain specialist should be consulted before surgery. If psychological comorbidity is present, it should be optimized preoperatively.[20]

Perioperatively, it is strongly recommended to use individualized multimodal pain management strategies, with analgesic drugs from different classes and analgesic techniques that target different mechanisms being combined.[20] Nonopioid analgesics, such as paracetamol and NSAIDs, should be routinely prescribed—if there is no contraindication. Several nonopioid analgesics can also be used as part of a comprehensive multimodal analgesia, and these include ketamine and lidocaine infusion, anticonvulsants, α-2 agonists, and nefopam. Strong evidence shows that regional anesthesia is superior to the use of opioid analgesia and usually reduces opioid consumption during the perioperative period.[21,22] Regional anesthesia techniques commonly used for head and neck surgery include blockade of the trigeminal nerve, maxillary nerve, mandibular nerve, and cervical plexus. Nonpharmacological methods, such as TENS, distraction therapy, and hypnosis, may be considered postoperatively in some patients.

Regarding perioperative opioid management, it is recommended to use the lowest effective dose of opioid during the perioperative period, while avoiding opioid dose escalation postoperatively. A patient's typical dose of prescribed opioid should be continued on the morning of surgery. Although opioid-free anesthesia is possible, there is insufficient data to recommend this method.[20]

For patients receiving medication-assisted therapy, such as methadone or buprenorphine, careful analgesic regimens may be required. It is suggested that methadone should be continued on the same dose throughout the perioperative period. For buprenorphine, perioperative management depends on several factors, including the extent of surgery, elective or emergency surgery, buprenorphine preparation, and indication for buprenorphine therapy. Several strategies have been proposed. Generally, for patients expected to have mild-to-moderate pain, buprenorphine should be continued, while supplementing with a titrated high affinity pure μ-opioid receptor agonist (such as fentanyl) or buprenorphine itself for acute postoperative pain control. Alternatively, switching to a full opioid agonist before surgery is recommended for patients expected to have moderate-to-severe pain. For these patients, buprenorphine should be discontinued 3—5 days before the operation, and a pure opioid agonist may be needed for the management of withdrawal symptoms.[23]

Postoperatively, the dosage of opioids should be deescalated to the preoperative dose. Physicians should limit opioid prescriptions to the expected duration of pain that is severe enough to require opioids. If opioid use is continued beyond the expected duration of acute pain, consultation with a pain specialist and coordination with the patient's outpatient provider may be necessary.

Chronic pain in otolaryngology

Chronic pain is the pain that persists past the normal healing time and usually lasts or recurs for more than 3 months.[24] In the United States, the prevalence of chronic pain ranges from 19% to 43% of the population,[25] which often results in patients' suffering, demoralization, and functional impairment and has led to a national economic burden. However, the difference between acute and chronic pain is not only time but also the pathophysiology, goal of treatment, and prognosis (Table 2.4).

Chronic pain itself can be classified into cancer and noncancer pain. The important difference is not only the cause of pain but also the role of strong opioids as a treatment.

Opioids are strong analgesics, and long-term use inevitably produces physical tolerance; opioids are indispensable for the relief of severe pain during short-lived painful events such as postoperative periods and at the end of life such as advanced cancer.[26] However, the long-term benefit of strong opioids for chronic noncancer pain is still unclear, but the risk of abuse, overdose, and death is evident from the "opioid crisis" in North America. The role of strong opioids for a long-lived painful event such as chronic noncancer pain is very limited in current practice.[5]

In otolaryngology, patients may present with various types of chronic pain, for example, chronic orofacial pain, chronic otalgia, and chronic neck pain. Even though the data about the exact prevalence of chronic pain in otolaryngology is still lacking, this problem is commonly encountered in otolaryngology clinics. Therefore, an understanding of pathophysiology, presentation, and management of these conditions is extremely beneficial for otolaryngologists.

Chronic noncancer pain

Chronic postsurgical pain

The majority of the patients who undergo surgery recover without consequences. However, up to 40% of these patients, can develop persistent pain beyond the healing period.[27] Moreover, in some procedures (such as thoracotomy, mastectomy, amputation), 5%−10% of patients reported severe pain 1 year after the surgery and had impacted quality of life, psychological and social function, and led to

Table 2.4 The differences between acute and chronic pain.

	Acute pain	Chronic pain
Pathophysiology	Tissue, nerve injuries	Sensitization
Response	Physiology	Pathology
Prognosis	Tends to improve over time	Persists more than 3−6 months
Goal of treatment	Pain intensity reduction	Improve function with multidisciplinary approach

disability.[28] The persistent pain beyond the period of wound healing is now recognized as a disease by itself called chronic postsurgical pain syndrome (CPSP).[29] Even though it can be a common consequence of surgery and can have a considerable negative impact on the patients' quality of life, CPSP is still underdiagnosed and undertreated.[27]

Definition of chronic postsurgical pain

The official definition of CPSP was defined by the International Association for the Study of Pain (IASP) in 2017 as "chronic pain developing or increasing in intensity after a surgical procedure and persisting beyond the healing process, i.e., at least 3 months after surgery. The pain is either localized to the surgical field, projected to the innervation territory of a nerve situated in this area, or referred to a dermatome (after surgery/injury to deep somatic or visceral tissues). Other causes of pain including infection, malignancy, etc. need to be excluded as well as pain continuing from a preexisting pain problem".[29] As a disease by itself, in the upcoming version of the International Classification of Diseases (ICD-11), CPSP has its own code as MG30.21 (chronic postsurgical pain).[30] CPSP is a growing area of study within pain medicine due to the increasing number of patients undergoing surgery each year.[31] Amplified by the variable reported incidence depending on the operation (5%−85%), producing an increased number of patients with new chronic pain. A survey of the prevalence of CPSP in a large tertiary care pain center found this diagnosis in 8% of total visits, the fourth ranked of the most common out-patient diagnoses in their pain clinic.[32]

Pathophysiology of chronic postsurgical pain

The mechanism by which CPSP develops is not completely understood, but a likely mechanism includes the maladaptation of acute pain to chronic pain (neuroplasticity), nerve injuries, and opioid-induced hyperalgesia. The neuroplasticity change is believed to be the result of inflammation and intense nociceptive stimuli from surgery leading to the alteration of the gene expression involving molecular and cellular level changes from the peripheral to central nerve pathways. This change in the somatosensory pathway leads to hyperalgesia, central sensitization, and chronic pain, the maladaptive version of sensitization.[28] This concept is supported by the clinical evidence that poor acute postoperative pain control is associated with a higher incidence of CPSP.[33] As such, it is important that there is a strategy to control pain early and in a proactive way to prevent central sensitization.[34] Additional strategies to prevent CPSP according to pathophysiology includes the modification of surgical technique to lessen nerve injuries[18] and the application of opioid-sparing strategies to prevent opioids induced hyperalgesia.[35]

Risk factors of chronic postsurgical pain

Risk factors for CPSP include surgical factors (type of surgery especially thoracotomy and mastectomy have the highest incidence of CPSP), patients' characteristics (younger age, presence of preoperative pain either at the surgical site or other sites), psychological factors[36] (lower SF-12 mental score, presence of depression, or catastrophizing ideas), and poor postoperative pain control.[37] As CPSP is common and has a high impact on patients' quality of life, the identification of patients at risk, to discuss the risks of CPSP as part of the consent for surgery, is necessary for all surgeons. Additionally, recognizing the risk factors to help stratify risk and tailor preventive measures for the high-risk patients including the following: changing the surgical technique to minimally invasive surgery, aggressive acute postoperative pain control, and preventive analgesia. Moreover, the administration of some analgesics such as ketamine, lidocaine infusion, or the application of regional anesthesia may be beneficial for the prevention of CPSP.[18]

Persistent postoperative opioid use

One of the most concerning long-term effects after surgery is persistent postoperative opioids use, which is defined as the use of opioids for more than 90 days after surgery in opioid-naïve patients.[38] The prevalence of new persistent opioid use was 5.9% for minor surgeries and 6.5% for major surgeries. The similar prevalence between minor and major surgeries (OR 1.04, [0.93, 1.18])[38] suggests that prolonged opioid use after surgery cannot be simply explained by the extent of surgical injury. The multivariable analysis found that significant risk factors for persistent opioid use included tobacco use, alcohol and substance abuse disorders, mood disorder, anxiety and preoperative chronic pain.[38] Similar to the risk of CPSP, the risk of persistent postoperative opioid use should be addressed and discussed before the operation.

Clinical evidence shows opioid use for acute pain, after even minor surgical procedures[39] is associated with long-term opioid use, and that a greater amount of early opioid exposure is associated with greater risk for long-term use.[5] Preventive measures, especially for high-risk patients include minimizing postdischarge opioid use with a multimodal analgesic care plan[40] and prescribing the lowest effective dose of immediate-release opioids, with no greater quantity than needed for the expected duration of pain that is severe enough to require opioids.[5]

Management of chronic postsurgical pain

CPSP is categorized as chronic noncancer pain, the principal of management includes patient education and using a multidisciplinary approach with the surgeon, pain physician, psychiatrist, and rehabilitation medicine physician. As the majority of the patients with common types of CPSP suffer from neuropathic pain (45%, 65%, and 80% in thoracotomy, mastectomy, and amputation, respectively), the commonly used analgesics for CPSP are those used for neuropathic pain.

The first line recommended analgesics for neuropathic pain are tricyclic antidepressants, serotonin-norepinephrine reuptake inhibitors, and gabapentinoids (Table 2.5). Neuropathic pain is generally difficult to treat by itself. The number needed to treat among the first-line medication range from 3.6 (tricyclic antidepressant) to 7.7 (pregabalin)[41] and a combination of the first-line medications is quite common in practice.

Table 2.5 The first line recommended analgesics for chronic noncancer neuropathic pain.[41]

Drug class	Example	Mechanism of actions	Precautions	Side effects
Tricyclic antidepressants (TCAs)	Amitriptyline Nortriptyline	Inhibit catecholamine reuptake (increases serotonin and norepinephrine in descending inhibitory pathway).	Precaution in elderly due to risk of fall, delirium, urinary retention (avoid dose more than 25 mg/day in elderly)	Anticholinergic effect (dry mouth, difficult urination, sedation, increase risk of delirium), cardiac arrhythmia
Serotonin and norepinephrine reuptake inhibitors (SNRIs)	Duloxetine Venlafaxine Desvenlafaxine	Increase norepinephrine in descending inhibitory pathway	- Coadministration with TCAs can increase the risk of serotonin syndrome - Precaution for duloxetine in a patient with hepatic disorder	Fewer than TCAs, but includes dry mouth, nausea, and hypertension (high-dose venlafaxine)
Gabapentinoids	Gabapentin Pregabalin	Blocks calcium channels, alpha2-delta subunit. (No interaction with GABA receptors)	Need dose adjustment in patients with renal impairment	Dizziness, sedation, peripheral edema, weight gain

There is no evidence of the long-term benefit of strong opioids for chronic non-cancer conditions, and both weak and strong opioids are not recommended as first line. Opioids may be considered as second- and third-line medications for chronic noncancer neuropathic pain;[41] however, the initiation of opioids in chronic non-cancer patients needs careful consideration of the risks and benefits, screening for potential abuse and close monitoring.[5] Opioids should be stopped if there is evidence of abuse, overdose, or no clinically meaningful improvement in pain and function.

Chronic orofacial pain

Orofacial pain (OFP) is considered one of the major problems in otolaryngology[42] that has a significant impact on quality of life. It is defined as pain occurring mainly or exclusively under the orbitomeatal line, anterior to the pinnae, and above the neck, including the oral cavity.[43] It can be caused by disorders of the orofacial structures, by dysfunction of the nervous system, or through a referral from distant sources. Dental issues are considered common causes of acute or subacute OFP, and these are well managed by dentists. However, chronic OFP can originate from a wide range of etiologies, which can be either odontogenic or nonodontogenic causes.

From a survey in the United Kingdom, about a quarter of the general population reported OFP during the 1-month period before the interview. The prevalence was higher in women than in men.[44] The reported prevalence of chronic OFP varies from 10% to 62% of the patients affected with OFP, depending on study populations.[44,45]

Chronic OFP can be classified in several ways. According to the IASP and the ICD-11, it can be either primary or secondary. Chronic primary OFP is defined as OFP that occurs on at least 15 days per month for longer than 3 months, where the pain is not better accounted for by another condition.[45] One of the common causes of chronic primary OFP is associated with temporomandibular joint disorders, accounting for almost 5% of the US population.[46] In contrast, chronic secondary OFP is pain that may be conceived as a symptom secondary to an underlying disease, such as cranial and regional neuralgias and neuropathies.[45]

In 2020, the comprehensive, internationally accepted classification of OFP was published as the first edition of the International Classification of Orofacial Pain (ICOP).[43] This classification is modeled on the third edition of the International Classification of Headache Disorders (ICHD-3), joining the ICHD-3 and the ICD-11 in establishing clear terminology that will allow better communication and data sharing. Additionally, the criterion of a 4-hour duration per day has been added when defining chronicity in OFP. In this system, OFP is classified according to Table 2.6. Apart from OFP diagnosis, the ICOP committee also recommends integrating a psychosocial assessment to understand and manage OFP more comprehensively.[43]

The diagnosis and management of OFP should begin with a careful history and physical examination. Pain history needs to include location, quality, severity, timing, relieving and aggravating factors, associated symptoms, and pain impact.

Table 2.6 International Classification of Orofacial Pain (ICOP).[43]

Classification of orofacial pain
1. Orofacial pain attributed to disorders of dentoalveolar and anatomically related structures
2. Myofascial orofacial pain
3. Temporomandibular joint pain
4. Orofacial pain attributed to lesion or disease of the cranial nerves
5. Orofacial pains resembling presentations of primary headaches
6. Idiopathic orofacial pain

Table 2.7 Common etiologies of chronic orofacial pain.[47–51]

Continuous pain or near-continuous pain	Unilateral pain	- Postherpetic neuralgia - Painful trigeminal neuropathy - Central poststroke pain - Chronic migraine - Giant cell arteritis - Temporomandibular joint disorders - Persistent orofacial muscle pain - Persistent idiopathic dentoalveolar pain - Chronic cancer-related pain - Cervicogenic headache - Referred pain
	Bilateral pain	- Burning mouth syndrome - Giant cell arteritis - Temporomandibular joint disorders - Persistent orofacial muscle pain - Persistent idiopathic facial pain
Episodic pain	Unilateral pain	- Trigeminal neuralgia - Glossopharyngeal neuralgia - Nervus intermedius neuralgia - Neck-tongue syndrome - Trigeminal autonomic cephalalgias (TACs) - Episodic migraine
	Bilateral pain	- Tension-type headache - Medication-overuse headache

Usually, characteristics of pain can provide some clues for possible differential diagnosis. Table 2.7 summarizes common etiologies of chronic orofacial pain classified by typical pain characters. Laboratory investigation can be ordered to confirm a diagnosis or exclude other conditions. Increased erythrocyte sedimentation rate (ESR) and C-reactive protein (CRP) can be found in cranial arteritis and autoimmune disorders. Imaging studies are indicated in some conditions. For instance, radiographs are particularly helpful for dental pain, and ultrasound imaging may be useful for salivary gland diseases. In addition, magnetic resonance imaging (MRI) and computerized tomography (CT) are beneficial when intracranial causes are suspected.

Generally, management of these pain conditions is usually based on the treatment of primary causes. For example, patients diagnosed with giant cell arteritis, which is a form of vasculitis, should be treated with steroids or other immunosuppressive drugs. Although pain control is often necessary and can reduce patients' suffering from these conditions, it is considered only symptomatic treatment. Nevertheless, in some conditions when their pathology cannot be completely cured, or in some patients who are refractory to primary treatment, pain management might be the mainstay of treatment. These patients need multidisciplinary treatment and are usually referred to a pain clinic. In this chapter, common chronic orofacial pain encountered in clinical practice will be discussed in detail.

Pain attributed to a lesion or disease of the trigeminal nerve

According to the ICHD-3, pain attributed to a lesion or disease of the trigeminal nerve is classified into two groups: trigeminal neuralgia (TN) and painful trigeminal neuropathy.[52] The former is characterized by unilateral brief stabbing pain, which is abrupt in onset and termination. In contrast, the latter usually presents with continuous or near-continuous pain, which is described as burning, squeezing, or pins and needles. For painful trigeminal neuropathy, brief paroxysms can also be superimposed, but they are not the main components.

Trigeminal neuralgia TN is one of the well-known causes of neuropathic orofacial pain. The lifetime prevalence of TN varies between 0.16% and 0.3%.[53,54] According to the database of the Dutch health care system from 1996 to 2006, after diagnosis by experts, the overall incidence rate was 12.6 per 100,000 persons annually with a slight female predominance. The incidence increased with age, with a mean of 51.5 years.[55]

TN is usually characterized by recurrent unilateral brief electric shock-like pain, which is abrupt in onset and termination. The pain is limited to the distribution of the trigeminal nerve and may be triggered by some activities of daily life or specific movements, for example, talking, washing the face, chewing, or light touch. Following a painful paroxysm, there is usually a refractory period when the pain cannot be evoked, although 14.2%−49% of patients also have concomitant continuous pain.[56,57] Commonly, the second or third division of the trigeminal nerve is affected.[58] It is more common on the right side, and bilateral involvement is rare. In severe cases, the pain may stimulate the forceful contraction of the ipsilateral facial muscles (tic convulsif). Mild autonomic symptoms, such as conjunctival injection, or lacrimation, may be present in 16.9% of patients,[56] especially when the ophthalmic division is involved. In this case, physicians have to distinguish from trigeminal autonomic cephalalgias (TACs).

Besides the triggering phenomenon, sensory examination within the trigeminal distribution is normal in most patients unless advanced methods, such as quantitative sensory testing (QST), are used. Subtle sensory abnormalities, such as mild

Table 2.8 Diagnostic criteria for trigeminal neuralgia.[52]

A. Recurrent paroxysms of unilateral facial pain in the distribution(s) of one or more divisions of the trigeminal nerve, with no radiation beyond, and fulfilling criteria B and C

B. Pain has all of the following characteristics:
  1. lasting from a fraction of a second to 2 minutes[a]
  2. severe intensity
  3. electric shock-like, shooting, stabbing, or sharp in quality

C. Precipitated by innocuous stimuli within the affected trigeminal distribution
D. Not better accounted for by another ICHD-3 diagnosis

[a] *Duration can change over time, with paroxysms becoming more prolonged. A minority of patients will report attacks predominantly lasting for more than 2 minutes.*

hypoesthesia, may be present in some patients. However, any abnormal neurological findings should give rise to further investigations to explore serious etiologies. The diagnostic criteria for TN are summarized in Table 2.8.

It should be noted that TN is a clinical diagnosis. Investigations are performed only to identify a possible cause. MRI is considered the most helpful imaging technique to determine the presence of lesions, such as neurovascular compression, tumors, vascular malformations, and evidence of multiple sclerosis.

According to possible etiologies, TN is categorized into three subtypes: classical, secondary, and idiopathic, as demonstrated in Table 2.9.[52] This classification system assists physicians by providing guidance toward differential patient management.

Table 2.9 Classification of trigeminal neuralgia.[52]

Type of trigeminal neuralgia	Criteria for diagnosis
Classical trigeminal neuralgia	**A.** Recurrent paroxysms of unilateral facial pain fulfilling criteria for trigeminal neuralgia **B.** Demonstration on MRI or during surgery of neurovascular compression (not simply contact), with morphological changes in the trigeminal nerve root
Secondary trigeminal neuralgia	**A.** Recurrent paroxysms of unilateral facial pain fulfilling criteria for trigeminal neuralgia, either purely paroxysmal or associated with concomitant continuous or near-continuous pain **B.** An underlying disease has been demonstrated that is known to be able to cause and explain the neuralgia **C.** Not better accounted for by another ICHD-3 diagnosis
Idiopathic trigeminal neuralgia	**A.** Recurrent paroxysms of unilateral facial pain fulfilling criteria for trigeminal neuralgia, either purely paroxysmal or associated with concomitant continuous or near-continuous pain **B.** Neither classical trigeminal neuralgia nor secondary trigeminal neuralgia has been confirmed by adequate investigation, including electrophysiological tests and MRI **C.** Not better accounted for by another ICHD-3 diagnosis

Classical TN is a TN with a demonstration on MRI or during surgery of neurovascular compression, which is defined as neurovascular contact with morphological changes of the trigeminal nerve root. Some studies have shown that the presence of a neurovascular contact has less clinical significance, as it appears to be equally prevalent on the asymptomatic side. Nevertheless, neurovascular compression with morphological changes is highly associated with the symptomatic side (odds ratio 13.3).[59]

The location of neurovascular compression is usually at the root entry zone, with compression in its superomedial portion. The most common offending vessel is the superior cerebellar artery, which features in 75% of patients undergoing microvascular decompression.[60] Morphological changes can demonstrate atrophy or displacement of the nerve root. Atrophic changes include focal demyelination, decreased nerve diameter or cross-sectional area, changes in microvasculature, and other morphological changes. Some studies suggest that demonstration of neurovascular compression may predict a good outcome following microvascular decompression.[59]

As well as neurovascular compression, TN can also have secondary causes such as identifiable neurologic diseases, tumor in the cerebellopontine angle, arteriovenous malformation, and multiple sclerosis. This group accounts for about 15% of total presentations. Unlike classical TN, clinical examination shows sensory changes in a significant proportion of these cases. The underlying neurologic conditions are usually detected by MRI. For patients with a contraindication for MRI, other investigations may include neurophysiological recording of trigeminal reflexes and trigeminal evoked potentials.

Of note, other recognized causes of TN are cranial base abnormalities, connective tissue diseases, dural arteriovenous fistula, and genetic abnormalities of sodium channels. An abnormal expression of some voltage-gated sodium channels and a gain-of-function mutation in the sodium channel $Na_v1.6$ have also been demonstrated in TN.

Management of trigeminal neuralgia In TN, pharmacological treatment is considered first-line treatment. Although it is classified as neuropathic pain, treatment of TN differs from that of other neuropathic pain syndromes. Carbamazepine is the first option for long-term treatment, with a number-needed-to-treat of 1.7−1.8.[61] Adverse effects include drowsiness, dizziness, ataxia, liver damage, skin rash, and the potential for multiple drug interactions. Of note, carbamazepine hypersensitivity may occur in up to 10% of patients and is related to the patient's ethnicity and HLA type. In Asians, there is a correlation between HLA-B*1502 and the risk of Stevens−Johnson syndrome and toxic epidermal necrolysis. The evidence for this gene type in Caucasians is still lacking. In Northern European populations, some studies have demonstrated the association between the HLA-A*3101 allele and carbamazepine-induced hypersensitivity reactions.

An alternative to carbamazepine is oxcarbazepine, which is better tolerated but with little evidence to support its effectiveness. Other medications which can be used for medium-term to long-term treatment are lamotrigine, gabapentin, pregabalin, baclofen, phenytoin, and botulinum toxin type A. These drugs may be used either as monotherapy or add-on therapy when the first-line drugs fail due to either efficacy or side effects.[59]

In an acute exacerbation, intravenous infusion of fosphenytoin or lidocaine can be effective. However, this should be administered under specialist supervision and close cardiac monitoring.

In medically refractory patients, surgical intervention should be offered, and patients should be informed early of this possibility. Microvascular decompression (MVD) is the most effective option for classical TN, with about 62%–89% of the patients being pain free at long-term follow-up (ranging from 3 to 10.9 years after surgery) with a relatively low recurrence rate (about 4% per year).[59] Although there are reported complications of MVD, most of them are transitory and severe, permanent adverse effects are rare.

For idiopathic TN, it remains controversial which surgical technique should be offered. Apart from MVD, other options include stereotactic gamma knife surgery, radiofrequency thermocoagulation, balloon compression, and glycerol rhizotomy. These techniques are neuroablative treatments, which mean sensory fibers may be damaged. A common side effect is a facial and corneal numbness, which tends to be associated with a better long-term response.[59] It is suggested that neuroablative treatments should be preferred when MRI does not show any neurovascular contact.

Painful trigeminal neuropathy According to ICHD-3, painful trigeminal neuropathy is defined as orofacial pain in the distribution of one or more branches of the trigeminal nerve caused by another disorder and indicative of neural damage.[52] Several causes of painful trigeminal neuropathy have been recognized as shown in Table 2.10. In contrast to TN, the pain in trigeminal neuropathy is usually persistent, moderate in intensity, and generally described as burning, squeezing, or pins and needles. Occasional paroxysms, that are more severe, may be present, but they are not the main characteristics. Physical examination usually demonstrates sensory deficits within the trigeminal distribution, mechanical allodynia, and cold hyperalgesia. It should be noted that allodynic areas are much larger than the trigger zones present in TN.

Painful trigeminal neuropathy related to herpes zoster Herpes zoster (HZ) is a well-recognized cause of painful trigeminal neuropathy. It results from the reactivation of the latent varicella-zoster virus (VZV) acquired during previous episodes of VZV infection (chickenpox). The reactivated VZV then causes vesicular eruptions confined to a dermatome, with neuropathic pain features. HZ affects the trigeminal ganglion in about 10%–15% of total cases. Among these, the ophthalmic division is frequently involved, accounting for 80% of patients, and may be associated with third, fourth, or sixth cranial nerve palsies.

Although herpetic eruptions are usually self-limited, resolving within 1 month, the pain in HZ may persist longer. In about 20% of patients, the pain will persist or recur for more than 3 months. This is called "postherpetic neuralgia" (PHN). Risk factors of PHN include the elderly, having prodromal pain, severe rash, severe acute HZ pain, ophthalmic involvement, severe immunosuppression, and diabetes mellitus.

Table 2.10 Potential causes of trigeminal neuropathy.[62–65]

Trauma	Maxillofacial fracture, dental implant, dental extraction (mandibular third molars), endodontic treatment, orthognathic surgery, local anesthetic injection (inferior alveolar and lingual nerve blocks), neuroablative procedure, radiation
Tumor	Meningioma, trigeminal schwannoma, vestibular schwannoma, nasopharyngeal carcinoma, odontoma, perineural spread of tumor, metastasis
Autoimmune disease	Systemic lupus erythematosus (SLE), rheumatoid arthritis, dermatomyositis, progressive systemic scleroderma, Sjögren's syndrome, multiple sclerosis, undifferentiated and mixed connective tissue disease
Infection	Varicella-zoster virus, herpes simplex virus, syphilis, leprosy, lyme disease, actinomycosis
Vascular	Pontomedullary ischemia or hemorrhage, vascular malformation
Congenital	Congenital trigeminal anesthesia, skull base anomalies
Others	Sarcoidosis, amyloidosis, sickle cell disease, Kennedy's disease, diabetes mellitus, toxin (stilbamidine, trichloroethylene, oxaliplatin)
Idiopathic	Idiopathic trigeminal neuropathy

In the acute period, besides antiviral therapy (acyclovir, valacyclovir, or famciclovir), it is reasonable to follow the principles of acute pain management; paracetamol or NSAIDs alone or in combination with weak opioids for mild to moderate pain, and strong opioids for severe pain. Tricyclic antidepressants (TCAs) and anticonvulsants may be considered as adjuvants. Neural blockades, such as supraorbital, infraorbital, or mental nerve block, may be performed in patients with inadequate pain control. Systemic corticosteroids have been shown to reduce acute pain, but they do not lower the incidence of PHN and should be used with caution. Currently, the only reliable method for preventing PHN is the prevention of HZ. A study showed that the zoster vaccination reduced the incidence of HZ by 51.3% and the incidence of PHN by 66.5%.[66] According to the Centers for Disease Control and Prevention's (CDC) recommendations, the recombinant zoster vaccine should be given to immunocompetent adults age 50 years and older.[67]

Regarding PHN, pain management strategies should follow guidelines for neuropathic pain. The first-line drugs include TCAs and gabapentinoids (gabapentin and pregabalin). Serotonin–norepinephrine reuptake inhibitors (SNRI) can be an alternative for TCA due to its low risk of serious side effects. However, the evidence about the effectiveness of SNRI in PHN is limited. Also, topical analgesics such as lidocaine patch 5% and capsaicin patch 8% have been demonstrated to be effective against PHN. Strong opioids are considered a third-line treatment for PHN. Opioids should be considered only if expected benefits for both pain and function are anticipated to outweigh the risks to the patient. Table 2.5 summarizes the pharmacological treatments for neuropathic pain.

Several interventions have been shown to be effective against acute HZ pain and PHN. Makharita and colleagues reported that early stellate ganglion blockades decreased the intensity of acute pain, shortened its duration, and reduced the incidence of PHN during a 6-month period.[68] Also, pulsed radiofrequency (PRF) of gasserian ganglion and peripheral nerve (supraorbital, infraorbital, or mental nerve) was demonstrated to be effective for PHN, with gasserian ganglion PRF being more effective than peripheral nerve PRF.[69] The other methods include cryoablation of the peripheral nerve, retrobulbar block, deep brain stimulation, and intrathecal drug delivery. However, further studies about the long-term efficacy and complications of these techniques are needed.

Painful posttraumatic trigeminal neuropathy Painful posttraumatic trigeminal neuropathy is orofacial pain caused by trauma (mechanical, thermal, chemical, or radiation) to the branch of the trigeminal nerve. As stated in the ICHD-3, the pain has to persist or recur for more than 3 months, and the onset must be within 6 months after the injury.[52] Common causes of injury include maxillofacial fractures, dental procedures, and neuroablative procedures. The pain characteristics can be varied in several ways (episodic, continuous, or combination). Somatosensory abnormalities in the same distribution are usually present, and these can be either positive signs (hyperalgesia, allodynia) or negative signs (hypoalgesia, hypoesthesia).

Several investigations can be used to confirm the diagnosis, including QST, imaging, nerve conduction study, laser-evoked potentials, blink reflex, or skin biopsy. However, this information needs to be correlated with clinical features.

The mainstays of pharmacologic treatment of painful posttraumatic trigeminal neuropathy are gabapentinoids, TCAs, and SNRIs. These drugs can be used either as a monotherapy or a combined therapy. Opioids should be reserved for patients whom first-line therapy fails.

Even though the role of surgery for improving numbness in nonpainful trigeminal neuropathies is well-documented, the efficacy of surgery in these painful conditions remains inconclusive. Of note, psychological treatment such as cognitive behavioral therapy might be helpful for some patients.

Glossopharyngeal neuralgia

Glossopharyngeal neuralgia (GPN) is a rare condition characterized by a sudden brief severe stabbing pain in the distributions not only of the glossopharyngeal nerve but also of the auricular and pharyngeal branches of the vagus nerve. Compared with the TN, GPN is much less common, occurring approximately 0.2–0.8 per 100,000 populations per year, with a mean age of 54 years.[55,70] It is more common on the left side, with left to right ratio of 3:2.[71]

Patients with GPN commonly present with pain located in the ear, base of the tongue, tonsillar fossa, or beneath the angle of the mandible, pain may radiate to the eye, nose, chin, or shoulder. The pain can be severe and may remit and relapse in the same manner as trigeminal neuralgia. It can be triggered by swallowing, talking, or coughing.

Table 2.11 Diagnostic criteria for glossopharyngeal neuralgia.[52]

A. Recurring paroxysmal attacks of unilateral pain in the distribution of the glossopharyngeal nerve and fulfilling criterion B
B. Pain has all of the following characteristics:
1. lasting from a few seconds to 2 minutes
2. severe intensity
3. electric shock-like, shooting, stabbing, or sharp in quality
4. precipitated by swallowing, coughing, talking, or yawning
C. Not better accounted for by another ICHD-3 diagnosis

Occasionally, attacks of pain are associated with vagal symptoms such as cough, hoarseness, syncope, bradycardia, asystole, and seizure. Some have suggested using the term "vago-glossopharyngeal neuralgia" when pain is accompanied by these symptoms.

Physical examination usually demonstrates no gross neurological deficits. Although mild sensory impairment can be present in some patients, major changes or a reduced gag reflex should prompt further investigations. As per ICHD-3, the diagnostic criteria for GPN are shown in Table 2.11.

Similar to trigeminal neuralgia, GPN is classified into three types: classical, secondary, and idiopathic.[52] Classical GPN is defined as GPN with a demonstration of neurovascular compression of the glossopharyngeal nerve on MRI or during surgery. Secondary GPN is in patients who have an underlying disease known to be able to cause, and explain, the neuralgia, such as multiple sclerosis, brain tumor, and Arnold-Chiari malformation. Lastly, GPN with no evidence of either neurovascular compression or causative underlying disease is termed idiopathic GPN.

Imaging studies, such as MRI or CT, have been used to identify etiologies of GPN. As an example, the elongated styloid process visualized on CT or plain radiograph may suggest GPN secondary to Eagle's syndrome, although this is a controversial diagnosis. These imaging techniques may demonstrate neurovascular compression, which can be caused by the posterior inferior cerebellar artery.

Management of glossopharyngeal neuralgia Due to the low prevalence of the condition, data about effective treatment are still lacking. Hence, treatment is based on case series and relies on comparisons with TN. Patients with GPN usually respond well to pharmacological treatment. First-line drugs are carbamazepine or oxcarbazepine. In addition, topical analgesia by application of local anesthetic to the affected area can be effective in preventing attacks. Cardiac pacing may be required in patients with related syncope.

A glossopharyngeal nerve block can be used as a rescue treatment due to its rapid onset. It can be performed using local anesthetic agents such as lidocaine 2% or bupivacaine 0.5% with or without steroids. Several techniques have been described, including an ultrasound-guided technique.[72] Even if bilateral glossopharyngeal neuralgia is extremely rare, it should be noted that performing bilateral proximal glossopharyngeal nerve block should be advised against since the vagus nerve lies in proximity with the glossopharyngeal nerve, and the blockade may cause airway compromise.

Surgical procedures may be considered when the pain is refractory to medications. MVD is the best option when neurovascular compression is present, with over 76% of the cases showing significant improvement.

Nevertheless, it should be noted that microvascular decompression for GPN is technically more difficult than that for TN. The major complications include dysphonia, dysphagia, hoarseness, hypoacusis, and facial paresis. Other techniques include direct surgical neurotomy, open trigeminal tractotomy-nucleotomy, radiofrequency thermorhizotomy, and stereotactic radiosurgery. However, the long-term efficacy of these techniques is still lacking.

Burning mouth syndrome

Burning mouth syndrome (BMS) (previously known as glossodynia, glossopyrosis, oral dysesthesia, or stomatodynia) is defined as an idiopathic, intraoral burning or dysesthetic sensation in the context of clinically normal oral mucosa, which recurs daily for more than 2 h per day for more than 3 months. The prevalence of BMS varies between 0.01% and 3.7%, with a female predisposition. Affected women are most often menopausal or postmenopausal, with a mean age of around 60 years.[73] This condition has been shown to substantially affect the quality of life.

Patients typically present with bilateral burning sensations felt superficially in the oral mucosa. The most common site is the tip and anterior two-thirds of the tongue, accounting for about 50% of patients. Other commonly affected sites include the anterior palate, gingivae, lower lips, and pharynx. Generally, the pain is spontaneous and fluctuates, usually worsening during the daytime. In some cases, pain can be triggered by certain foods, particularly spicy or acidic foods, and psychological factors such as stress and fatigue.

Dry mouth (xerostomia) and altered taste sensation (dysgeusia) are frequently present, affecting about two-thirds of the patients. These might be related to changes in salivary flow or composition and alterations in taste threshold, respectively. Many BMS patients also have psychiatric comorbidities, such as anxiety, depression, and personality disorders, which should be managed in collaboration with a psychiatrist.

Careful history taking, particularly medication history and physical examination, should be performed. Physicians should look for signs of disease, such as oral cancer, candidiasis, lichen planus, immunobullous conditions, orofacial granulomatosis, allergic contact dermatitis, and Sjögren's syndrome. A mucosal biopsy is unlikely to be useful if careful oral examination reveals normal mucosa. Sialometry should be performed when hyposalivation is suspected.

Despite the fact that the diagnosis of BMS is predominantly clinical, laboratory investigations should be done to exclude identifiable causes, including deficiencies in iron, zinc, folic acid and vitamin B12, anemia, diabetes mellitus, and hypothyroidism.

Management of burning mouth syndrome Although a number of therapies have been employed to treat BMS, currently, there is no clear evidence-based standard treatment for BMS. As the BMS may have a neuropathic mechanism, a pharmacological treatment used for neuropathic pain may be effective.

From the Cochrane Database of Systematic Reviews in 2016, topical benzodiazepines and anticonvulsants can be useful for short-term symptom relief, while topical capsaicin and benzodiazepines may be used for long-term symptom relief.[74] Medications shown to be beneficial include topical local anesthetics, systemic benzodiazepines, antidepressants, and α-lipoic acid. Nevertheless, the effectiveness of these drugs is still uncertain.

Several nonpharmacological methods have been demonstrated to be effective in BMS. These include electromagnetic radiation, physical barriers (tongue protectors), and psychological therapy. The evidence shows that individual or small-group cognitive-behavioral therapy can reduce the pain intensity of BMS. Also, a meta-analysis has confirmed the effectiveness of photobiomodulation (the therapy that applies red or near-infrared light to tissue) in pain reduction and quality of life improvement.[75]

Opioid use for chronic noncancer pain

Opioid medications have been frequently used as analgesic drugs and seen as effective for both chronic noncancer pain and chronic cancer pain. It is believed that opioids exert their actions mainly on opioid receptors located in the dorsal horn of the spinal cord and supraspinal centers, leading to potent analgesia, although several studies also demonstrate peripheral opioid analgesic mechanisms. In otolaryngology, some evidence shows that opioid pathways are also involved in the descending inhibitory control of trigeminal nociceptive transmission from the brainstem, which is one of the mechanisms hypothesized to contribute to OFP.[76]

In the general population, a meta-analysis reported that the prevalence of short-term opioid use (less than 3 months) was 8.1%, and the prevalence of long-term opioid use (more than 3 months) was 2.3%. The prevalence was higher among men, younger people, people with more chronic pain conditions, smokers, and patients without insurance or with noncommercial insurance.[77] In the United States, it was estimated that about 3%−4% of the adult US population were prescribed long-term opioid treatment in 2005. A study also showed that the incidence and the prevalence of long-term opioid use increased significantly between 1997 and 2005.[78]

For chronic noncancer pain (CNCP), the short-term efficacy of opioids (less than 12 weeks) in pain reduction and improved function has been well demonstrated by several studies in both neuropathic and musculoskeletal pain conditions. However, there is very low-quality evidence supporting the long-term efficacy. Few studies have been performed to evaluate the long-term outcomes (more than 1 year) of opioids for CNCP related to pain, function, quality of life, opioid abuse, or addiction.[79]

Regarding the risks of opioids, evidence suggests that long-term opioid therapy is associated with increased risk for opioid overdose, opioid abuse, fractures, myocardial infarction, and sexual dysfunction, all in a dose-dependent fashion.[79] As stated in the Cochrane Database of Systematic Reviews 2017, the incidence of adverse events associated with the medium- and long-term use of opioids for CNCP was as high as 78%, with the incidence of 7.5% for any serious adverse events.[80] A meta-analysis also showed that the estimated prevalence of problematic use of opioids, such as abuse, misuse, addiction, dependence, and aberrant behavior, in patients with CNCP was 36.3%.[81]

In the United States, from the 2019 national survey on drug use and health, 1.6 million people had an opioid use disorder, and 10.1 million people misused prescription opioids in the past year. Furthermore, there were 48,006 deaths in a 12-month period attributed to overdosing on synthetic opioids other than methadone. The data highlight the seriousness of the current opioid epidemic situation.

Based on the data, it is suggested that the short-term use of opioids may be a safe and effective method for CNCP in appropriately screened patients, but there is limited evidence to support long-term opioid therapy for CNCP. In 2016, the CDC developed a guideline for prescribing opioids for CNCP, which was intended to improve the effectiveness of opioid treatment and reduce the risks associated with long-term opioid therapy. This guideline states that nonpharmacologic treatment and nonopioid analgesics are preferred for the management of CNCP. Physicians should only consider opioid therapy when benefits are expected to outweigh risks to the patient.[5]

Before starting opioid therapy, physicians should establish realistic treatment goals with all patients and advise patients about the adverse effects of opioids. The potential harm of opioid therapy should be assessed comprehensively. Risk factors of opioid overdose include a history of opioid overdose, history of substance use disorder, higher opioid dosages (more than 50 MME per day), or concurrent benzodiazepine use.[5] For high-risk patients, "take home" naloxone, which is a nonselective and competitive opioid receptor antagonist used for the treatment of opioid overdose, should be offered to the patients and caregivers. Urine drug testing should be considered before starting opioids and at least annually to assess for prescribed medications as well as other illicit drugs.

When starting opioid treatment, physicians should prescribe an immediate-release (IR) opioid rather than an extended-release or long-acting formulation and use the lowest effective dosage to minimize the risk of opioid overdose, especially for opioid-naïve patients. The dosage should be kept at the minimum dose that achieves the patient's treatment goals. When the dosage is more than 50 MME per day, physicians should carefully reassess the benefits and risks of opioid use and should avoid increasing dosage to greater than 90 MME per day due to the increased risk of opioid-related adverse events.[5]

After prescribing opioids, physicians should assess the benefits and harms within 1 month. At follow-up, prescription drug monitoring program data should be reviewed at least every 3 months. Importantly, physicians should avoid concurrently prescribing opioids, benzodiazepines, and other central nervous system depressants, such as hypnotics or skeletal muscle relaxants, to reduce the risk of drug overdose and counsel against the use of alcohol while taking opioids.

Chronic cancer-related pain

Chronic cancer-related pain is one of the most common symptoms associated with cancer, negatively affecting patients' quality of life. It can be divided into chronic cancer pain (chronic pain caused by cancer itself) and chronic postcancer treatment pain (chronic pain that may be the consequence of surgery, radiotherapy, and chemotherapy, such as chronic postsurgical pain syndrome (CPSP), radiation-induced neuropathy, chemotherapy-induced neuropathy). For head and neck cancer, due to its abundant nerve supply and the confinement of many structures to a limited space, the prevalence of pain is significantly higher, ranging from 40% to 84%, compared with other types of cancer. Predictive factors include age, gender, low education, less physical activity, poor sleep quality, functional impairment after treatment, anxiety, and depression. Shuman and colleagues also reported that patients with head and neck cancer who undergo neck dissections, complain of xerostomia, and require feeding tubes tend to have a greater pain sensation.[82]

Pharmacological management of cancer pain

In accordance with the National Comprehensive Cancer Network Guidelines for Adult Cancer Pain, pain management in cancer patients should be focused on five dimensions, frequently referred to as the "5As," which are analgesia, activities, adverse effects, aberrant drug taking, and affect.[83] Pain management should include pharmacological, nonpharmacological, and interventional treatment strategies.

The most widely accepted algorithm for cancer pain management is the WHO analgesic ladder, which was proposed in 1986.[84] It recommends treating pain in a stepwise approach according to pain intensity. This algorithm involves the use of NSAIDs with or without adjuvants for mild pain (step 1), weak opioids with or without NSAIDs and adjuvants for moderate pain (step 2), and strong opioids with or without NSAIDs and adjuvants for severe pain (step 3). In addition, it also recommends that analgesics should be administered by mouth, given at fixed intervals (by the clock), adapted to each individual (for the individual), and prescribed with a concern for detail (with attention to detail). This method has been reported to be effective in about 70% of cases.[85]

Several modifications of the WHO analgesic ladder have been made to improve its validity. Because many advanced interventional techniques have been shown to be effective for cancer pain management, it is recommended that these techniques should be integrated with the standard pharmacological treatment as a fourth step (Fig. 2.2).[86–88] These interventions include neurolytic/ablative therapy, intrathecal infusion, and spinal cord stimulation. Furthermore, some studies suggest that these interventions may be more beneficial when performed earlier in the disease trajectory.

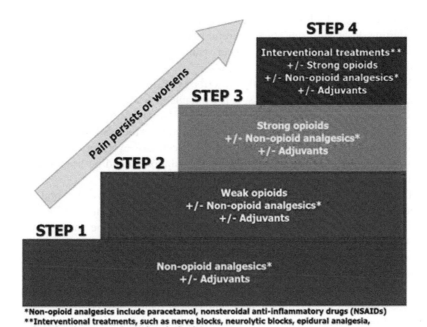

FIGURE 2.2

Modified WHO analgesic ladder for chronic cancer-related pain.[86,88,89]

Some authors have questioned the usefulness of step II, proposing the use of strong opioids instead of weak opioids when NSAIDs become ineffective. Some studies demonstrated a better therapeutic index of low-dose strong opioids compared to high-dose weak opioids. Compared with the WHO guidelines, patients receiving strong opioids have significantly better pain relief and reported greater satisfaction, without the development of tolerance or serious adverse events.[90,91] These data suggest that a direct move to the third step of the WHO analgesic ladder is possible without untoward serious complications. In fact, it may reduce the pain score and improve a patient's satisfaction.

At present, strong opioids are considered the mainstay of analgesic therapy for moderate to severe cancer-related pain. Although several kinds of opioids are available, there is no superiority of one opioid over another. Pure agonists (such as morphine, oxycodone, and fentanyl) are widely used medications because they have no ceiling effect. Opioids with a short half-life (such as fentanyl, hydromorphone, morphine, and oxycodone) are preferred as they can be more easily titrated than the long half-life opioids (such as methadone). As there might be differences between each type of opioid with regard to pharmacokinetics and adverse effects, the choice of opioid should be guided by its pharmacokinetics, contraindications, and the adverse effects in different patients. For instance, for patients with impaired renal function, morphine, oxymorphone, hydrocodone, and codeine should be used with caution, while hydromorphone, fentanyl, buprenorphine, or methadone given at low starting doses with subsequent careful titration may be more suitable. Meperidine is not recommended for cancer pain because of its toxic metabolite (normeperidine).[92]

Morphine is the most commonly prescribed first-line opioid treatment due to its accessibility and cost-effectiveness. It is available in a wide range of formulations, including intravenous (IV), immediate-release (IR), and slow-release (SR) forms. Both around-the-clock IR morphine and around-the-clock SR morphine can be effectively used for the background pain of cancer. However, for the treatment of breakthrough pain, the immediate-release formulation should be used as a rescue medicine.[93]

Despite the fact that oral medications are preferred whenever the oral route is possible, this may not be suitable for head and neck cancer patients as some patients may have difficulty with oral administration. Moreover, in some patients, medications need to be administered through a gastric tube. This may preclude the use of oral sustained-release formulation. In these cases, transdermal opioids, such as fentanyl or buprenorphine, may be used. Another benefit of the transdermal medication is that, at equianalgesic doses, they are both associated with less constipation.

Due to its rich innervation, neuropathic cancer pain is also commonly found in head and neck cancer. A study showed that neuropathic pain was present in about 25% of head and neck cancer patients, which resulted from both cancer itself and its treatment.[94] Antineuropathic medications, such as anticonvulsants, TCAs, or SNRIs, can be helpful in these patients. The pharmacotherapy for neuropathic pain is summarized in Table 2.5. Several studies have confirmed that these adjuvants improve pain control when combined with nonopioid and opioid analgesics. A recent study also found that high-dose gabapentin (2700 mg daily) increased the percentage of patients who required no opioid during chemoradiation for head and neck squamous cell cancer.[95] Additionally, corticosteroids may also be considered as adjuvant analgesics when neural structures are involved, for example, spinal cord compression.

Finally, topical agents can also effectively reduce pain intensity in some head and neck cancer patients, especially those with pain limited to oral mucosa and body surface, while possessing less systemic side effects. These agents comprise analgesic drugs, natural agents, antimicrobial agents, and growth factors. Due to the analgesic effect, topical analgesics may also improve patients' food and fluid intake, communication, and sleep. The evidence shows that effective agents for oral mucositis include mouthwash form of morphine 1% or 2%, phenytoin 0.5% or 1%, lidocaine viscous 2%, doxepin, and ketamine. However, the quality of evidence is still low, suggesting the need for further randomized clinical trials.

Adverse effects of opioids in cancer pain treatment

Despite the fact that opioids can be effectively used for cancer pain management, they also possess several drawbacks. A number of adverse effects associated with opioid analgesics have been reported, such as bowel dysfunction, pruritus, respiratory depression, central nervous system side effects (cognitive impairment, sedation, delirium, myoclonus, and opioid-induced hyperalgesia), especially when high doses of opioids are used. Some studies also reported that chronic opioid use may suppress the hypothalamic-pituitary axis and cause hypogonadism. These adverse effects remain an ongoing problem for the majority of patients and require careful assessment, preventive measures, and appropriate treatment strategies.

Opioid-induced bowel dysfunction is a major adverse effect of opioids, which includes a wide range of symptoms, such as constipation, nausea, vomiting, abdominal cramping, gastroesophageal reflux, and bloating. Among these symptoms, opioid-induced constipation (OIC) is the most frequently reported. It is mediated through the action on μ-receptors located in the enteric nervous system, which cause delayed gastrointestinal transit time, increased fluid absorption, and decreased water and electrolyte excretion. As patients do not develop tolerance to this side effect, prophylactic bowel regimens must be prescribed to almost all patients receiving opioids. Patients should be advised to intake adequate fluid and dietary fiber, together with maintaining their physical activities. Stimulant laxatives (such as sennosides or bisacodyl) are generally recommended for constipation prophylaxis.[96] Novel laxatives, such as prucalopride, and lubiprostone, have been shown to be effective for OIC; however, further studies are needed to confirm their efficacy. Supplemental bulk-forming agents, such as psyllium, are usually ineffective and may worsen constipation. Rectal enemas may be useful if constipation persists; however, they should be avoided in patients with neutropenia or thrombocytopenia. It is important to exclude other potential causes of constipation, such as bowel obstruction.

Several peripherally acting μ-opioid receptor antagonists are currently available, such as methylnaltrexone, naloxegol, or naldemedine. These can be used when patients poorly respond to standard laxative therapy. In addition, the combination of slow-release oral oxycodone and naloxone effectively decreases OIC while maintaining equal analgesia compared with oxycodone alone. Naloxone has extremely low systemic bioavailability, and it acts primarily on peripheral opioid receptors and spares central analgesia.

Nausea and vomiting are also major untoward effects of opioids, especially during the first week of treatment. When nausea develops, other possible causes should be ruled out, such as gut obstruction, intracranial pathology, hypercalcemia, chemotherapy, and radiation therapy. Effective treatments of opioid-induced nausea and vomiting include dopamine receptor antagonists, serotonin receptor antagonists, and corticosteroids.

As mentioned earlier, there is no single opioid suitable for all patients. When a selected opioid is ineffective, or causes intolerable adverse effects, changing to an alternative opioid may be appropriate. This approach is called "opioid rotation." The conversion ratios used for switching between different opioids are shown in Table 2.12. It is important to note that the dose of the new opioid should be reduced by approximately 25%–50% to account for incomplete cross-tolerance.

Table 2.12 Relative analgesic ratios for opioid switching.[83,93,97]

Opioid	Relative analgesic ratio	Strength of the recommendation for use
Oral morphine to oral codeine[83]	6.7:1	None
Oral morphine to oral tramadol[83]	10:1	None
Oral morphine to oral tapentadol[83]	2.5:1	None
Oral morphine to oral oxycodone	1:1.5	Strong
Oral oxycodone to oral hydromorphone	1:4	Strong
Oral morphine to oral hydromorphone	1:5	Weak
Oral morphine to oral methadone[a]	1:5–10	None
Oral morphine to TD buprenorphine	75:1	Weak
Oral morphine to TD fentanyl[b]	100:1	Strong

TD = transdermal.
[a] *The conversion ratio of methadone is varied. Therefore, it is recommended that pain specialists should be consulted for methadone conversion or dose adjustment.[93]*
[b] *Example: 60 mg oral morphine per day can be converted to TD fentanyl by dividing by 100 into 0.6 mg of TD fentanyl per 24 h (600 mcg/24 h), which is equivalent to TD fentanyl 25 mcg/h. Alternatively, the conversion can be quickly done by dividing mg of morphine per day by 2.4.*
Adapted with permission from Caraceni A, Hanks G, Kaasa S, et al. Use of opioid analgesics in the treatment of cancer pain: evidence-based recommendations from the EAPC. Lancet Oncol. 2012; 13(2):e58–e68, Copyright Elsevier (2012).

Interventions for head and neck cancer

Apart from pharmacological treatments, some interventions have also been shown to be useful for head and neck cancer patients and consequently may reduce opioid requirements. Somatic pain in the head and neck region may be benefit from a trigeminal or glossopharyngeal nerve block, depending on its location. If the nerve block is effective, a neurolytic block using alcohol or phenol may be considered for extended pain relief. A stellate ganglion block, which is a blockade of cervicothoracic sympathetic ganglia, may be appropriate for visceral pain (pain that results from the activation of nociceptors of the viscera organs) associated with head and neck cancer. For patients who are refractory to standard pharmacological treatment, intrathecal drug administration device implantation can allow for intrathecal administration of opioids and some other medications, such as ziconotide, to be offered. Regarding the cost-effectiveness of this method, a good candidate should have a life expectancy of at least 3 months. Nevertheless, the benefits of these procedures should be weighed against the risks of serious complications.

Acknowledgment

We would like to express our appreciation to Dr. Roger Goucke for the invaluable input, suggestion, and language editing of the manuscript.

References

1. Raja SN, Carr DB, Cohen M, et al. The revised International Association for the Study of Pain definition of pain: concepts, challenges, and compromises. *Pain*. 2020;161(9): 1976−1982.
2. Zinboonyahgoon N, Schreiber K. Acute pain: operative and post-operative pain, trauma, obstetric pain. In: Hogans B, Barreveld A, eds. *Pain Care Essentials*. Oxford University Press; 2020:241−258.
3. Fine PG. Long-term consequences of chronic pain: mounting evidence for pain as a neurological disease and parallels with other chronic disease states. *Pain Med*. 2011; 12(7):996−1004.
4. Cramer JD, Wisler B, Gouveia CJ. Opioid stewardship in otolaryngology: state of the art review. *Otolaryngol Head Neck Surg*. 2018;158(5):817−827.
5. Dowell D, Haegerich TM, Chou R. CDC guideline for prescribing opioids for chronic pain–United States, 2016. *J Am Med Assoc*. 2016;315(15):1624−1645.
6. Tompkins DA, Hobelmann JG, Compton P. Providing chronic pain management in the "Fifth Vital Sign" era: historical and treatment perspectives on a modern-day medical dilemma. *Drug Alcohol Depend*. 2017;173(Suppl 1):S11−S21.
7. National Quality Forum. *Surgery 2015−2017 Final Report*. Washington, DC: National Quality Forum; 2017. https://www.qualityforum.org/Publications/2017/04/Surgery_2015-2017_Final_Report.aspx. Accessed February 15, 2021.
8. Chou R, Gordon DB, de Leon-Casasola OA, et al. Management of postoperative pain: a clinical practice guideline from the American pain society, the American society of regional anesthesia and pain medicine, and the American society of anesthesiologists' committee on regional anesthesia, executive committee, and administrative council. *J Pain*. 2016;17(2):131−157.
9. Sommer M, Geurts JW, Stessel B, et al. Prevalence and predictors of postoperative pain after ear, nose, and throat surgery. *Arch Otolaryngol Head Neck Surg*. 2009;135(2): 124−130.
10. Morriss W, Goucke R, eds. *Essential Pain Management, Workshop Manual*. 2nd ed. Melbourne, Victoria: ANZCA & FPM; 2016. https://www.anzca.edu.au/safety-advocacy/global-health/essential-pain-management. Accessed February 15, 2021.
11. Schug SA, Palmer GM, Scott DA, Alcock M, Halliwell R, Mott JF, eds. *Acute Pain Management: Scientific Evidence*. 5th ed. Melbourne, Victoria: ANZCA & FPM; 2020.
12. Searle RD, Howell SJ, Bennett MI. Diagnosing postoperative neuropathic pain: a Delphi survey. *Br J Anaesth*. 2012;109(2):240−244.
13. Freynhagen R, Parada HA, Calderon-Ospina CA, et al. Current understanding of the mixed pain concept: a brief narrative review. *Curr Med Res Opin*. 2019;35(6): 1011−1018.
14. Blondell RD, Azadfard M, Wisniewski AM. Pharmacologic therapy for acute pain. *Am Fam Physician*. 2013;87(11):766−772.
15. Leung L. From ladder to platform: a new concept for pain management. *J Prim Health Care*. 2012;4(3):254−258.
16. Rosero EB, Joshi GP. Preemptive, preventive, multimodal analgesia: what do they really mean? *Plast Reconstr Surg*. 2014;134(4 Suppl 2):85S−93S.
17. Kehlet H. Postoperative opioid sparing to hasten recovery: what are the issues? *Anesthesiology*. 2005;102(6):1083−1085.

18. Zinboonyahgoon N, Chen YY, Schreiber K. Chronic postsurgical pain syndromes: prediction and preventive analgesia. In: Benzon H, Rathmell J, Wu C, Turk D, Argoff C, Hurley R, eds. *Practical Management of Pain*. 6th ed. Philadelphia, PA: Elsevier; 2021 (in press).

19. Menendez ME, Ring D, Bateman BT. Preoperative opioid misuse is associated with increased morbidity and mortality after elective orthopaedic surgery. *Clin Orthop Relat Res*. 2015;473(7):2402−2412.

20. Edwards DA, Hedrick TL, Jayaram J, et al. American society for enhanced recovery and perioperative quality initiative joint consensus statement on perioperative management of patients on preoperative opioid therapy. *Anesth Analg*. 2019;129(2):553−566.

21. Mayhew D, Sahgal N, Khirwadkar R, Hunter JM, Banerjee A. Analgesic efficacy of bilateral superficial cervical plexus block for thyroid surgery: meta-analysis and systematic review. *Br J Anaesth*. 2018;120(2):241−251.

22. Richman JM, Liu SS, Courpas G, et al. Does continuous peripheral nerve block provide superior pain control to opioids? A meta-analysis. *Anesth Analg*. 2006;102(1):248−257.

23. Jonan AB, Kaye AD, Urman RD. Buprenorphine formulations: clinical best practice strategies recommendations for perioperative management of patients undergoing surgical or interventional pain procedures. *Pain Physician*. 2018;21(1):E1−E12.

24. Treede RD, Rief W, Barke A, et al. Chronic pain as a symptom or a disease: the IASP classification of chronic pain for the international classification of diseases (ICD-11). *Pain*. 2019;160(1):19−27.

25. Pitcher MH, Von Korff M, Bushnell MC, Porter L. Prevalence and profile of high-impact chronic pain in the United States. *J Pain*. 2019;20(2):146−160.

26. International Association for the Study of Pain. *IASP Statement on Opioids*. Published February; 2018. https://www.iasp pain.org/Advocacy/Content.aspx?ItemNumber=7194. Accessed February 10, 2021.

27. Crombie IK, Davies HT, Macrae WA. Cut and thrust: antecedent surgery and trauma among patients attending a chronic pain clinic. *Pain*. 1998;76(1−2):167−171.

28. Kehlet H, Jensen TS, Woolf CJ. Persistent postsurgical pain: risk factors and prevention. *Lancet*. 2006;367(9522):1618−1625.

29. Schug SA, Bruce J. Risk stratification for the development of chronic postsurgical pain. *Pain Rep*. 2017;2(6):e627.

30. World Health Organization. ICD-11 Coding Tool. https://icd.who.int/ct11/icd11_mms/en/release. Accessed February 4, 2021.

31. Weiser TG, Haynes AB, Molina G, et al. Estimate of the global volume of surgery in 2012: an assessment supporting improved health outcomes. *Lancet*. 2015;385(Suppl 2):S11.

32. Zinboonyahgoon N, Luansritisakul C, Eiamtanasate S, et al. Comparing the ICD-11 chronic pain classification with ICD-10: how can the new coding system make chronic pain visible? A study in a tertiary care pain clinic setting. *Pain*. 2021;162(7):1995−2001. https://doi.org/10.1097/j.pain.0000000000002196 (Epub ahead of print).

33. Fletcher D, Stamer UM, Pogatzki-Zahn E, et al. Chronic postsurgical pain in Europe: an observational study. *Eur J Anaesthesiol*. 2015;32(10):725−734.

34. Clarke H, Poon M, Weinrib A, Katznelson R, Wentlandt K, Katz J. Preventive analgesia and novel strategies for the prevention of chronic post-surgical pain. *Drugs*. 2015;75(4):339−351.

35. Lavand'homme P, Estebe J-P. Opioid-free anesthesia: a different regard to anesthesia practice. *Curr Opin Anesthesiol*. 2018;31(5):556−561.

36. Montes A, Roca G, Sabate S, et al. Genetic and clinical factors associated with chronic postsurgical pain after hernia repair, hysterectomy, and thoracotomy: a two-year multi-center cohort study. *Anesthesiology.* 2015;122(5):1123−1141.

37. Althaus A, Hinrichs-Rocker A, Chapman R, et al. Development of a risk index for the prediction of chronic post-surgical pain. *Eur J Pain.* 2012;16(6):901−910.

38. Brummett CM, Waljee JF, Goesling J, et al. New persistent opioid use after minor and major surgical procedures in US adults. *JAMA Surg.* 2017;152(6):e170504.

39. Chou R, Wagner J, Ahmed AY, et al., eds. *Treatments for Acute Pain: A Systematic Review. Comparative Effectiveness Review No. 240.* Rockville, MD: Agency for Healthcare Research and Quality; 2020 (Prepared by the Pacific Northwest Evidence-based Practice Center under Contract No. 290-2015-00009-I.) AHRQ Publication No. 20(21)-EHC006.

40. Wu CL, King AB, Geiger TM, et al. American society for enhanced recovery and perioperative quality initiative joint consensus statement on perioperative opioid minimization in opioid-naïve patients. *Anesth Analg.* 2019;129(2):567−577.

41. Finnerup NB, Attal N, Haroutounian S, et al. Pharmacotherapy for neuropathic pain in adults: a systematic review and meta-analysis. *Lancet Neurol.* 2015;14(2):162−173.

42. Israel HA, Davila LJ. The essential role of the otolaryngologist in the diagnosis and management of temporomandibular joint and chronic oral, head, and facial pain disorders. *Otolaryngol Clin.* 2014;47(2):301−331.

43. The Orofacial Pain Classification Committee. International classification of orofacial pain, 1st edition (ICOP). *Cephalalgia.* 2020;40(2):129−221.

44. Macfarlane TV, Blinkhorn AS, Davies RM, Ryan P, Worthington HV, Macfarlane GJ. Orofacial pain: just another chronic pain? results from a population-based survey. *Pain.* 2002;99(3):453−458.

45. Benoliel R, Svensson P, Evers S, et al. The IASP classification of chronic pain for ICD-11: chronic secondary headache or orofacial pain. *Pain.* 2019;160(1):60−68.

46. Isong U, Gansky SA, Plesh O. Temporomandibular joint and muscle disorder-type pain in U.S. adults: the National Health Interview Survey. *J Orofac Pain.* 2008;22(4):317−322.

47. Benoliel R, Sharav Y. Chronic orofacial pain. *Curr Pain Headache Rep.* 2010;14(1):33−40.

48. Halpern L, Willis P. Orofacial pain: pharmacologic paradigms for therapeutic intervention. *Dent Clin.* 2016;60(2):381−405.

49. Okeson JP. The classification of orofacial pains. *Oral Maxillofac Surg Clin.* 2008;20(2):133−144.

50. Van Deun L, de Witte M, Goessens T, et al. Facial pain: a comprehensive review and proposal for a pragmatic diagnostic approach. *Eur Neurol.* 2020;83(1):5−16.

51. Zakrzewska JM. Differential diagnosis of facial pain and guidelines for management. *Br J Anaesth.* 2013;111(1):95−104.

52. Headache classification committee of the international headache society (IHS). The international classification of headache disorders, 3rd edition. *Cephalalgia.* 2018;38(1):1−211.

53. Sjaastad O, Bakketeig LS. The rare, unilateral headaches. Vågå study of headache epidemiology. *J Headache Pain.* 2007;8(1):19−27.

54. Mueller D, Obermann M, Yoon MS, et al. Prevalence of trigeminal neuralgia and persistent idiopathic facial pain: a population-based study. *Cephalalgia.* 2011;31(15):1542−1548.

55. Koopman JS, Dieleman JP, Huygen FJ, de Mos M, Martin CG, Sturkenboom MC. Incidence of facial pain in the general population. *Pain.* 2009;147(1−3):122−127.

56. Zakrzewska JM, Wu J, Mon-Williams M, Phillips N, Pavitt SH. Evaluating the impact of trigeminal neuralgia. *Pain.* 2017;158(6):1166−1174.

57. Maarbjerg S, Gozalov A, Olesen J, Bendtsen L. Concomitant persistent pain in classical trigeminal neuralgia–evidence for different subtypes. *Headache.* 2014;54(7):1173−1183.

58. Haviv Y, Khan J, Zini A, Almoznino G, Sharav Y, Benoliel R. Trigeminal neuralgia (part I): revisiting the clinical phenotype. *Cephalalgia.* 2016;36(8):730−746.

59. Bendtsen L, Zakrzewska JM, Abbott J, et al. European Academy of neurology guideline on trigeminal neuralgia. *Eur J Neurol.* 2019;26(6):831−849.

60. Barker FG, Jannetta PJ, Bissonette DJ, Larkins MV, Jho HD. The long-term outcome of microvascular decompression for trigeminal neuralgia. *N Engl J Med.* 1996;334(17):1077−1083.

61. Di Stefano G, Truini A, Cruccu G. Current and innovative pharmacological options to treat typical and atypical trigeminal neuralgia. *Drugs.* 2018;78(14):1433−1442.

62. Benoliel R, Teich S, Eliav E. Painful traumatic trigeminal neuropathy. *Oral Maxillofac Surg Clin.* 2016;28(3):371−380.

63. Flint S, Scully C. Isolated trigeminal sensory neuropathy: a heterogeneous group of disorders. *Oral Surg Oral Med Oral Pathol.* 1990;69(2):153−156.

64. Peñarrocha M, Cervelló MA, Martí E, Bagán JV. Trigeminal neuropathy. *Oral Dis.* 2007;13(2):141−150.

65. Smith JH, Cutrer FM. Numbness matters: a clinical review of trigeminal neuropathy. *Cephalalgia.* 2011;31(10):1131−1144.

66. Oxman MN, Levin MJ, Johnson GR, et al. A vaccine to prevent herpes zoster and postherpetic neuralgia in older adults. *N Engl J Med.* 2005;352(22):2271−2284.

67. Freedman MS, Ault K, Bernstein H. Advisory Committee on Immunization Practices recommended immunization schedule for adults aged 19 years or older - United States, 2021. *Morb Mortal Wkly Rep.* 2021;70(6):193−196.

68. Makharita MY, Amr YM, El-Bayoumy Y. Effect of early stellate ganglion blockade for facial pain from acute herpes zoster and incidence of postherpetic neuralgia. *Pain Physician.* 2012;15(6):467−474.

69. Ding Y, Hong T, Li H, Yao P, Zhao G. Efficacy of CT guided pulsed radiofrequency treatment for trigeminal postherpetic neuralgia. *Front Neurosci.* 2019;13:708.

70. Katusic S, Williams DB, Beard CM, Bergstralh EJ, Kurland LT. Epidemiology and clinical features of idiopathic trigeminal neuralgia and glossopharyngeal neuralgia: similarities and differences, Rochester, Minnesota, 1945−1984. *Neuroepidemiology.* 1991;10(5−6):276−281.

71. Rey-Dios R, Cohen-Gadol AA. Current neurosurgical management of glossopharyngeal neuralgia and technical nuances for microvascular decompression surgery. *Neurosurg Focus.* 2013;34(3):E8.

72. Ažman J, Stopar Pintaric T, Cvetko E, Vlassakov K. Ultrasound-guided glossopharyngeal nerve block: a cadaver and a volunteer sonoanatomy study. *Reg Anesth Pain Med.* 2017;42(2):252−258.

73. Jääskeläinen SK, Woda A. Burning mouth syndrome. *Cephalalgia.* 2017;37(7):627−647.

74. McMillan R, Forssell H, Buchanan JA, Glenny AM, Weldon JC, Zakrzewska JM. Interventions for treating burning mouth syndrome. *Cochrane Database Syst Rev.* 2016;11(11):CD002779.

75. Zhang W, Hu L, Zhao W, Yan Z. Effectiveness of photobiomodulation in the treatment of primary burning mouth syndrome-a systematic review and meta-analysis. *Laser Med Sci.* 2021;36(2):239−248.

76. Zubrzycki M, Stasiolek M, Zubrzycka M. Opioid and endocannabinoid system in orofacial pain. *Physiol Res.* 2019;68(5):705−715.

77. De Sola H, Dueñas M, Salazar A, Ortega-Jiménez P, Failde I. Prevalence of therapeutic use of opioids in chronic non-cancer pain patients and associated factors: a systematic review and meta-analysis. *Front Pharmacol.* 2020;11:564412.

78. Boudreau D, Von Korff M, Rutter CM, et al. Trends in long-term opioid therapy for chronic non-cancer pain. *Pharmacoepidemiol Drug Saf.* 2009;18(12):1166−1175.

79. Chou R, Turner JA, Devine EB, et al. The effectiveness and risks of long-term opioid therapy for chronic pain: a systematic review for a National Institutes of Health Pathways to Prevention Workshop. *Ann Intern Med.* 2015;162(4):276−286.

80. Els C, Jackson TD, Kunyk D, et al. Adverse events associated with medium- and long-term use of opioids for chronic non-cancer pain: an overview of Cochrane reviews. *Cochrane Database Syst Rev.* 2017;10(10):CD012509.

81. Silva C, Jantarada C, Guimarães-Pereira L. Prevalence of problematic use of opioids in patients with chronic non-cancer pain: a systematic review with meta-analysis. *Pain Pract.* 2021;21(6):715−729. https://doi.org/10.1111/papr.13001 (Epub ahead of print).

82. Shuman AG, Terrell JE, Light E, et al. Predictors of pain among patients with head and neck cancer. *Arch Otolaryngol Head Neck Surg.* 2012;138(12):1147−1154.

83. Swarm RA, Paice JA, Anghelescu DL, et al. Adult cancer pain, version 3.2019, NCCN clinical practice guidelines in oncology. *J Natl Compr Canc Netw.* 2019;17(8): 977−1007.

84. World Health Organization. *Cancer Pain Relief.* Geneva: World Health Organization; 1986.

85. Meuser T, Pietruck C, Radbruch L, Stute P, Lehmann KA, Grond S. Symptoms during cancer pain treatment following WHO-guidelines: a longitudinal follow-up study of symptom prevalence, severity and etiology. *Pain.* 2001;93(3):247−257.

86. Miguel R. Interventional treatment of cancer pain: the fourth step in the World Health Organization analgesic ladder? *Cancer Control.* 2000;7(2):149−156.

87. Tay W, Ho KY. The role of interventional therapies in cancer pain management. *Ann Acad Med Singapore.* 2009;38(11):989−997.

88. Vargas-Schaffer G. Is the WHO analgesic ladder still valid? Twenty-four years of experience. *Can Fam Physician.* 2010;56(6):514−517. e202-e205.

89. Pergolizzi JV, Raffa RB. *The WHO Pain Ladder: Do We Need Another Step?*; 2015. Published 2014. Updated April 14 https://www.practicalpainmanagement.com/resources/who-pain-ladder-do-we-need-another-step. Accessed March 17, 2021.

90. Vielvoye-Kerkmeer AP, Mattern C, Uitendaal MP. Transdermal fentanyl in opioid-naive cancer pain patients: an open trial using transdermal fentanyl for the treatment of chronic cancer pain in opioid-naive patients and a group using codeine. *J Pain Symptom Manag.* 2000;19(3):185−192.

91. Marinangeli F, Ciccozzi A, Leonardis M, et al. Use of strong opioids in advanced cancer pain: a randomized trial. *J Pain Symptom Manag.* 2004;27(5):409−416.

92. Davison SN. Clinical pharmacology considerations in pain management in patients with advanced kidney failure. *Clin J Am Soc Nephrol.* 2019;14(6):917−931.

93. World Health Organization. *WHO Guidelines for the Pharmacological and Radiotherapeutic Management of Cancer Pain in Adults and Adolescents.* Geneva: World Health Organization; 2018.

94. Grond S, Zech D, Lynch J, Diefenbach C, Schug SA, Lehmann KA. Validation of World Health Organization guidelines for pain relief in head and neck cancer. A prospective study. *Ann Otol Rhinol Laryngol.* 1993;102(5):342−348.

95. Hermann GM, Iovoli AJ, Platek AJ, et al. A single-institution, randomized, pilot study evaluating the efficacy of gabapentin and methadone for patients undergoing chemoradiation for head and neck squamous cell cancer. *Cancer.* 2020;126(7):1480−1491.

96. Müller-Lissner S, Bassotti G, Coffin B, et al. Opioid-induced constipation and bowel dysfunction: a clinical guideline. *Pain Med.* 2017;18(10):1837−1863.

97. Caraceni A, Hanks G, Kaasa S, et al. Use of opioid analgesics in the treatment of cancer pain: evidence-based recommendations from the EAPC. *Lancet Oncol.* 2012;13(2): e58−e68.

Perioperative pain management in rhinology and anterior skull base surgery

Nyssa Fox Farrell, MD [1]**, Timothy Smith, MD, MPH** [2]

[1]*Washington University in St. Louis School of Medicine, Department of Otolaryngology-Head and Neck Surgery, St. Louis, MO, United States;* [2]*Oregon Health & Science University, Department of Otolaryngology-Head and Neck Surgery, Portland, OR, United States*

Introduction

The nasal cavity exists to warm, humidify, and sample air for olfaction as we inspire. The role of the paranasal sinuses is not as clear, though it is hypothesized that they exist, at least in part, to lighten the skull and provide a source of protection for the intracranial and orbital contents as a sort of "crash zone" in the case of head trauma. While these roles are important, many pathologies can also manifest within the nose and paranasal sinuses.

Many pathologies involving the nose and paranasal sinuses can be managed with minimally invasive surgery—termed endoscopic sinus or endoscopic skull base surgery (Table 3.1). One of the most common pathologies within the paranasal sinuses is chronic rhinosinusitis, which is the presence of objective sinus inflammation for >12 weeks with associated symptoms such as mucopurulent drainage, nasal obstruction, and facial pain or pressure. Other common surgically managed pathologies include nasal airway obstruction and benign and malignant neoplasms. Many intracranial pathologies can involve the anterior and medial skull base, which can be managed through extended endoscopic endonasal approaches rather than external craniotomies.

Surgical injuries, whether external or endoscopic, initiate an acute inflammatory reaction that manifests as pain. Postoperative pain is expected after most surgical procedures, and it is essential that surgeons understand and prepare patients for the pain that they will experience. Some people even go as far as to say that one of the primary goals of surgery is the appropriate management of the resultant pain.[1]

Although endoscopic sinus and skull base surgeries are minimally invasive, it would be expected that they induce postoperative pain. Inadequate postoperative pain management adversely affects both the patient and the healthcare industry. Uncontrolled pain can result in surgical complications such as atelectasis from

Opioid Use, Overuse, and Abuse in Otolaryngology. https://doi.org/10.1016/B978-0-323-79016-1.00001-5

Table 3.1 Examples of pathologies managed with endoscopic sinus or skull base surgery.

Anatomic abnormalities
Septal deviation
Inferior turbinate hypertrophy
Concha bullosa
Inflammatory/infectious
Recurrent acute sinusitis
Chronic rhinosinusitis
Invasive fungal rhinosinusitis
Benign sinonasal neoplasms
Inverted papilloma
Juvenile nasopharyngeal angiofibroma
Osteoma
Hemangioma
Malignancy sinonasal neoplasms
Squamous cell carcinoma
Adenocarcinoma
Mucosal melanoma
Chondrosarcoma
Salivary gland tumors
Intracranial/skull base pathology
Pituitary adenoma
Craniopharyngioma
Chordoma
Rathke's cleft cyst
Meningioma

poor pulmonary toilet, thromboembolism from immobilization, and cardiovascular morbidity due to catecholamine release. These complications ultimately delay the patient's return to normal functional status.[2,3] Studies have also demonstrated that inadequate pain management after surgery results in decreased patient quality of life, decreased satisfaction, increased hospital readmission rates, increased length of hospital stay, and increased healthcare costs.[3,4]

A commonly cited source of surgical hesitation is the fear of severe or uncontrolled pain.[1] In the realm of the opioid crisis, many patients are also concerned about opioid addiction and fear the use of opioids after surgery. By having a better understanding of the expected postoperative pain, surgeons can improve patient counseling, allowing patients to mentally prepare for their recovery and potentially improving postoperative outcomes.

Endoscopic sinus surgery
Pain after endoscopic sinus surgery

Endoscopic sinus surgery (ESS) is utilized to manage pathologies of the nose and paranasal sinuses. Currently, ESS is one of the most commonly performed procedures in the United States, with greater than 250,000 performed annually.[5] Despite the prevalence of ESS, to date, there are no specialty-specific guidelines for the management of pain after surgery. Of those performed, approximately 3.7% result in readmission for pain.[6] While 3.7% is low overall, this corresponds to nearly 10,000 patients per year who are readmitted for poorly controlled pain after ESS. There are also likely many more patients whose pain is poorly controlled but do not require readmission.

To appropriately counsel patients on pain expectations after ESS, it is important to first understand the painfulness of ESS. Many studies have been performed evaluating the severity of ESS-induced pain, all with similar results: ESS is not associated with severe pain. Utilizing a visual analog scale of 0–10, with 10 being the most severe pain, most studies have demonstrated that the peak of pain after ESS is approximately 2–4 on postoperative day 1 and rapidly declines over the course of the first week.[1,7–10] One study of 64 patients found that only nine patients (14.1%) reported pain greater than five out of 10 within the first week of ESS.[8]

Many attempts have been made to identify features associated with increased pain after ESS. There is a general consensus that the severity of sinus disease, the presence or absence of nasal polyps, use of nasal packing, and extent of surgery do not significantly impact postoperative pain.[1,4] There are conflicting data regarding the impact of septoplasty on postoperative pain, with some studies demonstrating that the inclusion of a septoplasty at the time of ESS may increase pain, while other studies have not found a correlation.[8,11,12] Although evaluations of pain after nonrhinologic surgery have demonstrated an impact of age, gender, and mental illness of postoperative pain, unpublished data from our group show that only the presence of anxiety adversely impacted the severity of postoperative pain (Smith Unpublished Data).

As a first step in mitigating pain after ESS, surgeons should counsel patients on the expectation of mild to moderately severe pain. Surgeons should also evaluate their patients preoperatively for anxiety and ensure that any comorbid anxiety is appropriately managed. Often patients with anxiety also require additional counseling regarding expectations of pain after surgery. By optimizing the surgeon–patient relationship and providing more extensive counseling preoperatively, patients may have more realistic expectations for pain after ESS, resulting in improved outcomes.

Preemptive pain control

Acute tissue injury modulates the central nervous system, ultimately sensitizing patients to pain. Preemptive pain control, the application of regional or systemic medications before the initial surgical injury, diminishes the central nervous system response, ultimately mitigating the severity of perceived postoperative pain.[13] For ESS, many options have been proposed for preemptive pain control (Table 3.2).

Table 3.2 Preemptive pain control options.[14]

Drug	Dose/concentration	Risks
Acetaminophen	1000 mg PO	Nausea Headache Hepatotoxicity
Anticonvulsants		
Gabapentin Pregabalin	600–1200 mg PO 75–300 mg PO	Increased intraoperative bleeding Drowsiness Dizziness Nausea Anxiety Confusion Dry mouth
Glucocorticoids		
Dexamethasone	8–10 mg IV	Hyperglycemia Impaired wound healing
Alpha agonists		
Dexmedetomidine Clonidine	1 μg/kg IV bolus, 0.2 μg/kg/h infusion 2–5 μg/kg IV bolus, 0.3 μg/kg infusion	Sedation Dry mouth Nausea Vomiting Bradycardia Hypotension Loss of smell
Locoregional anesthetics		
Lidocaine Bupivacaine Levobupivacaine	1%–2% submucosal injection 0.25%–0.5% submucosal injection 0.5% submucosal injection	Dizziness Headache Blurred vision Twitching muscles Prolonged numbness

Acetaminophen

Acetaminophen is a common, inexpensive analgesic. The exact mechanism of acetaminophen is unknown, though it is believed to work via the inhibition of cyclooxygenase (COX) enzymes with simultaneous modulation of the serotonergic and cannabinoid pathways.[15] Overall, acetaminophen is well tolerated, though it has a known risk of hepatotoxicity, especially in those with a history of liver dysfunction.

Acetaminophen has been utilized for preemptive analgesia in nonrhinologic surgery, but there has only been limited research evaluating the role of preemptive acetaminophen for the prevention of ESS-induced pain. One study of otolaryngologic surgeries not limited to sinus surgery showed that the preoperative administration of acetaminophen resulted in a trend toward decreased pain after surgery, though the impact was not significant.[16] Bjoja et al. evaluated the impact of a preoperative dose of 1000 mg oral acetaminophen administered preoperatively against 1000 mg of intravenous acetaminophen administered at the end of ESS and found no significant difference in postoperative pain, indicating that a single preemptive oral dose is likely equivalent to a postoperative intravenous dose.[17]

Although the data are limited for ESS, acetaminophen has a long history of use in conjunction with surgery and is overall safe and well tolerated. Oral acetaminophen is significantly less expensive than parenteral acetaminophen, indicating that it is likely preferable to give a preoperative oral dose than to give an intravenous dose at the time of surgery. In patients in whom there is no contraindication, a preemptive dose of acetaminophen has little risk and the potential of significant benefit.

Gabapentinoids

The gabapentinoids gabapentin and its lipophilic analog pregabalin interact with neuron voltage-gated calcium channels, decreasing calcium influx and reducing neurotransmitter release.[14] They were first introduced as antiepileptic drugs but have also been found to have antihyperalgesic and antiallodynic properties via the reduction of neuron hyperexcitability in injured tissue.[18] The analgesic properties of gabapentinoids were first noted for neuropathic pain conditions such as diabetic neuropathy and postherpetic neuralgia. However, as gabapentinoids decrease neuronal excitability, there has been increased interest in their utilization for the prevention of central nervous system sensitization and postoperative pain.

Many studies outside of otolaryngology have evaluated the utility of a preemptive dose of gabapentin and pregabalin and have demonstrated their utility. One systematic review of 28 studies found that a preoperative dose of gabapentin significantly reduced postoperative analgesic requirements and pain for nonrhinologic surgeries.[19] While those studies are promising, there is one potential drawback of preemptive gabapentinoids that may limit their utility for preemptive analgesia—gabapentinoids are known to inhibit platelet aggregation via the phospholipase C-inositol 1,4,5-triphosphate thromboxane A(2)-Ca(2+) pathway. Platelet inhibition could potentially increase bleeding during surgery. Although the studies for nonrhinologic surgery do not note significant changes in operative bleeding, small changes in hemostasis can significantly impact ESS. As ESS is reliant upon endoscopic visualization, poor hemostasis intraoperatively can result in limited visibility and thus increase the risk of complications and increase operative times.

To date, very few studies have evaluated the impact of preoperative gabapentinoids on postoperative pain and analgesic use for ESS. In a recent meta-analysis of sinus and nasal surgery, only three studies that evaluated the impact after ESS were identified.[20] Those studies evaluated a range of preoperative gabapentin (600–1200 mg) and found that preemptive gabapentin significantly decreased analgesic requirements postoperative as well as lengthened the time until the first analgesic was required after ESS. Interestingly, despite the known side effects of nausea and vomiting, those that received gabapentin preoperatively had less postoperative nausea and vomiting.[21] Although the data were limited, on meta-analysis, subjects in the ESS subgroup were noted to have increased operative blood loss after gabapentinoid administration than the septoplasty subgroup, but operative field visibility was not found to be significantly impaired.[20]

Currently, there are no studies that have evaluated the use of pregabalin before ESS. However, pregabalin has been utilized before open septoplasty with promising results. Doses ranging from 75 to 300 mg have been administered, all of which significantly decreased pain within the first 24 h of surgery. Higher doses of pregabalin yielded more profound reductions in pain without apparent increases in adverse effects.[22–24]

Preoperative gabapentinoids have promising results for the mitigation of postoperative pain. However, their utility for pain management may be limited by the potential impact on intraoperative hemostasis. Additional studies will need to be performed to determine the overall impact of preoperative gabapentinoids on ESS. If intraoperative hemostasis and visibility are not adversely impacted, the gabapentinoids may serve as a viable adjunct for preemptive analgesia.

Glucocorticoids

Glucocorticoids are potent antiinflammatory agents that have strong antiemetic properties and have been long utilized perioperatively for the prevention of postoperative nausea and vomiting. They are also known to improve vascular tone that provides a distinct advantage during ESS—decreased blood loss and improved visualization. When utilized long-term, glucocorticoids have the potential of causing significant morbidity—weight gain, hyperglycemia, insomnia, glaucoma, and osteonecrosis of the hip. However, a one-time preoperative dose of corticosteroid, most commonly dexamethasone, is generally safe and well tolerated.

Preemptive pain mitigation with glucocorticoids, most commonly dexamethasone, has been suggested for many nonrhinologic procedures based off the hypothesis that the potential antiinflammatory response can reduce central and peripheral inflammation and pain sensitization. There is abundant evidence in the nonrhinologic literature supporting this hypothesis. Some have even demonstrated that a single dose of dexamethasone at the beginning of a procedure can result in a greater than 10% reduction in opioid consumption within the first 24 h of surgery.[25]

There are many benefits of preoperative glucocorticoids for ESS: decreased operative time, decreased blood loss, and improved visibility.[26] While there are strong data supporting the preemptive use of glucocorticoids for the reduction of postoperative pain in other fields, there are minimal data for or against the role of glucocorticoids in the prevention of postoperative pain in ESS. Only one randomized controlled trial has been performed, which was unable to identify any significant impact of a preemptive dose of dexamethasone compared to placebo.[27] Although the results of that study are not encouraging, a retrospective review of risk factors for opioid refills after ESS did note that a preoperative dose of glucocorticoid was associated with significantly decreased odds of requiring a refill of opioids. Although opioid refills are an indirect measure of pain, the decreased odds of requesting a refill do raise the question as to whether a preoperative dose of gluco-corticoids may be beneficial for the prevention of pain after ESS.

Although glucocorticoids have not been shown to directly decrease pain after ESS, a preoperative dose of dexamethasone is generally safe and well tolerated. The significant impact on the reduction of postoperative nausea and vomiting as well as improved visualization during ESS supports the use of glucocorticoids at the time of ESS.

Alpha agonists

When performing endoscopic sinus surgery, hemostasis is of the utmost importance as excess bleeding decreases visibility increasing the operative risks and length of the procedure. Alpha-2 agonists, such as clonidine and dexmedetomidine, have a central nervous system effect, reducing neural activity through the inhibition of adenylyl cyclase.[14] This results in vasoconstriction, which aids in intraoperative hemostasis, as well as sympatholytic, sedative, and allodynic changes, which may positively impact postoperative pain.

Dexmedetomidine is a highly selective alpha-2 agonist with hypotensive, sedative, and analgesic properties. It does so by modulating the alpha-2 receptors within the central nervous system while simultaneously inhibiting the release of inflammatory cytokines centrally and peripherally. The blockade of inflammatory mediators is thought to prevent central and peripheral sensitization, thus decreasing postoperative pain. A recent meta-analysis of 20 trials evaluating the effects of dexmedetomidine during nasal surgery demonstrated that intraoperative use of dexmedetomidine was associated with decreased postoperative pain and decreased intraoperative bleeding, suggesting that it would be a useful adjunct during ESS.[28]

Clonidine is another alpha-2 agonist that has been theorized to be beneficial for the management of postoperative pain. On meta-analysis, eight studies evaluating the impact of clonidine on nasal surgery were identified.[28] Overall, clonidine was found to lower intraoperative bleeding, but to a lesser extent than dexmedetomidine and was not associated with any decrease in postoperative pain.[28] Thus, dexmedetomidine would be preferential if an alpha-2 agonist were to be utilized during ESS.

Unfortunately, while there have been many studies evaluating alpha-agonists, there is no consistent drug administration guideline, and many studies include only small cohorts of patients, limiting the generalizability of the results. Additionally, an adverse effect of smell loss has been observed in up to 15% has been noted.[29] A known risk factor of ESS is olfactory loss, which can significantly impact patient quality of life. As such, anything that could increase the risk of olfactory loss, such as alpha-2 agonists, should be used with great caution in this patient population. However, if ESS is being performed on a patient with known long-standing anosmia, alpha-2 agonists may serve as a useful adjunct.

Locoregional anesthetics

The role of regional anesthesia has been well established throughout the surgical literature. Local anesthetics block nociceptive input at the time of tissue injury through the inhibition of voltage-gated sodium channels of neurons.[14] When utilized, topical and regional anesthetics can act to inhibit both peripheral and central sensitization of pain, limiting the release of inflammatory cytokines, and ultimately limiting the severity of postoperative pain.[30] The addition of epinephrine to the local anesthetic can potentiate these effects through vasoconstriction limiting drug clearance.

The sphenopalatine ganglion contains a large group of neurons that have somatosensory, parasympathetic, and sympathetic effects. The somatosensory component, via the trigeminal and facial nerves, supplies the majority of the sinonasal mucosa. Inhibition of these neurons has the potential to mitigate intraoperative nociceptive input, postoperative inflammatory responses, and the central processing of pain.[31]

Located within the pterygopalatine fossa, the sphenopalatine ganglion can be accessed through multiple routes. Regional blockade can be obtained through direct infiltration of the ganglion either through a transoral or transnasal injection (Fig. 3.1). Transoral injections utilize local anesthetic infiltrated through the greater palatine foramen. An alternative option for the sphenopalatine ganglion regional block is the transnasal injection. To perform the transnasal injection, the surgeon must visualize and inject an anesthetic into the region of the sphenopalatine foramen adjacent to the lateral attachment of the middle turbinate under endoscopic guidance. Both injections of local anesthetic, whether applied transorally or transnasally, can be technically challenging and have a steep learning curve. Additionally,

A.
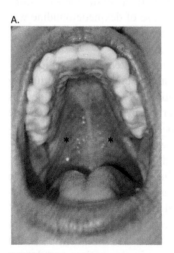

B.
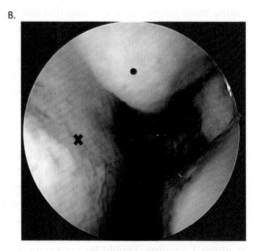

FIGURE 3.1

Sphenopalatine ganglion block. (A) Transoral injection via the greater palatine foramen. The greater palatine foramen (*) exists at the junction of the maxillary and palatine bones within the lateral oral cavity at the level of the third molar. (B) The sphenopalatine foramen is located on the lateral nasal wall, at the posterior superior portion of the maxillary sinus, anterior to the attachment of the horizontal attachment of the middle turbinate. X: nasal septum, dot: middle turbinate, *: region of the sphenopalatine foramen.

injection of the sphenopalatine ganglion is not without risk. Given the local connections to the internal carotid plexus, injection into the pterygopalatine fossa can lead to systemic absorption of local anesthetic. This can result in seizures from lidocaine toxicity or cardiovascular compromise if the local anesthetic is mixed with epinephrine.

Multiple studies have evaluated the efficacy of sphenopalatine blockage on postoperative pain. Meta-analysis of these has demonstrated that sphenopalatine ganglion blockade is both safe and effective. Regardless of the type of local anesthetic utilized, a preoperative block can decrease both the severity of postoperative pain as well as the amount of analgesic utilized after surgery. While the transoral approach has been associated with some adverse effects (dental numbness and retroocular pressure), no major or minor adverse effects were identified after transnasal blockade on meta-analysis.[30] During ESS, surgeons are already comfortable with sinonasal anatomy and utilization of endoscopes, making transnasal injection a simple and efficacious adjunct.

Postoperative pain control

Even after utilizing preemptive pain management strategies, it is expected that patients will have some pain after ESS. As such, it is important to know and understand the various options available to practitioners (Table 3.3).

Topical anesthetic

As discussed previously, regional blockade of the sphenopalatine ganglion can provide significant pain relief after ESS. Similarly, topical application of anesthetic has been demonstrated to be efficacious for the management of pain after endoscopic sinus surgery. Historically, nonabsorbable nasal packing was utilized for hemostasis after ESS. The presence of nonabsorbable packing can be uncomfortable, so multiple studies have evaluated the impact of the installation of anesthetic into the packing at the conclusion of ESS. These studies demonstrated that installation of any local anesthetic into nonabsorbable packing significantly reduced pain and analgesic consumption during the first 24 h after ESS.[32,33]

Modern ESS does utilize nasal packing, but there has been a shift away from nonabsorbable nasal packing and toward absorbable packings, such as chitin sponges, for improved hemostasis in most cases. These absorbable packs often require liquid for them to expand within the sinonasal cavity. As local infiltration of nonabsorbable packing significantly improves pain, it is reasonable to expect that infiltration of nonabsorbable packs with local anesthetic could similarly improve pain control after ESS. Additional studies need to be performed to determine if such a use does, in fact, mitigate postoperative pain and analgesic use.

Acetaminophen

Acetaminophen is an excellent option for both preemptive pain control and postoperative pain control. Acetaminophen is readily available, inexpensive, and can be

Table 3.3 Postoperative pain control options.[14]

Drug	Dose/ concentration	Risks
Topical anesthetic infiltrated into nasal packing		
Lidocaine Bupivacaine Levobupivacaine	1%–2% 0.25%–0.5% 0.5%	Dizziness Headache Blurred vision Twitching muscles Prolonged numbness
Acetaminophen	500–1000 mg PO	Nausea Headache Hepatotoxicity
Nonsteroidal antiinflammatories (NSAIDs)		
Ibuprofen Ketorolac Celecoxib	200–800 mg PO 10–30 mg IV, IM, or PO 200–400 mg PO	Renal dysfunction, bleeding, gastrointestinal ulcers, tinnitus
Anticonvulsants		
Gabapentin Pregabalin	600–1200 mg PO 75–300 mg PO	Increased intraoperative bleeding Drowsiness Dizziness Nausea Anxiety Confusion Dry mouth
Opioids		
Hydrocodone-Acetaminophen Oxycodone Oxycodone-Acetaminophen Tramadol	5–325 mg PO 5 mg PO 5–325 mg PO 50–100 mg PO	Constipation Somnolence Dizziness Nausea Pruritus Headache

given by mouth, intravenous, or rectally after surgery. As such, general surgical guidelines published by the American Pain Society and American Society of Anesthesiologists recommend the use of acetaminophen postoperative, except when contraindicated.[34] Despite these recommendations, a survey of otolaryngologists in 2018 found that only 73% of otolaryngologists prescribe acetaminophen postoperatively.[35] While patients may still be advised to take over-the-counter acetaminophen, many patients do not take medications that are not prescribed after surgery.

The role of acetaminophen after ESS has been well described. The first study analyzing the impact of acetaminophen after ESS compared the efficacy of a one-time dose of 1000 mg acetaminophen at the conclusion of surgery to placebo and found that the number of patients requiring rescue analgesics in the first 4 h after ESS decreased from 71% in the placebo group to 25% in the acetaminophen group.[36] A follow-up study by the same group evaluated the impact of scheduled acetaminophen versus medication taken on an as-needed basis. They evaluated postoperative pain for 30 days after ESS and found that patients who were given scheduled acetaminophen for the first 5 days after ESS noted the cessation of pain on average within 4.7 days, while those who only took acetaminophen as needed noted an average of 6.5 days until the cessation of pain. Only 18% of patients in the "scheduled acetaminophen" group noted moderate or severe pain, while 43% of the "as-needed acetaminophen" group had moderate or severe pain within the first postoperative week.[37]

Given the availability, low cost, and efficacy of acetaminophen, it should be utilized after ESS in patients who do not have contraindications. Common doses of acetaminophen postoperatively are 500–1000 mg every 6 h, which can be given either by mouth or intravenously.[14] The primary contraindication for acetaminophen use is liver dysfunction, and providers should be cognizant of patient comorbidities when prescribing acetaminophen. Additionally, providers should counsel patients not to exceed 4000 mg per day, to avoid hepatotoxicity.

Nonsteroidal antiinflammatories

Nonsteroidal antiinflammatories (NSAIDs), such as ibuprofen and ketorolac, are well known for their antiinflammatory and analgesic effects. They act by blocking cyclooxygenase (COX)-1 and 2, preventing the production of prostacyclins, prostaglandins, and thromboxanes. Their use has been recommended by the American Pain Society and American Society of Anesthesiologists as part of a multimodal strategy for the management of postoperative pain for general surgery.[34] However, while NSAIDs are excellent for postoperative analgesia, they also result in platelet dysfunction, which can potentially increase the risk of epistaxis after ESS. This fear of postoperative epistaxis has historically limited the use of NSAIDs after ESS. In fact, in a survey of otolaryngologists performing ESS, less than 50% of providers prescribed NSAIDs after ESS.[35]

Ibuprofen is the most commonly prescribed NSAID after ESS. Common doses of ibuprofen are 200–800 mg every 6 h after surgery. A recent multiinstitutional study of 175 patients evaluated the impact of low-dose ibuprofen (200 mg) given in addition to acetaminophen after ESS. Their cohort demonstrated significantly lower pain at all time points in those that received ibuprofen. The group that received ibuprofen also utilized significantly less opioid over the course of the first week after ESS.[38] Another small study of 39 patients evaluated the impact of 400 mg ibuprofen in addition to scheduled acetaminophen after ESS. They found that within the first week after ESS, subjects who received ibuprofen reported consistently lower pain than those without ibuprofen and utilized less oxycodone, though the differences were not significant. Importantly, there was no significant difference in postoperative bleeding between groups.[39] Multiple additional small studies have also been performed evaluating the potential role of oral NSAIDs with similar results: a decreased requirement for rescue analgesics.[14,29]

In an attempt to limit the use of postoperative opioids, one group evaluated the efficacy of 30 mg ketorolac to 25 μg fentanyl in the immediate postoperative period. Within the first hour after surgery, they did not find any significant difference in pain between the two groups, indicating that ketorolac provides equivalent analgesia. Most importantly, on self-assessment, there were no significant differences in epistaxis at postoperative day 1 or 7.[40] While ketorolac should likely be avoided preoperatively, due to its impact on platelet function, this study supports the potential use of ketorolac over opioids in the immediate postoperative period.

Another NSAID option includes celecoxib. Unlike ibuprofen and ketorolac, celecoxib is a COX-2 inhibitor. As a more selective NSAID, celecoxib does not cause inhibition of thromboxanes or prostaglandins. As such, the use of celecoxib should not result in platelet dysfunction, reducing concerns for postoperative bleeding. Celecoxib has not been evaluated for the management of ESS-induced pain but does present another potential option for opioid-sparing pain control in this patient population.

To date, there is no consensus on the ideal dose of NSAIDs or the timing of administration, but, in appropriate patients, NSAIDs can be used successfully as part of a multimodal pain management strategy. There are certain circumstances in which providers should not prescribe NSAIDs, however. First, NSAIDs should not be utilized in patients with a history of bleeding disorders, renal disease, or peptic ulcer disease. Second, there is also a subset of patients with chronic rhinosinusitis, deemed aspirin exacerbated respiratory disease, in whom NSAIDs trigger an exaggerated inflammatory response that manifests with respiratory symptoms. Despite these limitations, there is an abundance of evidence to support the use of NSAIDs in the management of pain after ESS and they should be included within the otolaryngologist's armamentarium.

Gabapentinoids

The gabapentinoids gabapentin and pregabalin have been extensively studied in non-rhinologic surgery and have demonstrated significant reductions in postoperative opioid analgesic use.[19] To date, the role of gabapentinoids for ESS-induced pain control has only been evaluated in one study. Thus, it is not surprising that a survey of American otolaryngology prescribing patterns did not identify a single otolaryngologist that prescribed gabapentin or pregabalin after ESS.[35]

As noted previously, gabapentinoids have analgesic, anticonvulsant, and anxiolytic properties, which may make them beneficial for the management of postoperative pain. Given the preponderance of data supporting the use of gabapentinoids in other surgical specialties, gabapentinoids may play a role after ESS. One trial did evaluate the efficacy of pregabalin 50 mg three times daily versus acetaminophen 500 mg every 6 h after ESS in 70 patients with chronic rhinosinusitis with nasal polyps. Pain scores and patient satisfaction were monitored for 3 days after surgery. At all timepoints, the authors found that the pregabalin group had significantly less pain than the acetaminophen group. Interestingly, subjects that received pregabalin had lower rates of postoperative nausea, vomiting, headache, and bleeding. However, they did have higher rates of dizziness and drowsiness, known side effects of gabapentinoids.[41]

Although there are limited data, gabapentinoids may serve as an adjunct for the management of pain after ESS. Additional studies will need to be performed before any definitive recommendations can be made regarding this class of medication and its optimal dosing. If utilized, providers should counsel patients on the risk of sedation and dizziness after administration of gabapentinoids.

Opioids

Opioids are one of the most commonly utilized medications for the management of pain after surgery, especially after ESS. However, opioids are potentially dangerous medications, with known risks of respiratory depression, constipation, nausea, headaches, and somnolence. In addition to the short-term side effects, opioids are commonly abused and misused. The prevalence of this abuse and misuse surged during the 21st century, culminating in the declaration of the opioid crisis in 2017.

While opioid abuse and misuse are not limited to the postoperative period, there is extensive evidence demonstrating that prescription opioids are a major contributor to the opioid crisis, with surgeons providing over a third of all opioid prescriptions per year.[42] A survey of American otolaryngologists showed that 94% of otolaryngologists prescribe opioids after ESS, with hydrocodone-acetaminophen being the most common. Given the high prevalence of ESS, this is not an insignificant contribution to annual opioid prescriptions within the United States.

Despite their potential negatives, opioids do play a role in pain management after ESS. However, it is vital that surgeons prescribe them appropriately. To that end, multiple studies have been performed with the goal of determining the optimal number of opioids that should be prescribed postoperatively. All studies have demonstrated similar results: only a minimum number of opioids are necessary after ESS, with most studies finding that patients used less than 10 pills in the postoperative period, regardless of the type of opioid prescribed.[9,43−45] Even more importantly, one study demonstrated that over 70% of patients kept leftover pills, which could ultimately lead to diversion and misuse of medication.[45]

Despite the minimal opioid requirement noted in the literature, many otolaryngologists overprescribe opioids after ESS, often providing greater than double the amount needed.[35] This is likely due to a combination of factors: fear of uncontrolled postoperative pain, avoidance of postoperative phone calls about poor pain control, and/or lack of knowledge about the typical pain experienced after ESS. Regardless of the rationale, it is vital that the otolaryngologist be cognizant of this common mistake and only prescribe the minimum number of opioids necessary for pain control after ESS. In our practice, patients are only prescribed 10 pills of 5 mg oxycodone and rarely require additional prescriptions.

It is important to identify patients that may require additional opioids so that they can be counseled appropriately. Our group, as well as others, have demonstrated that the extent of ESS, placement of nasal packing, and placement of nasal splints do not impact opioid use after ESS. Instead, increased opioid use appears to be more significantly influenced by the presence of anxiety preoperatively, current tobacco use, and a history of opioid use before ESS (Smith Unpublished Data).[44] Recognition of these risk factors can allow for otolaryngologists to appropriately counsel their patients on postoperative pain expectations and allow for more judicious prescribing of opioids after ESS. We also advocate for the utilization of the opioid-sparing discussed previously in this chapter as part of a multimodal pain strategy in all patients, especially those at increased risk of persistent opioid use.

Endoscopic skull base surgery
Pain after endoscopic skull base surgery

Over the past 2 decades, the management of anterior skull base pathology, both benign and malignant, has transitioned from an open neurosurgical approach to an endoscopic endonasal approach. This endoscopic approach allows for minimally invasive resection of midline skull base lesions from the clivus, pterygopalatine fossa, sella and parasellar regions, cribriform, and frontal sinus. Endoscopic skull base approaches often include removal of significant amounts of nasal mucosa, septectomies, bony removal, and manipulation of mucosal tissue through the creation of free and vascularized mucosal flaps.

There is little information regarding the severity of pain after endoscopic skull base surgery. However, given that extensive sinonasal manipulation is often required, it would not be surprising if endoscopic skull base surgery resulted in significant postoperative pain. In particular, the use of a nasoseptal flap, which requires significant mucosal manipulation and often results in significant nasal crusting during remucosalization, may influence pain after endoscopic skull base surgery.

One study did evaluate pain after expanded endoscopic approaches for pituitary lesions, which require bony removal, wide sphenoidotomies, and a posterior septectomy, and found that the average pain score was approximately 3 on a 10-point scale, which is only slightly higher than that which has been noted after ESS.[46] Unpublished data from our group, which evaluated all skull base surgeries, noted that pain after endoscopic skull base surgery was approximately twice that of ESS, with an average score of 5.2 on a 10 point scale. While both studies support that endoscopic skull base surgery is more painful than ESS, it is also important to note that the pain is still only moderately severe. Additional studies will need to be performed to identify risk factors for increased pain after endoscopic skull base surgery.

Pain management options for endoscopic skull base surgery

To date, very few studies have been performed describing pain management strategies or evaluating the efficacy of various techniques for the prevention and management of pain after endoscopic skull base surgery. Many surgeons rely on general principles for pain management and extrapolate from their experiences with ESS.

There has also been increased interest in the utilization of NSAIDs after endoscopic skull base surgery, given the demonstrated safety after ESS. One evaluation of pain management after transsphenoidal pituitary surgery supports the use of NSAIDs after pituitary surgery. In their randomized controlled trial, Shepherd et al. evaluated the impact of scheduled ibuprofen versus placebo to a standard regimen of scheduled acetaminophen and breakthrough opioid. Although the study was small, only evaluating a total of 62 subjects, the authors did note a 43% reduction in postoperative pain scores, from 3.0 to 1.7 out of 10 points. They also found a 58% reduction in opioid use in subjects who received scheduled ibuprofen. No bleeding complications were noted.[46] This study is promising for the use of NSAIDs, though they should be used cautiously, especially when intracranial dissection is performed, as the potential morbidity of an intracranial hematoma can be devastating.

In our group, acetaminophen and opioids remain the mainstay for pain management after endoscopic skull base surgery. NSAIDs are also utilized except in cases for which there is a concern for increased risk of bleeding or contraindications for NSAIDs, such as renal disease. Additional studies should be performed evaluating the impact of gabapentinoids, corticosteroids, α-blockers, and local anesthetic, as they may also serve as useful adjuncts for pain management.

Conclusions

There is increasing interest in nonopioid strategies for pain control after ESS and endoscopic skull base surgery. Although data are limited, neither ESS nor skull base surgery appears to result in significant postoperative pain. As such, opioids are likely overutilized and surgeons should consider nonopioid alternatives for improved pain management. Preemptive strategies, such as a preoperative dose of acetaminophen, gabapentinoid, or dexamethasone may mitigate the central sensitization of pain, decreasing the perception of postoperative pain. Operative strategies such as α-blockers and infiltration of local anesthetic may also decrease pain after surgery.

Patients should be counseled extensively on the expectation of pain after ESS and skull base surgery, with the understanding that, for most, pain is only moderate. Nonopioid options such as acetaminophen, ibuprofen, and gabapentinoids may spare the patient from requiring opioids. However, opioids may still be utilized in a judicious fashion for breakthrough pain control.

References

1. Friedman M, Venkatesan TK, Lang D, Caldarelli DD. Bupivacaine for postoperative analgesia following endoscopic sinus surgery. *Laryngoscope*. November 1996;106(11): 1382−1385. https://doi.org/10.1097/00005537-199611000-00014.
2. Gottschalk A, Ochroch EA. Preemptive analgesia: what do we do now? *Anesthesiology*. January 2003;98(1):280−281. https://doi.org/10.1097/00000542-200301000-00047. Author reply 281.

3. Gan TJ. Poorly controlled postoperative pain: prevalence, consequences, and prevention. *J Pain Res*. 2017;10:2287−2298. https://doi.org/10.2147/JPR.S144066.

4. Chowdhury NI, Turner JH, Dorminy C, Wu J, Chandra RK. Preoperative quality-of-life measures predict acute postoperative pain in endoscopic sinus surgery. *Laryngoscope*. 06 2019;129(6):1274−1279. https://doi.org/10.1002/lary.27763.

5. Bhattacharyya N. Ambulatory sinus and nasal surgery in the United States: demographics and perioperative outcomes. *Laryngoscope*. March 2010;120(3):635−638. https://doi.org/10.1002/lary.20777.

6. Bhattacharyya N. Unplanned revisits and readmissions after ambulatory sinonasal surgery. *Laryngoscope*. September 2014;124(9):1983−1987. https://doi.org/10.1002/lary.24584.

7. Badash I, Lui CG, Hur K, Acevedo JR, Ference EH, Wrobel BB. Quantifying the use of opioids in the immediate postoperative period after endoscopic sinus surgery. *Laryngoscope*. May 2020;130(5):1122−1127. https://doi.org/10.1002/lary.28178.

8. Ndon S, Spock T, Torabi SJ, Manes RP. Patterns in pain and opiate use after endoscopic sinus surgery. *Otolaryngol Head Neck Surg*. June 2020;162(6):969−978. https://doi.org/10.1177/0194599820915472.

9. Dodhia S, Patel S, Beghal G, Pandey K, Hopkins C. A study of the use of post-operative opioid analgesics following rhinology surgery in 35 patients. *J Laryngol Otol*. December 2019;133(12):1050−1052. https://doi.org/10.1017/S0022215119002251.

10. Wise SK, Wise JC, DelGaudio JM. Evaluation of postoperative pain after sinonasal surgery. *Am J Rhinol*. September−October 2005;19(5):471−477.

11. Jordan JW, Spankovich C, Stringer SP. Feasibility of implementing opioid stewardship recommendations for sinonasal surgery. *Otolaryngol Head Neck Surg*. April 2021; 164(4):895−900. https://doi.org/10.1177/0194599820969155.

12. Raikundalia MD, Cheng TZ, Truong T, et al. Factors associated with opioid use after endoscopic sinus surgery. *Laryngoscope*. August 2019;129(8):1751−1755. https://doi.org/10.1002/lary.27921.

13. Grape S, Tramèr MR. Do we need preemptive analgesia for the treatment of postoperative pain? *Best Pract Res Clin Anaesthesiol*. March 2007;21(1):51−63. https://doi.org/10.1016/j.bpa.2006.11.004.

14. Nguyen BK, Svider PF, Hsueh WD, Folbe AJ. Perioperative analgesia for sinus and skull-base surgery. *Otolaryngol Clin*. October 2020;53(5):789−802. https://doi.org/10.1016/j.otc.2020.05.008.

15. Oscier CD, Milner QJ. Peri-operative use of paracetamol. *Anaesthesia*. January 2009; 64(1):65−72. https://doi.org/10.1111/j.1365-2044.2008.05674.x.

16. Issioui T, Klein KW, White PF, et al. The efficacy of premedication with celecoxib and acetaminophen in preventing pain after otolaryngologic surgery. *Anesth Analg*. May 2002;94(5):1188−1193, Table of contents. https://doi.org/10.1097/00000539-2002050 00-00025.

17. Bhoja R, Ryan MW, Klein K, et al. Intravenous vs oral acetaminophen in sinus surgery: a randomized clinical trial. *Laryngoscope Investig Otolaryngol*. June 2020;5(3):348−353. https://doi.org/10.1002/lio2.375.

18. Dahl JB, Mathiesen O, Møiniche S. 'Protective premedication': an option with gabapentin and related drugs? A review of gabapentin and pregabalin in in the treatment of postoperative pain. *Acta Anaesthesiol Scand*. October 2004;48(9):1130−1136. https://doi.org/10.1111/j.1399-6576.2004.00484.x.

19. Mathiesen O, Møiniche S, Dahl JB. Gabapentin and postoperative pain: a qualitative and quantitative systematic review, with focus on procedure. *BMC Anesthesiol.* July 2007;7: 6. https://doi.org/10.1186/1471-2253-7-6.

20. Park IJ, Kim G, Ko G, Lee YJ, Hwang SH. Does preoperative administration of gabapentin/pregabalin improve postoperative nasal surgery pain? *Laryngoscope.* 10 2016; 126(10):2232−2241. https://doi.org/10.1002/lary.25951.

21. Mohammed MH, Fahmy AM, Hakim KYK. Preoperative gabapentin augments intraoperative hypotension and reduces postoperative opioid requirements with functional endoscopic sinus surgery. 2012;28(3):189−192.

22. Sagit M, Yalcin S, Polat H, Korkmaz F, Cetinkaya S, Somdas MA. Efficacy of a single preoperative dose of pregabalin for postoperative pain after septoplasty. *J Craniofac Surg.* March 2013;24(2):373−375. https://doi.org/10.1097/SCS.0b013e31827fece5.

23. Kim JH, Seo MY, Hong SD, et al. The efficacy of preemptive analgesia with pregabalin in septoplasty. *Clin Exp Otorhinolaryngol.* June 2014;7(2):102−105. https://doi.org/10.3342/ceo.2014.7.2.102.

24. Demirhan A, Akkaya A, Tekelioglu UY, et al. Effect of pregabalin and dexamethasone on postoperative analgesia after septoplasty. *Pain Res Treat.* 2014;2014:850794. https://doi.org/10.1155/2014/850794.

25. Waldron NH, Jones CA, Gan TJ, Allen TK, Habib AS. Impact of perioperative dexamethasone on postoperative analgesia and side-effects: systematic review and meta-analysis. *Br J Anaesth.* February 2013;110(2):191−200. https://doi.org/10.1093/bja/aes431.

26. Pundir V, Pundir J, Lancaster G, et al. Role of corticosteroids in functional endoscopic sinus surgery–a systematic review and meta-analysis. *Rhinology.* March 2016;54(1): 3−19. https://doi.org/10.4193/Rhin15.079.

27. Al-Qudah M, Rashdan Y. Role of dexamethasone in reducing pain after endoscopic sinus surgery in adults: a double-blind prospective randomized trial. *Ann Otol Rhinol Laryngol.* April 2010;119(4):266−269. https://doi.org/10.1177/000348941011900410.

28. Kim DH, Lee J, Kim SW, Hwang SH. The efficacy of hypotensive agents on intraoperative bleeding and recovery following general anesthesia for nasal surgery: a network meta-analysis. *Clin Exp Otorhinolaryngol.* August 2020;14(2):200−209. https://doi.org/10.21053/ceo.2020.00584.

29. Svider PF, Nguyen B, Yuhan B, Zuliani G, Eloy JA, Folbe AJ. Perioperative analgesia for patients undergoing endoscopic sinus surgery: an evidence-based review. *Int Forum Allergy Rhinol.* July 2018;8(7):837−849. https://doi.org/10.1002/alr.22107.

30. Kim DH, Kang H, Hwang SH. The effect of sphenopalatine block on the postoperative pain of endoscopic sinus surgery: a meta-analysis. *Otolaryngol Head Neck Surg.* February 2019;160(2):223−231. https://doi.org/10.1177/0194599818805673.

31. Cho DY, Drover DR, Nekhendzy V, Butwick AJ, Collins J, Hwang PH. The effectiveness of preemptive sphenopalatine ganglion block on postoperative pain and functional outcomes after functional endoscopic sinus surgery. *Int Forum Allergy Rhinol.* May−June 2011;1(3):212−218. https://doi.org/10.1002/alr.20040.

32. Mo JH, Park YM, Chung YJ. Effect of lidocaine-soaked nasal packing on pain relief after endoscopic sinus surgery. *Am J Rhinol Allergy.* November−December 2013;27(6): e174−e177. https://doi.org/10.2500/ajra.2013.27.3942.

33. Haytoğlu S, Kuran G, Muluk NB, Arıkan OK. Different anesthetic agents-soaked sinus packings on pain management after functional endoscopic sinus surgery: which is the

most effective? *Eur Arch Oto-Rhino-Laryngol*. July 2016;273(7):1769—1777. https://doi.org/10.1007/s00405-015-3807-2.

34. Chou R, Gordon DB, de Leon-Casasola OA, et al. Management of postoperative pain: a clinical practice guideline from the American pain society, the American society of regional anesthesia and pain medicine, and the American society of Anesthesiologists' committee on regional anesthesia, executive committee, and administrative council. *J Pain*. February 2016;17(2):131—157. https://doi.org/10.1016/j.jpain.2015.12.008.

35. Gray ML, Fan CJ, Kappauf C, et al. Postoperative pain management after sinus surgery: a survey of the American Rhinologic Society. *Int Forum Allergy Rhinol*. October 2018; 8(10):1199—1203. https://doi.org/10.1002/alr.22181.

36. Kemppainen T, Kokki H, Tuomilehto H, Seppä J, Nuutinen J. Acetaminophen is highly effective in pain treatment after endoscopic sinus surgery. *Laryngoscope*. December 2006;116(12):2125—2128. https://doi.org/10.1097/01.mlg.0000239108.12081.35.

37. Kemppainen TP, Tuomilehto H, Kokki H, Seppä J, Nuutinen J. Pain treatment and recovery after endoscopic sinus surgery. *Laryngoscope*. August 2007;117(8):1434—1438. https://doi.org/10.1097/MLG.0b013e3180600a16.

38. Wu AW, Walgama ES, Genç E, et al. Multicenter study on the effect of nonsteroidal anti-inflammatory drugs on postoperative pain after endoscopic sinus and nasal surgery. *Int Forum Allergy Rhinol*. April 2020;10(4):489—495. https://doi.org/10.1002/alr.22506.

39. Miller C, Humphreys IM, Davis GE. Effect of over the counter ibuprofen dosing after sinus surgery for chronic rhinosinusitis: a prospective cohort pilot study. *Ann Otol Rhinol Laryngol*. July 2020;129(7):677—683. https://doi.org/10.1177/0003489420906179.

40. Moeller C, Pawlowski J, Pappas AL, Fargo K, Welch K. The safety and efficacy of intravenous ketorolac in patients undergoing primary endoscopic sinus surgery: a randomized, double-blinded clinical trial. *Int Forum Allergy Rhinol*. July—August 2012;2(4): 342—347. https://doi.org/10.1002/alr.21028.

41. Rezaeian A. Administering of pregabalin and acetaminophen on management of postoperative pain in patients with nasal polyposis undergoing functional endoscopic sinus surgery. *Acta Otolaryngol*. December 2017;137(12):1249—1252. https://doi.org/10.1080/00016489.2017.1358464.

42. Levy B, Paulozzi L, Mack KA, Jones CM. Trends in opioid analgesic-prescribing rates by specialty, U.S., 2007—2012. *Am J Prev Med*. September 2015;49(3):409—413. https://doi.org/10.1016/j.amepre.2015.02.020.

43. Sethi RKV, Miller AL, Bartholomew RA, et al. Opioid prescription patterns and use among patients undergoing endoscopic sinus surgery. *Laryngoscope*. May 2019; 129(5):1046—1052. https://doi.org/10.1002/lary.27672.

44. Jafari A, Shen SA, Bracken DJ, Pang J, DeConde AS. Incidence and predictive factors for additional opioid prescription after endoscopic sinus surgery. *Int Forum Allergy Rhinol*. May 2018;8(8):883—889. https://doi.org/10.1002/alr.22150.

45. Newberry CI, Casazza GC, Pruitt LC, Meier JD, Skarda DE, Alt JA. Prescription patterns and opioid usage in sinonasal surgery. *Int Forum Allergy Rhinol*. March 2020;10(3): 381—387. https://doi.org/10.1002/alr.22478.

46. Shepherd DM, Jahnke H, White WL, Little AS. Randomized, double-blinded, placebo-controlled trial comparing two multimodal opioid-minimizing pain management regimens following transsphenoidal surgery. *J Neurosurg*. February 2018;128(2):444—451. https://doi.org/10.3171/2016.10.JNS161355.

Perioperative pain management in facial plastic and reconstructive surgery

4

Yanjun Xie, MD, Andrew W. Joseph, MD, MPH

Department of Otolaryngology—Head and Neck Surgery, University of Michigan Medical School,
Ann Arbor, MI, United States

Introduction

Pain management is a major concern for many patients who contemplate undergoing facial plastic and reconstructive surgeries. Numerous over-the-counter and prescription pain medications have been used to address this important and universal patient issue. The treatment of acute postoperative pain commonly includes the administration of nonopioid analgesics, opioids, and injectable anesthetics.[1] Over time, the large variety of available medications have led to differences in prescribing patterns and at times, inconsistency in pain management approaches.

Inadequate analgesia negatively affects recovery, length of stay, and quality of life.[2] While many medications provide analgesia, maintaining a judicious balance between the risks and benefits of each pharmacologic modality is paramount in preventing misuse, overdose, or abuse. Opioids have historically been prescribed for many facial plastic procedures, but their potential for abuse and drug diversion rendered increased scrutiny into finding safer and more effective alternatives.[3–6] Previous studies showed that patients had an increased risk of chronic dependence even after a short-term exposure to prescription opioids.[6–8] However, most pain management guidelines focus on the treatment of chronic rather than acute postprocedural pain.[8] As such, there is a critical need to examine provider prescribing trends after facial plastic and reconstructive surgeries.

Facial plastic and reconstructive procedures, particularly aesthetic facial surgeries, account for a large number of operations performed in the United States.[9] A comprehensive review of pain management strategies after common surgeries is useful in informing clinical decision-making for providers who perform these types of operations. The purpose of this chapter is to integrate current literature on pain management for common facial plastic and reconstructive surgeries. To mitigate the risk of medication abuse, we propose that all facial surgeons remain vigilant about minimizing opioid misuse and overprescription while maintaining adequate pain control.

Analgesic pharmacology

The head and neck region contains a dense network of nociceptive receptors, which are responsible for high sensitivity and discomfort that patients may experience after facial surgeries.[10] Perioperative analgesics can be classified as topical, local, or systemic; systemic drugs exist in an oral, intramuscular, or intravenous (IV) form.[11] Regardless of the mode of delivery, a comprehensive understanding of pharmacology can guide facial surgeons in selecting the most appropriate modalities for their patients. In this section, we review clinically relevant pharmacology of dermal analgesia, local anesthetics, and systemic medications.

Dermal analgesia

A commonly used topical analgesic in facial plastic surgery is the eutectic mixture of local anesthetics (EMLA) cream. EMLA cream is a water and oil emulsion mixture that contains 2.5% lidocaine and 2.5% prilocaine.[12] EMLA cream has been shown to provide pain relief on intact and nonintact skin, making it useful for a variety of applications including chemodenervation, skin grafts, and laser treatments.[11,12] The onset, depth, and duration of analgesia are dependent on the timing of medication application. EMLA cream should ideally be applied to the targeted area for at least 1 h before the procedure.[12] This medication can achieve a penetration depth of 3—12 mm and lasts for up to 2 h.[12] Inadequate analgesia occurs secondary to insufficient application or short waiting time for the medication to achieve its maximal effect. The side effects of EMLA include local allergic reactions or sensitivity, but this medication is generally well tolerated. Topical lidocaine alone or in combination with benzocaine and tetracaine may also be considered, which can be supplied in a variety of concentrations and formulations. However, the surgeon should be aware of the potential for adverse outcomes in some compounded products with high anesthetic concentrations.[13]

Local anesthetics

Local anesthetics are another modality for delivering perioperative analgesia. The biochemical structures of local anesthetics determine their potency, duration of action, and metabolism.[14] In facial surgery, local anesthetics can be used to block branches of the trigeminal nerve to provide regional anesthesia. Regional nerve blocks are a powerful tool for pain control and are frequently utilized for in-office procedures, such as laser resurfacing, cutaneous surgeries, or hair transplant. Fig. 4.1 demonstrates the distribution of head and neck cutaneous nerves and potential sites of local anesthetic injections.[15] Furthermore, dilute epinephrine solutions of 1:100,000 or 1:200,000 concentrations are frequently mixed with local anesthetics to provide vasoconstriction on top of analgesia, which can prolong the duration of action.[14]

Toxicities of local anesthetics have the potential to be greater than those of topical agents. Systemic toxicity is dose-dependent and relates to cardiovascular

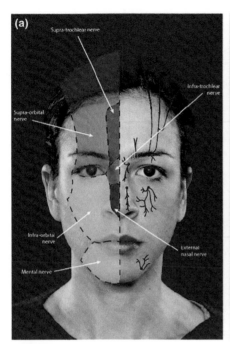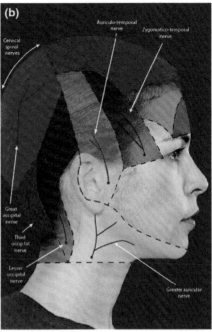

FIGURE 4.1

Cutaneous innervation of the face and scalp and potential sites of head and neck regional anesthesia.

Reproduced under creative commons license from Davies T, Karanovic S, Shergill B. Essential regional nerve blocks for the dermatologist: part 1. Clin Exp Dermatol. *2014;39(7):777–784.*

side effects and neurotoxicity, including arrhythmias, convulsions, coma, and central nervous system depression or collapse.[14–16] Additionally, local adverse effects, such as injection site pain, nerve injury, burning, intravascular injections, or tissue necrosis, have all been reported.[14] Before using an injectable anesthetic, it is imperative that the surgeon be mindful of the maximal dosing and drug-specific side effects. Examples of pharmacologic characteristics of commonly used local anesthetics are provided in Table 4.1.[16]

The process of injecting local anesthetics can cause discomfort and distress to the patient. Various methods to reduce injection-related pain have been proposed, including the application of ice, cool air, and vibration devices. Nestor et al. demonstrated the efficacy of a contact cooling device in alleviating pain and ecchymosis after small gel particle hyaluronic acid dermal filler injections.[17] Similarly, vibrotactile devices have been used for decreasing injection-related pain in many office-based procedures. Although the underlying physiology is incompletely understood, vibration devices are thought to reduce pain by stimulating large nerve fibers and suppressing pain stimuli transmitted by small A-δ and C nerve fibers.[18] At the

Table 4.1 Pharmacologic characteristics of common local anesthetics.

	Structural classification	Molecular weight	Onset	Elimination half-life (min)	Maximum dose without vasoconstrictor (mg kg^{-1})	Maximum dose with vasoconstrictor (mg kg^{-1})
Cocaine	Ester	311	Fast	100	1.5 (topical)	–
Chloroprocaine	Ester	271	Fast	6	11	14
Prilocaine	Ester	220	Fast	100	6	8
Lidocaine	Amide	234	Fast	100	3	7
Mepivacaine	Amide	246	Fast	115	5	7
Bupivacaine	Amide	288	Moderate	210	2	2
Ropivacaine	Amide	274	Moderate	120	3	3
Levobupivacaine	Amide	288	Moderate	210	2	2

Reproduced under creative commons license from Taylor A, McLeod G. Basic pharmacology of local anaesthetics. BJA Educ. 2020;20(2):34–41.

time of anesthetic injections, the operator simply applies the vibratory stimuli in an area adjacent to the target area for needle injections. Several studies confirmed the effectiveness of vibration devices, such as the Buzzy device and Vibration Anesthesia Device, in reducing needle- or injection-associated pain for adult and pediatric applications.[19,20]

Systemic analgesics

Systemic medications are available in oral or IV forms and include a variety of over-the-counter and prescription analgesics, such as acetaminophen, nonsteroidal drugs, and narcotics. Over-the-counter acetaminophen and nonsteroidal antiinflammatory drugs (NSAIDs) are typically first-line medications in this category due to their high tolerability, ease of access, and safety profile.[21] Both acetaminophen and NSAIDs are available in the IV form, although their use is limited to the perioperative setting due to a need for IV access. From a side effect perspective, acetaminophen can cause hypersensitivity, hepatotoxicity, and metabolic derangement.[21] Similarly, excessive NSAIDs can lead to nephropathy, gastrointestinal bleeding, or cardiovascular compromise.[22] NSAIDs also decrease the formation of prostaglandins and thromboxane A2 and can lead to platelet dysfunction.[22] Thus, the use of NSAIDs in a postsurgical setting remains controversial and will be further discussed later in this chapter.

Opioids are commonly prescribed as an adjunct to over-the-counter medications.[23] There is a large variety of opioids available for prescription use, ranging from oxycodone to hydromorphone and opioids that are combined with acetaminophen. Morphine milligram equivalent (MME) is a standardized measurement to approximate the amount and potency of different types of opioids and can be calculated as a product of dose, quantity, and opioid-specific conversion factor.[24] Common side effects of opioids include reduction in gastric motility leading to bloating, nausea, vomiting, and sedation, which can lead to cardiopulmonary depression and collapse.[23]

In addition, opioids have the potential for abuse and can lead to drug diversion.[25] Prescription opioid use has contributed to the rising opioid epidemic in the United States.[8] Studies have shown that postsurgical opioid prescription, even for a short course, can be associated with conversion to long-term dependence.[7,8,26] More recent studies demonstrated a general trend of overprescription by clinicians, and as such, there has been a nationwide push to examine prescribing patterns of opioids after all surgical procedures.[7,8]

Contemporary strategies for managing postoperative pain focus on reducing opioid prescriptions and advocacy for a multimodal pain treatment regimen, including the use of nonopioid analgesics, injectable anesthetics, topical medications, and a combination of these options.[4,11,14,23] This approach has been shown to increase patient satisfaction and reduce narcotic use in a large variety of surgical procedures.[4,8] In the following sections, studies on pain after common facial plastic and reconstructive surgeries are discussed in the context of each operation.

Procedure-specific pain management
Septorhinoplasty

Rhinoplasty and septoplasty are two of the most commonly performed operations by facial surgeons.[27] Establishing clear management guidelines is important and has been the subject of numerous studies. For these operations, nonopioid medications have been shown to decrease or even eliminate the need for opioids among some patients.[4] Nguyen et al. conducted a systematic review on nonopioid analgesic use after septorhinoplasty and concluded that of all the modalities studied, local anesthetics provide highly effective analgesia and were associated with decreased pain scores and lower rescue analgesic consumption.[1] Although some local anesthetics have short half-lives and rapid clearance, their effects were found to extend beyond the duration of action for up to 24 h.[28,29] The utility of local anesthetics in facial surgeries is further supported by the American Society of Anesthesiologists practice guidelines.[30] Thus, they remain a workhorse for pain control among patients who undergo septorhinoplasty.

Acetaminophen and NSAIDs are also highly effective for providing postoperative analgesia.[1] In several randomized controlled trials, NSAIDs use after septoplasty was shown to decrease pain and consumption of rescue analgesics.[31,32] In another randomized control study of 150 patients who underwent open septoplasty with concurrent rhinoplasty, Celik et al. studied patients who received IV paracetamol versus IV ibuprofen and concluded that IV ibuprofen provided more analgesia than paracetamol in the first 12 h after surgery.[33] All of these studies considered bleeding as a potential complication due to the platelet-altering effect of NSAIDs; however, none reported an elevated incidence of hematoma or other bleeding-related complications.[1,31-35] The safety of acetaminophen and NSAIDs were further established by the American Academy of Otolaryngology—Head and Neck Surgery Clinical Practice Guideline, which advocated the use of acetaminophen and NSAIDs as first-line agents for pain after rhinoplasty and septoplasty.[4]

Opioids were commonly prescribed after septoplasty and rhinoplasty. However, recent studies actually suggested overprescription and underutilization of these medications. In a case series of 62 patients undergoing a combination of open septoplasty, open rhinoplasty, and endonasal rhinoplasty, Patel et al. (2018) demonstrated that patients used a median of 8.7 out of 20—30 hydrocodone-acetaminophen tablets prescribed.[36] Patient age, sex, septoplasty or turbinate resection, use of osteotomy, or a history of prior rhinoplasty was not associated with the number of opioid tablets used.[36] In this study, only one patient underwent endonasal rhinoplasty. Postoperative pain between the open versus endonasal approach was not specifically queried. In another retrospective study, Rock et al. reported similar findings in a cohort of 75 patients and noted that the mean number of opioids consumed after septorhinoplasty was 14.7 out of 42.4 tablets prescribed. Sex, procedure performed, use of nasal splints, or surgeon was not associated with the number of opioids prescribed.[3] In a prospective study, Scalafani et al. (2019) demonstrated that most patients experienced only mild pain for 2—3 days.[5] About 90% of their patients required fewer than 11 opioid tablets. The total MMEs were compared and found to be similar between septoplasty and rhinoplasty.[5] In this study, both open and endonasal techniques were included, but the authors detected no differences in MME, opioids consumed, or pain scores between the open or closed approaches. Based on their data, Scalafani et al. concluded that pain control after septorhinoplasty would require 10–11 opioid doses of sufficient potency, or an equivalent of 71–80 MMEs.[5]

The abundance of literature on septorhinoplasty extended to other less commonly used modalities. One randomized control trial evaluated electro-acupuncture and morphine as adjunctive methods of pain control for septoplasty.[37] This study did not identify differences in pain scores or consumption of rescue opioid medications, but they reported a reduction in nausea and vomiting in the electro-acupuncture group compared to morphine users.[37] Additionally, two studies evaluated the use of dexamethasone as an adjunct to local anesthetics and gabapentin.[38,39] These studies demonstrated decreased pain and rescue analgesic use with steroid administration with no increases in side effects, though further prospective, controlled trials examining the efficacy of steroid administration as a pain control modality should be conducted.

Facial rejuvenation

In contrast to the breadth of studies on postoperative pain after septorhinoplasty, there are considerably fewer publications on pain management following facial rejuvenation. Facial rejuvenation procedures include an array of operations such as upper and lower blepharoplasty, brow lift, volume augmentation procedures, and cervicofacial rhytidectomy. In periorbital facial rejuvenation, postprocedural pain is generally reported as mild and managed by acetaminophen and/or NSAIDs.[40,41] In a study by Henrici, Clemens, and Tost, the application of EMLA cream to the eyelid before upper blepharoplasty was also shown to lower postoperative pain.[42] Similarly, Wei et al. evaluated preoperative use of a single dose of 150 mg pregabalin in patients undergoing upper eyelid surgery and showed lower pain scores in treated patients compared to controls.[43] In that study, patients who were treated with pregabalin consumed less acetaminophen in the first 48 h after surgery. In oculoplastic and orbital surgeries, information on opioid prescription had been limited until recently. A study in a cohort of 2660 patients who underwent oculoplastic and orbital surgeries demonstrated that the average MME of prescribed opioids was 73.2 for brow lifts, 64.7 for blepharoptosis repair, and 71.9 for upper blepharoplasty, but the authors did observe a decrease in prescribed opioids over time.[44] This study also evaluated other procedures and concluded that soft tissue surgeries in the periorbital region had lower MMEs than orbital surgeries.[44] This study did not specifically examine patient use of opioids or the adequacy of pain control.

For patients undergoing cervicofacial rhytidectomy, pain can be more significant due to a greater extent of tissue dissection. In a prospective randomized trial of 140 patients, Torgerson et al. investigated intraoperative ketorolac for analgesia following cervicofacial rhytidectomy.[45] In this study, patients who received local injections of ketorolac into the surgical field required less pain medications than those who had an intramuscular ketorolac injection and controls who received injectable anesthetics alone. Two patients in the control group developed a hematoma requiring surgical evacuation, while none of the 115 patients in the local ketorolac group developed bleeding complications. Aynehchi et al. evaluated the use of celecoxib in 50 patients undergoing deep-plane rhytidectomies.[46] In their study, patients who were treated with preoperative and postoperative celecoxib reported less pain compared to controls. No studies to date have examined postoperative pain between various rhytidectomy techniques.

Cutaneous reconstruction

Cutaneous reconstructive surgeries are another type of operation commonly performed by facial surgeons. Cutaneous reconstruction of defects from skin cancers is most commonly achieved through tissue rearrangement and local flaps. Because the reconstructive approach can vary depending on the size and location of the defect, patients often experience different amounts of discomfort.

In general, pain after cutaneous reconstruction is mild. A study from 2010 showed that only 7% of patients who underwent Mohs micrographic surgery consumed postoperative opioids.[47] Limthogkul, Samie, and Humphreys corroborated with these findings in 158 patients and concluded that the majority of patients did not require prescription analgesics.[48] Another subsequent study showed that opioids were prescribed to a minority (34%) of patients undergoing Mohs surgery; furthermore, 35% of patients did not consume any opioids that were prescribed to them.[49] In general, patients undergoing cutaneous procedures may be expected to do well with a combination of acetaminophen and NSAIDs, and at least one randomized controlled trial supports this approach.[50]

Several studies showed that the type of reconstruction for Mohs defect may be predictive of opioid prescriptions. Harris et al. identified increased odds of receiving opioid prescriptions in patients who underwent Mohs closure using local flaps compared to healing by secondary intention.[49] They also concluded that young age, female sex, and use of full-thickness skin graft for closure were associated with increasing pain scores. Firoz et al. found that patients who had full-thickness skin grafts and local flaps had higher mean pain scores and greater narcotic prescription use than those undergoing linear repair or healing by secondary intention.[47] These findings were redemonstrated in a study by Brahe et al.[51] Skin graft reconstruction of cutaneous defects portends a large extent of tissue dissection as well as a secondary donor site, which may contribute to increased postoperative pain. Prospective studies on analgesic requirements after Mohs reconstructive techniques are needed to understand the extent and severity of postoperative pain, as well as narcotic prescribing patterns after these reconstructive procedures.

Facial trauma

Maxillofacial fractures account for over 400,000 emergency room visits annually in the United States.[52] The management of pain after repair of facial trauma is an area of active investigation. A recently published study by Lapidus et al. shed light on opioid prescribing and use in postsurgical facial trauma patients.[53] In this large retrospective cohort of 20,191 patients who underwent repair of facial fractures, a majority of patients (78.6%) filled opioid prescriptions; within the subgroup of patients who filled their prescriptions, a majority (58.7%) also went to complete a refill of an opioid-containing medication. In this analysis, patients who suffered from nasal, naso-orbito-ethmoid, and Le Fort fractures most commonly filled their prescriptions. The authors also evaluated the appropriateness of opioid prescriptions and found that 39.3% of their cohort received inappropriate prescriptions characterized by overlapping opioid prescriptions, high morphine equivalents, or concurrent use of opioids and benzodiazepines.[53] Prior substance use, mental health disorders, number of procedures performed, and prescription of tramadol were associated with increased odds of opioid prescription refills.

Another recent study by Som et al. evaluated opioid use among adolescent patients seeking repair of facial trauma and similarly identified high percentages of opioid prescription and use.[54] In this study, older age, comorbidities, and multiple fractures were associated with persistent opioid use. Interestingly, their analysis identified that the rates of potentially inappropriate opioid prescribing differed based on the analgesic medication, with oxycodone, propoxyphene, and less commonly prescribed opioids being associated with higher odds of inappropriate use.[54]

Despite the high rates of opioid use identified in the previous studies, overall narcotic prescribing trends for facial trauma repair in the United States have remained stable. In a study by Shah et al. the authors assessed opioid prescribing trends for craniofacial trauma between 2006 and 2016 and identified relatively unchanged rates of opioid prescriptions, with 13.4% of all patient visits receiving opioid prescriptions.[55] Younger age (ages 18–44) and lower face trauma were associated with increased rates of opioid prescriptions, while there were no significant differences across geographical regions, ethnicity, or sex. Nonetheless, opioid prescription and use after trauma are substantially higher in comparison to other facial plastic and reconstructive surgeries discussed earlier. Future studies are needed to more accurately identify predictors of poor pain control and risk factors for inappropriate use in this patient cohort.

Conclusion

The treatment of acute postoperative pain after facial plastic and reconstructive surgery is a complex and evolving topic, involving throughout considerations of the specific type of procedures, the extent of surgery, and a host of underlying patient factors. In this review, we discussed several approaches to pain management following common facial plastic and reconstructive surgeries and reviewed recent evidence related to septoplasty, rhinoplasty, facial rejuvenation, cutaneous reconstruction, and repair of facial trauma. Throughout these discussions, we highlight the increasingly recognized national trends of opioid overuse and overprescription for patients undergoing facial plastic and reconstructive surgeries. Specifically, in our review of data in septorhinoplasty, opioids were routinely prescribed, but studies favored a more limited course of no more than 10—15 doses of narcotic medications.

We acknowledge that the field of facial plastic and reconstructive surgery encompasses a large variety of operations beyond those discussed here. The breadth of procedures can contribute to challenges in standardizing a universal pain management algorithm. For instance, while analgesic requirement after cutaneous reconstruction is low, patients who undergo free tissue transfers typically require multiple pain management approaches, including the use of a patient-controlled IV analgesics in addition to prescription opioids and nonopioid analgesics.[41] Thus, ongoing studies are needed to assess pain requirements following other cosmetic facial and reconstructive surgeries.

In the face of considerable risks of opioid abuse and chronic dependence, it is imperative that the facial surgeon prescribes all analgesic medications judiciously. Regardless of the type of operation, the efficacy of a multimodal pain management strategy must be considered by the facial surgeon.[4,30,41] Future clinical practice should emphasize preoperative counseling, education regarding the risks, benefits, and alternatives of opioids, and active postoperative surveillance of pain control and analgesic medication use. Future research efforts should continue to search for novel alternative modalities to mitigate the risk of iatrogenic medication abuse and dependency.

References

1. Nguyen BK, Yuhan BT, Folbe E, et al. Perioperative analgesia for patients undergoing septoplasty and rhinoplasty: an evidence-based review. *Laryngoscope*. 2019;129(6): E200—E212.
2. Gan TJ. Poorly controlled postoperative pain: prevalence, consequences, and prevention. *J Pain Res*. 2017;10:2287—2298.
3. Rock AN, Akakpo K, Cheresnick C, et al. Postoperative prescriptions and corresponding opioid consumption after septoplasty or rhinoplasty. *Ear Nose Throat J*. 2019, 145561319866824.
4. Anne S, Mims JW, Tunkel DE, et al. Clinical practice guideline: opioid prescribing for analgesia after common Otolaryngology operations executive summary. *Otolaryngol Head Neck Surg*. 2021;164(4):687—703.
5. Sclafani AP, Kim M, Kjaer K, Kacker A, Tabaee A. Postoperative pain and analgesic requirements after septoplasty and rhinoplasty. *Laryngoscope*. 2019;129(9):2020—2025.
6. Brummett CM, Waljee JF, Goesling J, et al. New persistent opioid use after minor and major surgical procedures in US adults. *JAMA Surg*. 2017;152(6):e170504.

7. Jiang X, Orton M, Feng R, et al. Chronic opioid usage in surgical patients in a large academic center. *Ann Surg*. 2017;265(4):722–727.

8. Kolodny A, Courtwright DT, Hwang CS, et al. The prescription opioid and heroin crisis: a public health approach to an epidemic of addiction. *Annu Rev Publ Health*. 2015;36:559–574.

9. Moayer R, Sand JP, Han A, Nabili V, Keller GS. The prevalence of cosmetic facial plastic procedures among facial plastic surgeons. *Facial Plast Surg*. 2018;34(2):220–226.

10. Duerr ER, Chang A, Venkateswaran N, et al. Resolution of pain with periocular injections in a patient with a 7-year history of chronic ocular pain. *Am J Ophthalmol Case Rep*. 2019;14:35–38.

11. Kundu S, Achar S. Principles of office anesthesia: part II. Topical anesthesia. *Am Fam Phys*. 2002;66(1):99–102.

12. Lycka BA. EMLA. A new and effective topical anesthetic. *J Dermatol Surg Oncol*. 1992;18(10):859–862.

13. Sobanko JF, Miller CJ, Alster TS. Topical anesthetics for dermatologic procedures: a review. *Dermatol Surg*. 2012;38(5):709–721.

14. Becker DE, Reed KL. Local anesthetics: review of pharmacological considerations. *Anesth Prog*. 2012;59(2):90–101. quiz 102-103.

15. Davies T, Karanovic S, Shergill B. Essential regional nerve blocks for the dermatologist: part 1. *Clin Exp Dermatol*. 2014;39(7):777–784.

16. Taylor A, McLeod G. Basic pharmacology of local anaesthetics. *BJA Educ*. 2020;20(2):34–41.

17. Nestor MS, Ablon GR, Stillman MA. The use of a contact cooling device to reduce pain and ecchymosis associated with dermal filler injections. *J Clin Aesthet Dermatol*. 2010;3(3):29–34.

18. Kuwahara H, Ogawa R. Using a vibration device to ease pain during facial needling and injection. *Eplasty*. 2016;16:e9.

19. Ballard A, Khadra C, Adler S, Trottier ED, Le May S. Efficacy of the Buzzy device for pain management during needle-related procedures: a systematic review and meta-analysis. *Clin J Pain*. 2019;35(6):532–543.

20. Ueki S, Yamagami Y, Makimoto K. Effectiveness of vibratory stimulation on needle-related procedural pain in children: a systematic review. *JBI Database System Rev Implement Rep*. 2019;17(7):1428–1463.

21. Gerriets V, Anderson J, Nappe TM. Acetaminophen. In: *StatPearls. Treasure Island (FL)*. 2020.

22. Harirforoosh S, Asghar W, Jamali F. Adverse effects of nonsteroidal antiinflammatory drugs: an update of gastrointestinal, cardiovascular and renal complications. *J Pharm Pharmaceut Sci*. 2013;16(5):821–847.

23. James A, Williams J. Basic opioid pharmacology - an update. *Br J Pain*. 2020;14(2):115–121.

24. Nielsen S, Degenhardt L, Hoban B, Gisev N. A synthesis of oral morphine equivalents (OME) for opioid utilisation studies. *Pharmacoepidemiol Drug Saf*. 2016;25(6):733–737.

25. Seth P, Scholl L, Rudd RA, Bacon S. Overdose deaths involving opioids, cocaine, and psychostimulants - United States, 2015-2016. *MMWR Morb Mortal Wkly Rep*. 2018;67(12):349–358.

26. Hooten WM, St Sauver JL, McGree ME, Jacobson DJ, Warner DO. Incidence and risk factors for progression from short-term to episodic or long-term opioid prescribing: a population-based study. *Mayo Clin Proc*. 2015;90(7):850–856.

27. Chuang J, Barnes C, Wong BJF. Overview of facial plastic surgery and current developments. *Surg J*. 2016;2(1):e17—e28.
28. Karaman E, Gungor G, Alimoglu Y, et al. The effect of lidocaine, bupivacaine and ropivacaine in nasal packs on pain and hemorrhage after septoplasty. *Eur Arch Oto-Rhino-Laryngol*. 2011;268(5):685—689.
29. Erkul E, Babayigit M, Kuduban O. Comparison of local anesthesia with articaine and lidocaine in septoplasty procedure. *Am J Rhinol Allergy*. 2010;24(5):e123—126.
30. American Society of Anesthesiologists Task Force on Acute Pain M. Practice guidelines for acute pain management in the perioperative setting: an updated report by the American Society of Anesthesiologists Task Force on Acute Pain Management. *Anesthesiology*. 2012;116(2):248—273.
31. Turan A, Emet S, Karamanlioglu B, Memis D, Turan N, Pamukcu Z. Analgesic effects of rofecoxib in ear-nose-throat surgery. *Anesth Analg*. 2002;95(5):1308—1311 (table of contents).
32. Sener M, Yilmazer C, Yilmaz I, et al. Efficacy of lornoxicam for acute postoperative pain relief after septoplasty: a comparison with diclofenac, ketoprofen, and dipyrone. *J Clin Anesth*. 2008;20(2):103—108.
33. Celik EC, Kara D, Koc E, Yayik AM. The comparison of single-dose preemptive intravenous ibuprofen and paracetamol on postoperative pain scores and opioid consumption after open septorhinoplasty: a randomized controlled study. *Eur Arch Oto-Rhino-Laryngol*. 2018;275(9):2259—2263.
34. Moeller C, Pawlowski J, Pappas AL, Fargo K, Welch K. The safety and efficacy of intravenous ketorolac in patients undergoing primary endoscopic sinus surgery: a randomized, double-blinded clinical trial. *Int Forum Allergy Rhinol*. 2012;2(4):342—347.
35. Newberry CI, McCrary HC, Cerrati EW. The efficacy of oral celecoxib following surgical rhinoplasty. *Facial Plast Surg Aesthet Med*. 2020;22(2):100—104.
36. Patel S, Sturm A, Bobian M, Svider PF, Zuliani G, Kridel R. Opioid use by patients after rhinoplasty. *JAMA Facial Plast Surg*. 2018;20(1):24—30.
37. Sahmeddini MA, Farbood A, Ghafaripuor S. Electro-acupuncture for pain relief after nasal septoplasty: a randomized controlled study. *J Alternative Compl Med*. 2010;16(1):53—57.
38. Demirhan A, Akkaya A, Tekelioglu UY, et al. Effect of pregabalin and dexamethasone on postoperative analgesia after septoplasty. *Pain Res Treat*. 2014;2014:850794.
39. Ma'somi A, Abshirini H, Hekmat Shoar M. Comparison of local anesthetic effect of bupivacaine versus bupivacaine plus dexamethasone in nasal surgery. *Iran J Otorhinolaryngol*. 2013;25(70):7—10.
40. Richards BG, Schleicher WF, Zins JE. Putting it all together: recommendations for improving pain management in plastic surgical procedures-surgical facial rejuvenation. *Plast Reconstr Surg*. 2014;134(4 Suppl 2):108S—112S.
41. Meraj TS, Bresler A, Zuliani GF. Acute pain management following facial plastic surgery. *Otolaryngol Clin*. 2020;53(5):811—817.
42. Henrici K, Clemens S, Tost F. [Application of EMLA creme before upper lid blepharoplasty]. *Ophthalmologe*. 2005;102(8):794—797.
43. Wei LA, Davies BW, Hink EM, Durairaj VD. Perioperative pregabalin for attenuation of postoperative pain after eyelid surgery. *Ophthalmic Plast Reconstr Surg*. 2015;31(2):132—135.
44. Xie Y, Joseph AW, Rudy SF, et al. Change in postoperative opioid prescribing patterns for oculoplastic and orbital procedures associated with state opioid legislation. *JAMA Ophthalmol*. 2021;139(2):157—162.

45. Torgerson C, Yoskovitch A, Cole AF, Conrad K. Postoperative pain management with ketorolac in facial plastic surgery patients. *J Otolaryngol Head Neck Surg.* 2008; 37(6):888−893.

46. Aynehchi BB, Cerrati EW, Rosenberg DB. The efficacy of oral celecoxib for acute postoperative pain in face-lift surgery. *JAMA Facial Plast Surg.* 2014;16(5):306−309.

47. Firoz BF, Goldberg LH, Arnon O, Mamelak AJ. An analysis of pain and analgesia after Mohs micrographic surgery. *J Am Acad Dermatol.* 2010;63(1):79−86.

48. Limthongkul B, Samie F, Humphreys TR. Assessment of postoperative pain after Mohs micrographic surgery. *Dermatol Surg.* 2013;39(6):857−863.

49. Harris K, Curtis J, Larsen B, et al. Opioid pain medication use after dermatologic surgery: a prospective observational study of 212 dermatologic surgery patients. *JAMA Dermatol.* 2013;149(3):317−321.

50. Sniezek PJ, Brodland DG, Zitelli JA. A randomized controlled trial comparing acetaminophen, acetaminophen and ibuprofen, and acetaminophen and codeine for postoperative pain relief after Mohs surgery and cutaneous reconstruction. *Dermatol Surg.* 2011;37(7): 1007−1013.

51. Brahe CA, Hardy CL, Miladi A. Postoperative pain after Mohs micrographic surgery is well tolerated regardless of psychological and pain-related comorbidities. *Dermatol Surg.* 2021;47(4):462−466.

52. Allareddy V, Allareddy V, Nalliah RP. Epidemiology of facial fracture injuries. *J Oral Maxillofac Surg.* 2011;69(10):2613−2618.

53. Lapidus JB, Santosa KB, Skolnick GB, et al. Opioid prescribing and use patterns in postsurgical facial trauma patients. *Plast Reconstr Surg.* 2020;145(3):780−789.

54. Som A, Santosa KB, Skolnick GB, Lapidus JB, Waljee JF, Patel KB. Opioid use among adolescents undergoing surgical repair of facial trauma. *Plast Reconstr Surg.* 2021; 147(3):690−698.

55. Shah J, Lesko RP, Lala B, Ricci J. Trends in opioid prescription for craniomaxillofacial trauma in the United States: an 11-year retrospective study of emergency room and office visits. *Surgery.* 2021;170(1):232−238. https://doi.org/10.1016/j.surg.2021.03.007.

Perioperative pain management in pediatric otolaryngology—head and neck surgery

Ruth J. Davis, MD, David E. Tunkel, MD

Department of Otolaryngology—Head and Neck Surgery, Johns Hopkins University School of Medicine, Baltimore, MD, United States

Introduction

The two most common pediatric surgeries in the United States, tympanostomy tube insertion and tonsillectomy, are both performed by otolaryngologists.[1] For this reason, a contemporary understanding of pediatric perioperative pain control is critical for otolaryngologists. The majority of these procedures are performed on an outpatient basis, with selected patients requiring one night of monitored observation after tonsillectomy. Anticipated postoperative pain and perioperative risks differ greatly between these two procedures, and the challenges of pain management usually take place after discharge. A variety of pharmacologic and nonpharmacologic strategies for perioperative pain management in children have been studied, with the goal of improving postoperative patient comfort while minimizing the likelihood of dangerous side effects. Commonly used medications include acetaminophen, nonsteroidal antiinflammatory drugs (NSAIDs), and opioids. This chapter discusses current issues and recommendations with the use of these analgesic classes and presents nonpharmacologic adjuncts for perioperative pain control in children. Although we focus on care after adenotonsillectomy or tympanostomy tube placement, the strategies discussed in this chapter can be adapted to other procedures in children, acknowledging that pharyngeal surgery usually causes significant pain with the need for aggressive management strategies.[2,3]

Special considerations for pain management in children

Pain control in pediatric patients requires several special considerations. Unlike adult patients undergoing otolaryngologic procedures, young children are not usually able to perform their own pain assessments, communicate pain severity, or administer their own pain medications. Instead, it falls upon parents or caregivers to both assess the child's pain level and administer appropriate types and dosages

Opioid Use, Overuse, and Abuse in Otolaryngology. https://doi.org/10.1016/B978-0-323-79016-1.00006-4

of analgesics. These caregivers must be educated to recognize the signs and symptoms of uncontrolled pain as well as early signs of overmedication to avoid potentially serious consequences from improper analgesic dosing.

The most obvious difference between pediatric and adult pain management is patient size. Given the variation in size and weight among children of all ages, ideal weight-based dosing is critical to achieving therapeutic effects. The smaller the patient, the narrower the margin of error to achieve levels within the therapeutic window. For example, a study of posttonsillectomy pain control in the United Kingdom, where over-the-counter acetaminophen and ibuprofen are dosed by age rather than weight, found that implementation of standardized weight-based dosing significantly improved the readmission rate for pain control without impacting postoperative hemorrhage rate.[4]

Many opioid medications are dependent upon the cytochrome P450 2D6 (CYP2D6) pathway for breakdown into their active metabolites (Table 5.1).

Table 5.1 Opioids, metabolism, FDA warnings.[7,8,47,114,115]

Opioid	Enzymes of metabolism	Metabolites	FDA warnings
Codeine	CYP 2D6; CYP 3A4; UGT 2B7	Morphine (active); norcodine; codeine-6-glucuronide (active)	Box warning against use in posttonsillectomy pain; contraindicated for treatment of pain or cough in age <12; warning against use in age 12–18 with obesity, OSA, or severe lung disease
Tramadol	CYP 2D6; CYP 3A4	O-desmethyl-tramadol (active)	Contraindicated for treatment of pain in age <12; Contraindicated for posttonsillectomy pain in age <18
Morphine	UGT 2B7	Morphine-6-glucuronide (active); morphine-3-glucuronide	
Hydromorphone	UGT 1A3; UGT 2B7	Hydromorphine-6-glucuronide (active); hydromorphine-3-glucuronide	
Oxycodone	CYP 3A4; CYP 2D6	Noroxycodone (active); oxymorphone (active)	
Hydrocodone	CYP 2D6; CYP 3A4	Hydromorphone (active); norhydrocodone (active)	

CYP, cytochrome P450; OSA, obstructive sleep apnea; UDP, uridine diphosphate; UGT, UDP-glucuronosyltransferase.

Well-described variation in CYP2D6 activity exists, leading to four phenotypes of poor metabolizers, intermediate metabolizers, extensive metabolizers (considered "normal"), and ultrarapid metabolizers.[5] Whereas ultrarapid metabolism and higher serum concentrations of an active metabolite may not exceed the wider therapeutic window in adults, this phenotype has been associated with respiratory depression and even death in young children after surgery.[6–8]

Given the role of caregivers in managing postoperative pediatric pain in the outpatient setting, education of these caregivers before discharge, and perhaps at the time of presurgical counseling, is essential. Parents can be taught to use behavioral pain scales to assess pain levels at routine intervals.[9] Studies demonstrate that although caregivers are able to recognize pain in children, they often underdose analgesics.[10,11] Pain management education starts preoperatively and should be incorporated into the discussion of risks and benefits of surgery. Perioperative staff, such as preoperative and postanesthesia care unit (PACU) nurses, play a central role in parental education and should reinforce analgesic dosing recommendations, teach parents the signs of pain, and detail the side effects of the prescribed medications. A standardized program including teaching in the PACU with an educational booklet, use of a timer to adhere to the analgesic regimen, instructions on how to accurately measure doses, use of a pain management diary, and reinforcement/coaching through telephone calls can be effective for parental education.[12] An educational booklet or video has been shown to increase parental knowledge about managing their children's pain.[13,14]

Caregiver education is particularly critical when opioids are prescribed. Evidence suggests that parents may not understand the risk of oversedation in children with obstructive sleep apnea syndrome (OSAS), and half of the parents in one study would give an opioid medication when their child exhibited signs of oversedation, demonstrating the need for improved education to recognize and manage signs of opioid toxicity.[16] Implementation of provider education to use nonopioid analgesics first in conjunction with a guideline reducing the number of oxycodone doses prescribed after tonsillectomy resulted in both decreased opioid prescription quantity and higher odds of good pain control.[15] Otolaryngologists should also recognize that cultural factors such as ethnicity may affect how caregivers assess and treat pain.[17] Such education should balance our efforts to improve pain control after uncomfortable procedures like tonsillectomy with the imperative to avoid adverse drug reactions.

Tympanostomy tube placement

Myringotomy with insertion of tympanostomy tubes is the most commonly performed pediatric surgical procedure in the United States.[18] Pain following tympanostomy tube placement is neither severe nor long lasting. Given the short duration and limited nature of the procedure, inhalational anesthetics are typically used and intravenous (IV) access is often not required. However, inhalational anesthetics are associated with higher rates of emergence delirium, which typically lasts 5–15 min. While this is usually limited in time and severity, it may result in injury to self or others. The mechanism of emergence delirium is not clear; however, pain, anxiety, and anesthetic choice are all thought to contribute.

Studies have evaluated varying approaches to preoperative, intraoperative, and postoperative analgesia for tympanostomy tube placement, both with regards to pain control and reduction of emergence delirium. No obvious benefit has been observed with one analgesic regimen compared to another, and most patients are managed postoperatively with acetaminophen and/or ibuprofen as needed. Prescription pain medications are typically not required. A randomized controlled trial (RCT) found no benefit in postoperative pain control when children were premedicated with acetaminophen and ibuprofen before tympanostomy tube placement.[19] A large retrospective study found superior analgesia when a combination of intramuscular fentanyl and ketorolac were administered.[20] However, another retrospective study found that choice of intraoperative analgesic among fentanyl, ketorolac, or a combination had no impact on postoperative pain control or time to discharge.[21] Intraoperative acupuncture has been shown to reduce postoperative pain and agitation following tympanostomy tube insertion; however, this has not been widely adopted or studied.[22]

Emergence delirium was reduced with the administration of a single IV dose of propofol and ketorolac at the conclusion of sevoflurane anesthetic for tympanostomy tube placement in a prospective observational study.[23] However, most children undergoing tympanostomy tube placement do not require IV access and such intervention may be neither practical nor time- and cost-effective. Although dexmedetomidine is used both in the management and prevention of pediatric emergence delirium, a retrospective study of intranasal dexmedetomidine before tympanostomy tube placement found no reduction in emergence delirium scores or duration of PACU stay with its use.[24]

Tonsillectomy and adenoidectomy

After myringotomy with insertion of tympanostomy tubes, tonsillectomy is the second most common pediatric surgical procedure performed in the United States.[1] Tonsillectomy and adenotonsillectomy, like other pharyngeal procedures, are associated with severe pain that is often poorly controlled. Pain after tonsillectomy has a stereotypic course with worsening later in the first postoperative week.[25–27] Pain after tonsillectomy appears to be more severe and long lasting than after orchiopexy or inguinal hernia repair in children.[26] In general, adenoidectomy alone causes significantly less pain than tonsillectomy, and our discussion in this chapter, like the bulk of the research, is focused on tonsillectomy or adenotonsillectomy.

Poorly controlled oropharyngeal pain is the primary cause of morbidity after tonsillectomy in children, and this may lead to a reduction in oral intake with subsequent dehydration or weight loss. Studies have found that dehydration, hemorrhage, and throat pain are the three most common reasons for unplanned posttonsillectomy emergency room (ER) presentations.[28,29] Additional reasons for presentation included nausea and vomiting, respiratory issues, and fever.[28,29] Poor pain control and choice of analgesic regimen are likely involved with each of these potential complications.

Opioids

OSAS represents the most common indication for tonsillectomy (or adenotonsillectomy) in children.[30] Patients with sleep apnea have a unique sensitivity to opioids with regard to respiratory depression, and this is further complicated by impaired upper airway function from postoperative swelling as well as the effects of general anesthesia. Administration of opioids, given their dose-dependent risk of sedation and respiratory depression, is particularly fraught in this high-risk population.[31−34] Although tonsillectomy usually improves and often cures OSAS in children, the improvement is not immediate, and in fact sleep-related airway obstruction may worsen transiently in the immediate postoperative period.[35−37]

This risk of respiratory depression with opioid use in "typical" OSAS patients after tonsillectomy is further compounded by the known variation in the rate of metabolism of certain opioid preparations. Several commonly used opioids, including codeine, are metabolized by the CYP2D6 pathway into active morphine metabolites (Table 5.1). Ultrarapid metabolizer phenotypes with duplication of the CYP2D6 allele can cause rapid accumulation of active metabolites to supratherapeutic levels, leading to accelerated sedation and respiratory depression even with standard opioid dosing.

Although respiratory depression is the most severe risk associated with opioid use in children, other side effects may make opioids intolerable for some. Gastrointestinal side effects such as nausea, vomiting, or constipation can compound pain-related difficulties with reduced oral intake and worsen dehydration.[38] Additional bothersome adverse effects include lightheadedness/dizziness, dry mouth, itching, and rash.[5]

Prescription opioids also have the potential for misuse and abuse in adolescents, who are thought to be even more susceptible than adults due to the sensitivity of reward centers in the adolescent brain.[39,40] An analysis of a large commercial claims database found that 4.8% of opioid-naïve patients aged 13−21 continued to refill opioid prescriptions 90−180 days after tonsillectomy.[39] Although older children and adolescents may be less vulnerable to respiratory depression, habit formation and potential for opioid misuse is an important consideration in this age group. Opioid prescriptions, even for children, should be accompanied by education regarding appropriate secure storage, cessation of medication when pain abates, and methods for disposal of unused medication.[3]

Codeine

Historically, codeine, usually combined with acetaminophen, was the most commonly prescribed medication used for the management of posttonsillectomy pain. However, in 2009, a report of the codeine-related posttonsillectomy death of a 2-year-old with obstructive sleep apnea (OSA) who had a duplication of the CYP2D6 allele raised awareness of the risk of codeine administration in patients with this ultrarapid metabolizer phenotype.[6] In 2013, after a review of similar cases, the FDA issued a new box warning (its strongest warning) against the use of codeine for posttonsillectomy pain management in children. In 2017, the FDA expanded this advisory to a contraindication against the use of codeine for the treatment of pain or cough in children under 12, and a warning against its use in adolescents age 12–18 with obesity, OSA, or severe lung disease.[8] A review of the FDA Adverse Event Reporting System (FAERS) from 1969 to 2015 identified 24 codeine-related deaths in children under 18, 21 of which occurred in children under the age of 12.[8] Many of these patients were ultrarapid or extensive metabolizers, leading to supratherapeutic morphine levels that can be especially dangerous in the posttonsillectomy OSAS population. Unfortunately, preprocedural screening for CYP2D6 polymorphisms would be impractical and has not been shown to correlate with clinical phenotype.[5]

On the other end of the spectrum, the subset of patients belonging to the "poor metabolizer" phenotype is unable to metabolize codeine to its active metabolite and therefore derive minimal analgesia from its administration. RCTs have found no difference in pain control with acetaminophen with codeine compared to either acetaminophen[38] or ibuprofen alone in children after tonsillectomy.[41] Codeine use was associated with increased nausea and decreased tolerance of a normal diet in these studies.[38,41] All of these data taken together indicate that the risks of codeine far outweigh the benefits in children, and codeine administration has decreased substantially in recent years.[42] However, despite the strongest FDA warnings, 1 in 20 children who underwent a tonsillectomy in 2015 still received a prescription for codeine.[43]

Tramadol

Tramadol is a synthetic codeine analog that is a weak opioid receptor agonist and has been proposed as a safer alternative to codeine for pediatric posttonsillectomy pain.[44–46] However, in a review of its FAERS database from 1969 to 2016, the FDA identified nine reports of respiratory depression in children under 18 including three deaths in children under 6. Based on this data, in 2017, the FDA released a contraindication against tramadol use for the treatment of all types of pain in children under 12 and against its specific use for posttonsillectomy pain in children under 18.[8] Similar to codeine, tramadol is also dependent upon CYP2D6 for conversation to its active metabolite, and ultra-rapid metabolizer status may contribute to tramadol-associated respiratory depression.[47]

Hydrocodone, oxycodone, and morphine

Oxycodone is metabolized largely by pathways other than CYP2D6, and morphine is an active agent without metabolism, and therefore these drugs have been proposed as safer opioids for treating posttonsillectomy pain in children. However, these narcotics are stronger opioid receptor agonists than codeine or tramadol, and they may cause serious side effects regardless of methods of metabolic breakdown and pharmacogenomic effects. Stronger opioid receptor stimulation may lead to more severe respiratory depression in high-risk OSAS patients.[33] An RCT comparing oral morphine to ibuprofen found increased desaturation events on the night of tonsillectomy/adenotonsillectomy in the morphine group, with improved oxygen saturations in only 14% of the morphine group compared to 68% of the ibuprofen group, and no difference in other side effects.[48] Brown et al. found that children with OSAS are more sensitive to both respiratory depression and analgesic effect of opioids, and therefore urge caution when dosing opioids in this group.[31]

There is no such thing as a "safe narcotic" for all children undergoing tonsillectomy. Each child's particular risk factors, such as the severity of OSAS, young age, and presence of comorbidities such as obesity or lung disease must be considered when making decisions regarding the use and dosing of opioids after tonsillectomy. Additionally, high-risk patients who appear to require opioids for successful pain control should have therapy started in a monitored setting with conservative dosing. These risks must be weighed against the ability to provide equivalent analgesia with nonopioid medications.

Acetaminophen

Acetaminophen is the most commonly used medication in children. Although generally considered to be one of the safest analgesics, acetaminophen is associated with the risk of hepatic injury with prolonged use, high doses, or in patients with preexisting liver conditions.[49] Although acetaminophen is commonly used after tonsillectomy, it is often inadequate to provide satisfactory pain control when used on its own.[50] The 2019 American Academy of Otolaryngology-Head and Neck Surgery (AAOHNS) clinical practice guideline on tonsillectomy in children included a strong recommendation for "ibuprofen, acetaminophen, or both for pain control after tonsillectomy."[1] Although IV acetaminophen is expensive, its use in the immediate postoperative period has been shown to reduce overall costs by decreasing side effects and time spent in PACU.[51]

Nonsteroidal antiinflammatory drugs

Ibuprofen is now commonly used as an effective alternative to opioids for posttonsillectomy analgesia, especially with the recognition of the risks of opioids in this setting. However, concerns regarding potential increased bleeding risk with NSAID use continue to stimulate debate.[52] The 2019 AAOHNS guideline strongly supports ibuprofen use after tonsillectomy but describes ketorolac use as controversial.[1] Both a Cochrane review and a meta-analysis of 18 RCTs found no association between NSAID use and posttonsillectomy hemorrhage.[53,54] Systematic reviews have also identified decreased risk of nausea and vomiting with NSAIDs compared to opioids.[41,54,55] Several single-center studies compared their tonsillectomy patients historically treated with codeine with those more recently treated with ibuprofen and found no change in the incidence of bleeding complications.[56−58]

On the other hand, a recent multicenter noninferiority RCT of 688 children randomized to ibuprofen or acetaminophen could not exclude a higher rate of severe bleeding requiring operative intervention in the ibuprofen group.[59] A meta-analysis of RCTs and cohort studies found a possible increased tendency to bleeding with ibuprofen use,[60] and a systematic review observed more reoperations due to bleeding in patients treated with NSAIDs.[55]

It has been suggested that dosing intervals may play a role in the risk of posttonsillectomy hemorrhage with NSAID use. A retrospective study found a reduction in posttonsillectomy hemorrhage rate and posttonsillectomy ER visits after spacing out alternating doses of acetaminophen and ibuprofen from every 3 h to every 4 h, without an increase in phone calls regarding pain.[61]

Ketorolac is not commonly used after tonsillectomy due to even greater concerns regarding hemorrhage risk. Bleeding rates of 4.4%−18% after tonsillectomy were observed in trials of ketorolac use, leading the 2011 AAOHNS clinical practice guideline to recommend against its use in children after tonsillectomy.[62−64] Although children have a smaller increase in bleeding risk with ketorolac use after tonsillectomy than adult patients,[65] and the 2019 updated guideline no longer explicitly recommends against ketorolac, its use remains highly controversial.[1]

Steroids

Steroids have been proposed as a nonnarcotic adjunct for pain control after tonsillectomy. The 2019 AAOHNS clinical practice guideline on tonsillectomy in children strongly recommends the administration of a single intraoperative dose of IV dexamethasone.[1] This practice decreases postoperative nausea and vomiting, which can contribute to postoperative dehydration.[66] An observed elevated bleeding risk with dexamethasone use in one study[67] has not been replicated in a number of other studies or substantiated by meta-analyses.[1,66,68−71] Although intraoperative steroid administration has become standard of care, there is conflicting evidence supporting postoperative steroid use. Two randomized double-blind, placebo-controlled trials found no benefit to a postoperative course of oral prednisolone,[72,73] whereas one nonblinded nonplacebo-controlled randomized trial found improved pain scores with its use.[74] A recent blinded RCT found improved pain control and fewer ER visits and phone calls with a single oral dose of dexamethasone administered on postoperative day 3, suggesting that choice of steroid and timing of administration may influence efficacy.[75]

Opioid sparing regimens

Most major centers have adopted NSAIDs and acetaminophen as the centerpiece of posttonsillectomy pain management in children. A retrospective review of 583 patients who received alternating doses of ibuprofen and acetaminophen after tonsillectomy found a 90.4% rate of adequate pain control without an increase in postoperative hemorrhage rate.[76] An RCT comparing oral morphine and acetaminophen to ibuprofen and acetaminophen found no difference in pain control.[48] Evaluation of oral morphine for breakthrough pain in addition to acetaminophen and ibuprofen also found no added benefit.[77] RCTs have shown no difference in pain control in children treated with acetaminophen with codeine compared with either acetaminophen[38] or ibuprofen alone.[41] A parental survey found no difference in parental satisfaction or inadequate pain control with acetaminophen and ibuprofen compared to hydrocodone and acetaminophen.[78] Interestingly, in an RCT of 152 children the combination of ibuprofen and acetaminophen did not provide superior pain control compared to either medication alone.[79] All of these studies indicate that equivalent pain control can be achieved with opioid-sparing regimens, while avoiding the known risks of opioid administration. Experienced clinicians recognize that some of the "equivalence" of opioid and opioid-sparing regimens may actually reflect inadequate pain relief for some of the postoperative periods no matter what medications are prescribed.

Enhanced recovery after surgery pathways have been implemented in a variety of settings to optimize perioperative outcomes in adults, but have not been widely used in pediatric perioperative management.[80] However, studies have demonstrated the advantages of standardized multimodal protocols for posttonsillectomy pain management.[76] A recent study of discharge order set implementation demonstrated a significant reduction in opioid prescriptions, ER visits for posttonsillectomy dehydration, and pain with a standardized regimen of acetaminophen, ibuprofen, and opioid.[81] An increase in readmission for posttonsillectomy hemorrhage was observed in this study; however, this finding has not been replicated in other studies of nonopioid regimens.[82,83]

At the Johns Hopkins Children's Center, we primarily use opioid-sparing protocols for children after tonsillectomy and adenotonsillectomy (Table 5.2). The decision to prescribe opioids is based on (1) *age*, where children younger than 6 years are prescribed acetaminophen and ibuprofen, and children 6 years and older can receive also an opioid prescription, and (2) *plan for postoperative care*, where any child who is scheduled for overnight observation or hospital admission does not receive opioids after the immediate perioperative period in the PACU. The decision to admit or observe after adenotonsillectomy is made based on the known clinical risk factors for respiratory compromise, and thus is a proxy for the severity of obstructive sleep apnea in a given patient.[34,84] We use oxycodone when an opioid is prescribed, to avoid combination medications and to provide an opioid that is not primarily metabolized with the CYP2D6 pathway.

Table 5.2 Analgesia after adenotonsillectomy at the Johns Hopkins Children's Center.

	Age <6 years	Age ≥6 years Ambulatory surgery	Age ≥6 years Surgery is planned as 23 h stay or overnight admission
Acetaminophen	12.5 mg/kg/dose q4h for 24 h, then q4h prn pain/fever	12.5 mg/kg/dose q4h for 24 h, then q4h prn pain/fever	12.5 mg/kg/dose q4h for 24 h, then q4h prn pain/fever
Ibuprofen	10 mg/kg/dose q6h prn pain	10 mg/kg/dose q6h prn pain	10 mg/kg/dose q6h prn pain
Oxycodone	**None**	0.1 mg/kg/dose[a] q4h prn pain not relieved by acetaminophen/ ibuprofen	**None** without the approval of attending

[a] Oxycodone dosing based on ideal body weight, maximum dose 5 mg.

Nonpharmacologic adjuncts

A variety of nonpharmacologic methods have been studied for posttonsillectomy pain control to decrease dependence on controversial analgesics. A recent review of these alternative modalities found the greatest support for honey and acupuncture for posttonsillectomy pain and nausea and recommended against hydrogen peroxide rinses and chewing gum.[85] A meta-analysis of four trials found significant improvement in pain on postoperative day 1 and decreased analgesic intake for the first 5 days in patients treated with honey compared to placebo.[86] Randomized trials have found that intraoperative acupuncture may also reduce postoperative pain[87,88] as well as nausea and vomiting.[88,89] Imagery has also been suggested to reduce posttonsillectomy pain.[90] Although initial data supporting these alternative approaches are promising, further study with larger trials is needed before recommending broader implementation.

Surgical technique

Instrument choice

A variety of instruments have been used for tonsillectomy, including cold/sharp tools, monopolar or bipolar cautery, microdebriders, coblation devices, lasers, harmonic scalpels, and others.[91] Historically, tonsillectomy was performed using "cold" instrumentation, which has been associated with decreased postoperative pain compared to "hot" techniques. However, cold dissection tonsillectomy is less popular now due to greater operative blood loss and longer operative times.[92,93]

Monopolar cautery is now the most popular instrument used in tonsillectomy, although coblation is increasing in popularity.[94,95] A coblator delivers bipolar radio-frequency energy through a saline field, resulting in less heat compared to traditional cautery, and has therefore been thought to result in less postoperative pain. However, a Cochrane review of nine studies found insufficient evidence to support this claim.[96]

Intracapsular tonsillectomy

Partial or "powered" intracapsular tonsillectomy (PITA) is a technique that spares the tonsillar pillars and pharyngeal constrictor muscles by removing tonsillar bulk without violating its capsule. Given the more limited dissection and sparing of muscular injury, it is generally thought to result in decreased pain compared to traditional tonsillectomy, with reduced secondary bleeding risk. At least in the short term, PITA does provide a cure for children with mild or moderate OSAS.[97] However, there is a small but finite risk of tonsillar regrowth with recurrent symptoms after intracapsular tonsillectomy. Studies have shown that PITA performed with microdebrider,[98] scissors,[99] radiofrequency,[100] or carbon dioxide (CO_2) laser[101] all resulted in decreased postoperative pain compared to traditional tonsillectomy. PITA performed with coblator or radiofrequency devices may be less painful than CO_2 laser.[102] Several systematic reviews and a meta-analysis have examined the growing literature on this topic, which generally supports better pain-related outcomes with PITA; however, firm conclusions are limited by the heterogeneity and quality of published studies.[103–106]

Operative adjuncts

There is no conclusive evidence to support the routine use of intraoperative adjunctive interventions to improve postoperative analgesia. Although some small studies of intraoperative injection of local anesthetic and/or dexamethasone[107–109] showed benefit, a Cochrane systematic review of six trials found no support for improved pain control with perioperative local anesthetic injections.[110] Small studies of intraoperative treatment of the tonsillar fossae with cold water irrigation[111,112] or coating with hyaluronic acid suggest that these interventions may reduce postoperative pain, but the application of polyglycolic acid sheeting to the operative sites was shown to exacerbate pain.[113]

Conclusions

Perioperative pain management in children after otolaryngology operations can be especially challenging for patients, caregivers, and clinicians. While some procedures, like tympanostomy tube placement, cause pain in children of short duration that can be managed quite effectively, pharyngeal procedures like tonsillectomy are associated with prolonged periods of pain that can be difficult to alleviate. Caregivers can be unprepared or even surprised by these difficulties, as tonsillectomy is considered "routine" by many. Additionally, the children who undergo tonsillectomy often have risk factors, some predictable and some less apparent, for poor pain control and side effects of the analgesics we prescribe. Pre- and postoperative caregiver education should be part of an integrated approach combining pharmacologic and nonpharmacologic modalities.

In recent years, the efficacy of opioid-sparing regimens has been demonstrated, while the risks of opioid use in children have come to the forefront. Codeine and tramadol should not be used in this population, and other opioids should be employed with appropriate caution and counseling. Although debate continues regarding the bleeding risk associated with NSAIDs, they appear to be a safe and effective opioid alternative. Choice of surgical techniques, such as intracapsular tonsillectomy for appropriate candidates, may also improve postoperative pain control. Ongoing research will shed additional light upon these controversies, as we continue to search for ideal perioperative pain management strategies in pediatric otolaryngology.

References

1. Mitchell RB, Archer SM, Ishman SL, et al. Clinical practice guideline: tonsillectomy in children (update). *Otolaryngol Head Neck Surg*. 2019;160(1_suppl):S1–S42. https://doi.org/10.1177/0194599818801757.
2. Kelley-Quon LI, Kirkpatrick MG, Ricca RL, et al. Guidelines for opioid prescribing in children and adolescents after surgery. *JAMA Surg*. 2020;156(1):76–90. https://doi.org/10.1001/jamasurg.2020.5045.
3. Anne S, Mims J, Tunkel DE, Rosenfeld RM, et al. Clinical practice guideline: opioid prescribing for analgesia after common otolaryngology operations. *Otolaryngol Head Neck Surg*. 2021;164(2S):S1–S42.
4. Shelton FR, Ishii H, Mella S, et al. Implementing a standardised discharge analgesia guideline to reduce paediatric post tonsillectomy pain. *Int J Pediatr Otorhinolaryngol*. 2018;111:54–58. https://doi.org/10.1016/j.ijporl.2018.05.020.
5. Prows CA, Zhang X, Huth MM, et al. Codeine-related adverse drug reactions in children following tonsillectomy: a prospective study. *Laryngoscope*. 2014;124(5):1242–1250. https://doi.org/10.1002/lary.24455.
6. Ciszkowski C, Madadi P, Phillips MS, Lauwers AE, Koren G. Codeine, ultrarapid-metabolism genotype, and postoperative death. *N Engl J Med*. 2009;361(8):827–828. https://doi.org/10.1056/nejmc0904266.
7. Research C for DE and Drug Safety and Availability - FDA Drug Safety Communication. *Safety Review Update of Codeine Use in Children; New Boxed Warning and Contraindication on Use after Tonsillectomy and/or Adenoidectomy*. 2013.
8. FDA Drug Safety Communication. *FDA Restricts Use of Prescription Codeine Pain and Cough Medicines and Tramadol Pain Medicines in Children; Recommends against Use in Breastfeeding Women*. FDA; 2017. https://www.fda.gov/drugs/drug-safety-and-

availability/fda-drug-safety-communication-fda-restricts-use-prescription-codeine-pain-and-cough-medicines-and.Published. Accessed December 8, 2020. Accessed.

9. Sutters KA, Holdridge-Zeuner D, Waite S, et al. A descriptive feasibility study to evaluate scheduled oral analgesic dosing at home for the management of postoperative pain in preschool children following tonsillectomy. *Pain Med*. 2012;13(3):472−483. https://doi.org/10.1111/j.1526-4637.2011.01324.x.

10. Lennon P, Amin M, Colreavy MP. A prospective study of parents' compliance with their child's prescribed analgesia following tonsillectomy. *Ear Nose Throat J*. 2013;92(3):134−140. https://doi.org/10.1177/014556131309200312.

11. Fortier MA, MacLaren JE, Martin SR, Perret-Karimi D, Kain ZN. Pediatric pain after ambulatory surgery: where's the medication? *Pediatrics*. 2009;124(4):e588−e595. https://doi.org/10.1542/peds.2008-3529.

12. Sutters KA, Savedra MC, Miaskowski C. The pediatric PRO-SELF©: pain control program: an effective educational program for parents caring for children at home following tonsillectomy. *J Spec Pediatr Nurs*. 2011;16(4):280−294. https://doi.org/10.1111/j.1744-6155.2011.00299.x.

13. Greenberg RS, Billett C, Zahurak M, Yaster M. Videotape increases parental knowledge about pediatric pain management. *Anesth Analg*. 1999;89(4):899. https://doi.org/10.1213/00000539-199910000-00015.

14. Chambers CT, Reid GJ, McGrath PJ, Finley GA, Ellerton ML. A randomized trial of a pain education booklet: effects on parents' attitudes and postoperative pain management. *Child Heal Care*. 1997;26(1):1−13. https://doi.org/10.1207/s15326888chc2601_1.

15. Harbaugh CM, Vargas G, Sloss KR, et al. Association of opioid quantity and caregiver education with pain control after pediatric tonsillectomy. *Otolaryngol Head Neck Surg*. 2020;162(5):746−753. https://doi.org/10.1177/0194599820912033.

16. Schymik FA, Lavoie Smith EM, Voepel-Lewis T. Parental analgesic knowledge and decision making for children with and without obstructive sleep apnea after tonsillectomy and adenoidectomy. *Pain Manag Nurs*. 2015;16(6):881−889. https://doi.org/10.1016/j.pmn.2015.07.003.

17. Donaldson CD, Jenkins BN, Fortier MA, et al. Parent responses to pediatric pain: the differential effects of ethnicity on opioid consumption. *J Psychosom Res*. 2020;138. https://doi.org/10.1016/j.jpsychores.2020.110251.

18. Rosenfeld RM, Schwartz SR, Pynnonen MA, et al. Clinical practice guideline: tympanostomy tubes in children. *Otolaryngol Head Neck Surg*. 2013;149(SUPPL.1):S1−S35. https://doi.org/10.1177/0194599813487302.

19. McHale B, Badenhorst CD, Low C, Blundell D. Do children undergoing bilateral myringotomy with placement of ventilating tubes benefit from pre-operative analgesia? A double-blinded, randomised, placebo-controlled trial. *J Laryngol Otol*. 2018;132(8):685−692. https://doi.org/10.1017/S0022215118001111.

20. Stricker PA, Muhly WT, Jantzen EC, et al. Intramuscular fentanyl and ketorolac associated with superior pain control after pediatric bilateral myringotomy and tube placement surgery: a retrospective cohort study. *Anesth Analg*. 2017;124(1):245−253. https://doi.org/10.1213/ANE.0000000000001722.

21. Riley B, Kawai K, Irace AL, Leung P, Adil E. Perioperative pain control and tympanostomy tube outcomes. *Int J Pediatr Otorhinolaryngol*. 2020;138:110337. https://doi.org/10.1016/j.ijporl.2020.110337.

22. Lin YC, Tassone RF, Jahng S, et al. Acupuncture management of pain and emergence agitation in children after bilateral myringotomy and tympanostomy tube insertion. *Paediatr Anaesth.* 2009;19(11):1096–1101. https://doi.org/10.1111/j.1460-9592.2009.03129.x.

23. d'Eon B, Hackmann T, Wright AS. The addition of intravenous propofol and ketorolac to a sevoflurane anesthetic lessens emergence agitation in children having bilateral myringotomy with tympanostomy tube insertion: a prospective observational study. *Children.* 2020;7(8):96. https://doi.org/10.3390/children7080096.

24. Santana L, Mills K. Retrospective study of intranasal dexmedetomidine as a prophylactic against emergence delirium in pediatric patients undergoing ear tube surgery. *Int J Pediatr Otorhinolaryngol.* 2017;100:39–43. https://doi.org/10.1016/j.ijporl.2017.06.023.

25. Wilson CA, Sommerfield D, Drake-Brockman TFE, von Bieberstein L, Ramgolam A, von Ungern-Sternberg BS. Pain after discharge following head and neck surgery in childrenVeyckemans F, ed. *Pediatr Anesth.* 2016;26(10):992–1001. https://doi.org/10.1111/pan.12974.

26. Stewart DW, Ragg PG, Sheppard S, Chalkiadis GA. The severity and duration of postoperative pain and analgesia requirements in children after tonsillectomy, orchidopexy, or inguinal hernia repair. *Paediatr Anaesth.* 2012;22(2):136–143. https://doi.org/10.1111/j.1460-9592.2011.03713.x.

27. Warnock FF, Lander J. Pain progression, intensity and outcomes following tonsillectomy. *Pain.* 1998;75(1):37–45. https://doi.org/10.1016/S0304-3959(97)00202-9.

28. Duval M, Wilkes J, Korgenski K, Srivastava R, Meier J. Causes, costs, and risk factors for unplanned return visits after adenotonsillectomy in children. *Int J Pediatr Otorhinolaryngol.* 2015;79(10):1640–1646. https://doi.org/10.1016/j.ijporl.2015.07.002.

29. Curtis JL, Harvey DB, Willie S, et al. *Causes and costs for ED visits after pediatric adenotonsillectomy.* In: *Otolaryngology - Head and Neck Surgery (United States).* Vol. 152. SAGE Publications Inc.; 2015:691–696. https://doi.org/10.1177/0194599815572123.

30. Patel HH, Straight CE, Lehman EB, Tanner M, Carr MM. Indications for tonsillectomy: a 10 year retrospective review. *Int J Pediatr Otorhinolaryngol.* 2014;78(12):2151–2155. https://doi.org/10.1016/j.ijporl.2014.09.030.

31. Brown KA, Laferrière A, Lakheeram I, Moss IR. Recurrent hypoxemia in children is associated with increased analgesic sensitivity to opiates. *Anesthesiology.* 2006;105(4):665–669. https://doi.org/10.1097/00000542-200610000-00009.

32. Brown KA, Morin I, Hickey C, Manoukian JJ, Nixon GM, Brouillette RT. Urgent adenotonsillectomy: an analysis of risk factors associated with postoperative respiratory morbidity. *Anesthesiology.* 2003;99(3):586–595. https://doi.org/10.1097/00000542-200309000-00013.

33. Waters KA, McBrien F, Stewart P, Hinder M, Wharton S. Effects of OSA, inhalational anesthesia, and fentanyl on the airway and ventilation of children. *J Appl Physiol.* 2002;92(5):1987–1994. https://doi.org/10.1152/japplphysiol.00619.2001.

34. McColley SA, April MM, Carroll JL, Naclerio RM, Loughlin GM. Respiratory compromise after adenotonsillectomy in children with obstructive sleep apnea. *Arch Otolaryngol Neck Surg.* 1992;118(9):940–943. https://doi.org/10.1001/archotol.1992.01880090056017.

35. De A, Waltuch T, Gonik NJ, et al. Sleep and breathing the first night after adenotonsillectomy in obese children with obstructive sleep apnea. *J Clin Sleep Med.* 2017;13(06): 805−811. https://doi.org/10.5664/jcsm.6620.

36. Helfaer MA, McColley SA, Pyzik PL, et al. Polysomnography after adenotonsillectomy in mild pediatric obstructive sleep apnea. *Crit Care Med.* 1996;24(8):1323−1327. https://doi.org/10.1097/00003246-199608000-00009.

37. Jamieson K, Soh HJ, Davey MJ, Rimmer J, Horne RS, Nixon GM. Continuous oximetry recordings on the first post-operative night after pediatric adenotonsillectomy-a case-control study. *Int J Pediatr Otorhinolaryngol.* 2020;138. https://doi.org/10.1016/j.ijporl.2020.110313.

38. Moir MS, Bair E, Shinnick P, Messner A. Acetaminophen versus acetaminophen with codeine after pediatric tonsillectomy. *Laryngoscope.* 2000;110(11):1824−1827. https://doi.org/10.1097/00005537-200011000-00011.

39. Harbaugh CM, Lee JS, Hu HM, et al. Persistent opioid use among pediatric patients after surgery. *Pediatrics.* 2018;141(1):e20172439. https://doi.org/10.1542/peds.2017-2439.

40. Schramm-Sapyta NL, Walker QD, Caster JM, Levin ED, Kuhn CM. Are adolescents more vulnerable to drug addiction than adults? Evidence from animal models. *Psychopharmacology.* 2009;206(1):1−21. https://doi.org/10.1007/s00213-009-1585-5.

41. Charles CSS, Matt BH, Hamilton MM, Katz BP. *A Comparison of Ibuprofen Versus Acetaminophen with Codeine in the Young Tonsillectomy Patient.* Los Angeles, CA: SAGE PublicationsSage CA; 1997. https://doi.org/10.1016/S0194-59989770211-0.

42. Goldman JL, Ziegler C, Burckardt EM. Otolaryngology practice patterns in pediatric tonsillectomy: the impact of the codeine boxed warning. *Laryngoscope.* 2018;128(1): 264−268. https://doi.org/10.1002/lary.26719.

43. Chua KP, Shrime MG, Conti RM. Effect of FDA investigation on opioid prescribing to children after tonsillectomy/adenoidectomy. *Pediatrics.* 2017;140(6). https://doi.org/10.1542/peds.2017-1765.

44. Hullett BJ, Chambers NA, Pascoe EM, Johnson C. Tramadol vs morphine during adenotonsillectomy for obstructive sleep apnea in children. *Paediatr Anaesth.* 2006;16(6): 648−653. https://doi.org/10.1111/j.1460-9592.2005.01827.x.

45. Benini F, Barbi E. Doing without codeine: why and what are the alternatives? *Ital J Pediatr.* 2014;40(1). https://doi.org/10.1186/1824-7288-40-16.

46. Friedrichsdorf SJ, Postier AC, Foster LP, et al. *Tramadol versus codeine/acetaminophen after pediatric tonsillectomy: a prospective, double-blinded, randomized controlled trial.* In: *Journal of Opioid Management.* Vol. 11. Weston Medical Publishing; 2015: 283−294. https://doi.org/10.5055/jom.2015.0277.

47. Smith HS. Opioid metabolism. *Mayo Clin Proc.* 2009;84(7):613−624. https://doi.org/10.1016/s0025-6196(11)60750-7.

48. Kelly LE, Sommer DD, Ramakrishna J, et al. Morphine or ibuprofen for post-tonsillectomy analgesia: a randomized trial. *Pediatrics.* 2015;135(2):307−313. https://doi.org/10.1542/peds.2014-1906.

49. Star K, Choonara I. How safe is paracetamol? *Arch Dis Child.* 2015;100(1):73−74. https://doi.org/10.1136/archdischild-2014-307431.

50. Rømsing J, Hertel S, Harder A, Rasmussen M. Examination of acetaminophen for outpatient management of postoperative pain in children. *Paediatr Anaesth.* 1998; 8(3):235−239. https://doi.org/10.1046/j.1460-9592.1998.00768.x.

51. Subramanyam R, Varughese A, Kurth CD, Eckman MH. Cost-effectiveness of intravenous acetaminophen for pediatric tonsillectomy. *Paediatr Anaesth*. 2014;24(5): 467−475. https://doi.org/10.1111/pan.12359.

52. Cramer JD, Barnett ML, Anne S, et al. Nonopioid, multimodal analgesia as first-line therapy after otolaryngology operations: primer on nonsteroidal anti-inflammatory drugs (NSAIDs). *Otolaryngol Head Neck Surg*. 2020. https://doi.org/10.1177/0194599820947013.

53. Riggin L, Ramakrishna J, Sommer DD, Koren G. A 2013 updated systematic review & meta-analysis of 36 randomized controlled trials; no apparent effects of non steroidal anti-inflammatory agents on the risk of bleeding after tonsillectomy. *Clin Otolaryngol*. 2013;38(2):115−129. https://doi.org/10.1111/coa.12106.

54. Lewis SR, Nicholson A, Cardwell ME, Siviter G, Smith AF. Nonsteroidal anti-inflammatory drugs and perioperative bleeding in paediatric tonsillectomy. *Cochrane Database Syst Rev*. 2013;2013(7). https://doi.org/10.1002/14651858.CD003591.pub3.

55. Møiniche S, Rømsing J, Dahl JB, Tramèr MR. Nonsteroidal antiinflammatory drugs and the risk of operative site bleeding after tonsillectomy: a quantitative systematic review. *Anesth Analg*. 2003;96(1):68−77. https://doi.org/10.1213/00000539-200301000-00015.

56. Pfaff JA, Hsu K, Chennupati SK. *The use of ibuprofen in posttonsillectomy analgesia and its effect on posttonsillectomy hemorrhage rate*. In: *Otolaryngology - Head and Neck Surgery (United States)*. Vol. 155. SAGE Publications Inc.; 2016:508−513. https://doi.org/10.1177/0194599816646363.

57. Mattos JL, Robison JG, Greenberg J, Yellon RF. Acetaminophen plus ibuprofen versus opioids for treatment of post-tonsillectomy pain in children. *Int J Pediatr Otorhinolaryngol*. 2014;78(10):1671−1676. https://doi.org/10.1016/j.ijporl.2014.07.017.

58. Bedwell JR, Pierce M, Levy M, Shah RK. Ibuprofen with acetaminophen for postoperative pain control following tonsillectomy does not increase emergency department utilization. *Otolaryngol Head Neck Surg*. 2014;151(6):963−966. https://doi.org/10.1177/0194599814549732.

59. Diercks GR, Comins J, Bennett K, et al. Comparison of ibuprofen vs acetaminophen and severe bleeding risk after pediatric tonsillectomy: a noninferiority randomized clinical trial. *JAMA Otolaryngol Head Neck Surg*. 2019;145(6):494−500. https://doi.org/10.1001/jamaoto.2019.0269.

60. Stokes W, Swanson RT, Schubart J, Carr MM. Postoperative bleeding associated with ibuprofen use after tonsillectomy: a meta-analysis. *Otolaryngol Head Neck Surg*. 2019;161(5):734−741. https://doi.org/10.1177/0194599819852328.

61. Mast G, Henderson K, Carr MM. The effect of ibuprofen dosing interval on post-tonsillectomy outcomes in children: a quality improvement study. *Ann Otol Rhinol Laryngol*. 2020;129(12):1210−1214. https://doi.org/10.1177/0003489420934843.

62. Baugh RF, Archer SM, Mitchell RB, et al. Clinical practice guideline: tonsillectomy in children. *Otolaryngol Head Neck Surg*. 2011;144(Suppl.1):S1−S30. https://doi.org/10.1177/0194599810389949.

63. Bailey R, Sinha C, Burgess LPA. Ketorolac tromethamine and hemorrhage in tonsillectomy: a prospective, randomized, double-blind study. *Laryngoscope*. 1997;107(2): 166−169. https://doi.org/10.1097/00005537-199702000-00006.

64. Judkins JH, Dray TG, Hubbell RN. Intraoperative ketorolac and posttonsillectomy bleeding. *Arch Otolaryngol Head Neck Surg*. 1996;122(9):937−940. https://doi.org/10.1001/archotol.1996.01890210017004.

65. Chan DK, Parikh SR. Perioperative ketorolac increases post-tonsillectomy hemorrhage in adults but not children. *Laryngoscope*. 2014;124(8):1789−1793. https://doi.org/10.1002/lary.24555.

66. Steward DL, Grisel J, Meinzen-Derr J. Steroids for improving recovery following tonsillectomy in children. *Cochrane Database Syst Rev*. 2011;2017(10). https://doi.org/10.1002/14651858.CD003997.pub2.

67. Czarnetzki C, Elia N, Lysakowski C, et al. Dexamethasone and risk of nausea and vomiting and postoperative bleeding after tonsillectomy in children: a randomized trial. *J Am Med Assoc*. 2008;300(22):2621−2630. https://doi.org/10.1001/jama.2008.794.

68. Mahant S, Keren R, Localio R, et al. Dexamethasone and risk of bleeding in children undergoing tonsillectomy. *Otolaryngol Head Neck Surg*. 2014;150(5):872−879. https://doi.org/10.1177/0194599814521555.

69. Gallagher TQ, Hill C, Ojha S, et al. Perioperative dexamethasone administration and risk of bleeding following tonsillectomy in children: a randomized controlled trial. *J Am Med Assoc*. 2012;308(12):1221−1226. https://doi.org/10.1001/2012.jama.11575.

70. Plante J, Turgeon AF, Zarychanski R, et al. Effect of systemic steroids on post-tonsillectomy bleeding and reinterventions: systematic review and meta-analysis of randomised controlled trials. *BMJ*. 2012;345(7873). https://doi.org/10.1136/bmj.e5389.

71. Geva A, Brigger MT. Dexamethasone and tonsillectomy bleeding: a meta-analysis. *Otolaryngol Head Neck Surg*. 2011;144(6):838−843. https://doi.org/10.1177/0194599811399538.

72. Palme CE, Tomasevic P, Pohl DV. Evaluating the effects of oral prednisolone on recovery after tonsillectomy: a prospective, double-blind, randomized trial. *Laryngoscope*. 2000;110(12):2000−2004. https://doi.org/10.1097/00005537-200012000-00003.

73. MacAssey E, Dawes P, Taylor B, Gray A. The effect of a postoperative course of oral prednisone on postoperative morbidity following childhood tonsillectomy. *Otolaryngol Head Neck Surg*. 2012;147(3):551−556. https://doi.org/10.1177/0194599812447776.

74. Park SK, Kim J, Kim JM, Yeon JY, Shim WS, Lee DW. Effects of oral prednisolone on recovery after tonsillectomy. *Laryngoscope*. 2015;125(1):111−117. https://doi.org/10.1002/lary.24958.

75. Greenwell AG, Isaiah A, Pereira KD. Recovery after adenotonsillectomy—do steroids help? Outcomes from a randomized controlled trial. *Otolaryngol Neck Surg*. November 2020;165(1):83−88. https://doi.org/10.1177/0194599820973250.

76. Liu C, Ulualp SO. Outcomes of an alternating ibuprofen and acetaminophen regimen for pain relief after tonsillectomy in children. *Ann Otol Rhinol Laryngol*. 2015;124(10):777−781. https://doi.org/10.1177/0003489415583685.

77. Oremule B, Johnson M, Sanderson L, Lutz J, Dodd J, Hans P. Oral morphine for pain management in paediatric patients after tonsillectomy and adenotonsillectomy. *Int J Pediatr Otorhinolaryngol*. 2015;79(12):2166−2169. https://doi.org/10.1016/j.ijporl.2015.09.040.

78. Adler AC, Mehta DK, Messner AH, Salemi JL, Chandrakantan A. Parental assessment of pain control following pediatric adenotonsillectomy: do opioids make a difference? *Int J Pediatr Otorhinolaryngol*. 2020;134:110045. https://doi.org/10.1016/j.ijporl.2020.110045.

79. Merry AF, Edwards KE, Ahmad Z, Barber C, Mahadevan M, Frampton C. Randomized comparison between the combination of acetaminophen and ibuprofen and each constituent alone for analgesia following tonsillectomy in children. *Can J Anesth*. 2013; 60(12):1180−1189. https://doi.org/10.1007/s12630-013-0043-3.

80. George JA, Koka R, Gan TJ, et al. Review of the enhanced recovery pathway for children: perioperative anesthetic considerations. *Can J Anesth.* 2018;65(5):569—577. https://doi.org/10.1007/s12630-017-1042-6.

81. Agamawi YM, Cass LM, Mouzourakis M, Pannu JS, Brinkmeier JV. Pediatric post-tonsillectomy opioid prescribing practices. *Laryngoscope.* October 2020;131(6): 1386—1391. https://doi.org/10.1002/lary.29157. lary.29157.

82. Luk LJ, Mosen D, MacArthur CJ, Grosz AH. *Implementation of a pediatric posttonsillectomy pain protocol in a large group practice.* In: *Otolaryngology - Head and Neck Surgery (United States).* Vol. 154. SAGE Publications Inc.; 2016:720—724. https://doi.org/10.1177/0194599815627810.

83. Chua KP, Harbaugh CM, Brummett CM, et al. Association of perioperative opioid prescriptions with risk of complications after tonsillectomy in children. *JAMA Otolaryngol - Head Neck Surg.* 2019;145(10):911—918. https://doi.org/10.1001/jamaoto.2019.2107.

84. Rosen GM, Muckle RP, Goding GS, Mahowald MW, Ullevig C. Postoperative respiratory compromise in children with obstructive sleep apnea syndrome: can it Be anticipated? *Pediatrics.* 1994;93(5):784—788.

85. Keefe KR, Byrne KJ, Levi JR. Treating pediatric post-tonsillectomy pain and nausea with complementary and alternative medicine. *Laryngoscope.* 2018;128(11): 2625—2634. https://doi.org/10.1002/lary.27231.

86. Hwang SH, Song JN, Jeong YM, Lee YJ, Kang JM. The efficacy of honey for ameliorating pain after tonsillectomy: a meta-analysis. *Eur Arch Oto-Rhino-Laryngol.* 2016; 273(4):811—818. https://doi.org/10.1007/s00405-014-3433-4.

87. Tsao GJ, Messner AH, Seybold J, Sayyid ZN, Cheng AG, Golianu B. Intraoperative acupuncture for posttonsillectomy pain: a randomized, double-blind, placebo-controlled trial. *Laryngoscope.* 2015;125(8):1972—1978. https://doi.org/10.1002/lary.25252.

88. Pouy S, Etebarian A, Azizi-Qadikolaee A, Saeidi S. The effect of acupuncture on postoperative pain, nausea and vomiting after pediatric tonsillectomy: a systematic review. *Int J Adolesc Med Health.* 2019:1. https://doi.org/10.1515/ijamh-2018-0285 (ahead-of-print).

89. Martin CS, Deverman SE, Norvell DC, Cusick JC, Kendrick A, Koh J. Randomized trial of acupuncture with antiemetics for reducing postoperative nausea in children. *Acta Anaesthesiol Scand.* 2019;63(3):292—297. https://doi.org/10.1111/aas.13288.

90. Huth MM, Broome ME, Good M. Imagery reduces children's post-operative pain. *Pain.* 2004;110(1):439—448. https://doi.org/10.1016/j.pain.2004.04.028.

91. Younis RT, Lazar RH. History and current practice of tonsillectomy. *Laryngoscope.* 2009;112(S100):3—5. https://doi.org/10.1002/lary.5541121403.

92. Leinbach RF, Markwell SJ, Colliver JA, Lin SY. Hot versus cold tonsillectomy: a systematic review of the literature. *Otolaryngol Neck Surg.* May 2016. https://doi.org/10.1016/S0194-5998(02)00729-0.

93. Aydin S, Taskin U, Altas B, et al. Post-tonsillectomy morbidities: randomised, prospective controlled clinical trial of cold dissection versus thermal welding tonsillectomy. *J Laryngol Otol.* 2014;128(2):163—165. https://doi.org/10.1017/S0022215113003253.

94. Walner DL, Parker NP, Miller RP. Past and present instrument use in pediatric adenotonsillectomy. *Otolaryngol Head Neck Surg.* 2007;137(1):49—53. https://doi.org/10.1016/j.otohns.2007.02.036.

95. Setabutr D, Adil EA, Adil TK, Carr MM. Emerging trends in tonsillectomy. *Otolaryngol Head Neck Surg.* 2011;145(2):223–229. https://doi.org/10.1177/0194599811401728.

96. Burton MJ, Doree C. Coblation versus other surgical techniques for tonsillectomy. *Cochrane Database Syst Rev.* 2007;3:CD004619. https://doi.org/10.1002/14651858.CD004619.pub2.

97. Tunkel DE, Hotchkiss KS, Carson KA, Sterni LM. Efficacy of powered intracapsular tonsillectomy and adenoidectomy. *Laryngoscope.* 2008;118(7):1295–1302. https://doi.org/10.1097/MLG.0b013e3181724269.

98. Lister MT, Cunningham MJ, Benjamin B, et al. Microdebrider tonsillotomy vs electrosurgical tonsillectomy: a randomized, double-blind, paired control study of postoperative pain. *Arch Otolaryngol Head Neck Surg.* 2006;132(6):599–604. https://doi.org/10.1001/archotol.132.6.599.

99. Vlastos IM, Parpounas K, Economides J, Helmis G, Koudoumnakis E, Houlakis M. Tonsillectomy versus tonsillotomy performed with scissors in children with tonsillar hypertrophy. *Int J Pediatr Otorhinolaryngol.* 2008;72(6):857–863. https://doi.org/10.1016/j.ijporl.2008.02.015.

100. Hultcrantz E, Ericsson E. Pediatric tonsillotomy with the radiofrequency technique: less morbidity and pain. *Laryngoscope.* 2004;114(5):871–877. https://doi.org/10.1097/00005537-200405000-00016.

101. Hultcrantz E, Linder A, Markström A. Tonsillectomy or tonsillotomy? - a randomized study comparing postoperative pain and long-term effects. *Int J Pediatr Otorhinolaryngol.* 1999;51(3):171–176. https://doi.org/10.1016/S0165-5876(99)00274-8.

102. Babademez MA, Yurekli MF, Acar B, Günbey E. Comparison of radiofrequency ablation, laser and coblator techniques in reduction of tonsil size. *Acta Otolaryngol.* 2011;131(7):750–756. https://doi.org/10.3109/00016489.2011.553244.

103. Acevedo JL, Shah RK, Brietzke SE. Systematic review of complications of tonsillotomy versus tonsillectomy. *Otolaryngol Head Neck Surg.* 2012;146(6):871–879. https://doi.org/10.1177/0194599812439017.

104. Wang H, Fu Y, Feng Y, Guan J, Yin S. Tonsillectomy versus tonsillotomy for sleep-disordered breathing in children: a meta analysis. In: Gao C-Q, ed. *PLoS One.* Vol. 10. 2015:e0121500. https://doi.org/10.1371/journal.pone.0121500, 3.

105. Walton J, Ebner Y, Stewart MG, April MM. Systematic review of randomized controlled trials comparing intracapsular tonsillectomy with total tonsillectomy in a pediatric population. *Arch Otolaryngol Head Neck Surg.* 2012;138(3):243–249. https://doi.org/10.1001/archoto.2012.16.

106. Sathe N, Chinnadurai S, McPheeters M, Francis DO. Comparative effectiveness of partial versus total tonsillectomy in children. *Otolaryngol Head Neck Surg.* 2017;156(3):456–463. https://doi.org/10.1177/0194599816683916.

107. Aysenur D, Mine C, Ozgur Y, et al. Pre-emptive peritonsillar dexamethasone vs levobupivacaine infiltration for relief of post-adenotonsillectomy pain in children: a controlled clinical study. *Int J Pediatr Otorhinolaryngol.* 2014;78(9):1467–1471. https://doi.org/10.1016/j.ijporl.2014.06.010.

108. Safavi M, Naghibi K, Attari M, et al. Preemptive peritonsillar infiltration with bupivacaine in combination with tramadol improves pediatric post-tonsillectomy pain better than using bupivacaine or tramadol alone: a randomized, placebo-controlled, double blind clinical trial. *Adv Biomed Res.* 2015;4(1):132. https://doi.org/10.4103/2277-9175.161518.

109. Basuni AS, Ezz HAA, Albirmawy OA. Preoperative peritonsillar infiltration of dexamethasone and levobupivacaine reduces pediatric post-tonsillectomy pain: a double-blind prospective randomized clinical trial. *J Anesth.* 2013;27(6):844–849. https://doi.org/10.1007/s00540-013-1638-0.

110. Hollis L, Burton MJ, Millar J. Perioperative local anaesthesia for reducing pain following tonsillectomy. *Cochrane Database Syst Rev.* 1999;4. https://doi.org/10.1002/14651858.cd001874.

111. Shin JM, Byun JY, Baek BJ, Lee JY. Effect of cold-water cooling of tonsillar fossa and pharyngeal mucosa on post-tonsillectomy pain. *Am J Otolaryngol Head Neck Med Surg.* 2014;35(3):353–356. https://doi.org/10.1016/j.amjoto.2014.01.005.

112. Raggio BS, Barton BM, Grant MC, McCoul ED. Intraoperative cryoanalgesia for reducing post-tonsillectomy pain: a systemic review. *Ann Otol Rhinol Laryngol.* 2018;127(6):395–401. https://doi.org/10.1177/0003489418772859.

113. Miyaguchi SI, Horii A, Kambara R, et al. Effects of covering surgical wounds with polyglycolic acid sheets for posttonsillectomy pain. *Otolaryngol Head Neck Surg.* 2016;155(5):876–878. https://doi.org/10.1177/0194599816660072.

114. Tan GX, Tunkel DE. Control of pain after tonsillectomy in children: a review. *JAMA Otolaryngol Head Neck Surg.* 2017;143(9):937–942. https://doi.org/10.1001/jamaoto.2017.0845.

115. Smith HS. The metabolism of opioid agents and the clinical impact of their active metabolites. *Clin J Pain.* 2011;27(9):824–838. https://doi.org/10.1097/AJP.0b013e31821d8ac1.

Approach to pain management in otology and neurotology

Abhishek Gami, BS [1], Daniel Q. Sun, MD [2]

[1]*Johns Hopkins University, School of Medicine, Baltimore, MD, United States;* [2]*Johns Hopkins University, Department of Otolaryngology-Head and Neck Surgery, Baltimore, MD, United States*

Overview

Otology and neurotology encompass a broad spectrum of procedures, from minor surgical procedures performed under local anesthesia in an outpatient setting (e.g., bone-anchored hearing aid placement), to complex intracranial surgeries involving critical neurovascular structures that require ICU admission (e.g., vestibular schwannoma excision). The patient population also encompasses the entire span of life, from infants to the elderly. The heterogeneity in procedural scope and patient demographics render pain management particularly challenging and require deliberate consideration for each patient and procedure.

Opioid overuse and misuse remain a significant challenge in medicine, especially in postsurgical care. Surgeons have the second highest rate of opioid prescribing and write 37% of all prescriptions, second only to pain medicine specialists.[1] Studies have demonstrated that surgeons poorly estimate postoperative opioid needs, with patients often using less than half of their prescribed course.[2] The need to manage a patient's pain postoperatively, variability in patient pain tolerance, and the broad spectrum of procedures performed make the standardization of pain medication regimens especially challenging in otology and neurotology.

Studies have evaluated trends in opioid prescribing specific to the field of otology. Gerbershagen et al. examined pain intensity the first day after surgery and found that middle and inner ear surgery ranked 155 out of 179 different procedures in terms of pain intensity. However, these surgeries were labeled as a "heterogenous surgical group," demonstrating the variation in otologic surgery.[3] Mohan et al. reviewed outpatient otolaryngology visits and found that although only a minority of visits resulted in the prescription of opioids, the ambulatory opioid prescription rate doubled between 2008 and 2011, with chronic otitis media and otitis externa ranking among the most common visit diagnoses associated with opioid prescription (8.7% and 6.2% of all diagnoses, respectively).[4] Separate studies have evaluated the opioid prescribing patterns within otolaryngology for procedures including tympanoplasty and mastoidectomy and showed there is high variability in prescribing patterns, especially when comparing prescriptions written by attending versus resident physicians, suggesting the need for standardized postoperative narcotic guidelines.[5,6] A study of opioid use also revealed that while a median number of 24 (IQR [20−45]) narcotic pills were prescribed by physicians to treat postsurgical pain following an otologic procedure, only a median number of 6 (IQR [2−15]) were actually consumed by patients.[7] This study highlighted another challenge in opioid prescribing—not only are opioids commonly overprescribed, this overprescription leads to leftover opioids that may not be disposed of properly, leading to a risk of misuse. Indeed, over 80% of respondents in this study had leftover opioids following surgery, with the majority keeping the excess instead of disposing it using designated medication boxes.[7]

It is clear that the variability in otologic surgery mandates tailored approaches to pain. As the emphasis on reducing opioid prescriptions grows, further subspecialty data will be needed to guide analgesic principles. Furthermore, with the advent of enhanced recovery after surgery (ERAS) pathways a strong understanding of pain management principles is needed. The objective of this chapter is to provide an overview of postoperative pain management in otology and neurotology with a view toward the role of multimodal analgesia and opioid-sparing approaches.

Otologic surgery

Most otologic surgeries are conducted on an outpatient basis and include both adult and pediatric patient populations. Otologic procedures are confined to the external and/or middle ear and do not intrude into major body cavities or involve extensive soft tissue work. Consequently, postoperative pain control is seldom a major issue for patients. Although the approach to pain management in this discipline is ostensibly simpler than in neurotologic surgery, where pain control must be considered in the setting of a craniotomy, specific considerations may be required for pediatric patients and for procedures performed under conscious sedation or local anesthesia alone for certain procedures. Assessment of pain control in the pediatric population is particularly challenging due to the variety of pain scales used in this population, such as the Global Mood Scale and pain visual analog scales, which may not be adequate in capturing the subjective experience of pain.

The procedural safety and pain levels associated with outpatient ear surgery have been previously evaluated: a recent retrospective review of 1368 patients undergoing outpatient otologic surgery showed that only 2.5% of patients required readmission or inpatient stay, mostly due to vertigo, pain, or dizziness.[8] Although ear surgery tends to be well tolerated, patients must be counseled preoperatively on expectations for pain management and made aware that the aim of analgesia is not to eliminate the pain but to decrease it to a manageable level. In the United States, nonopioid analgesics such as acetaminophen and nonsteroidal antiinflammatory drugs (NSAIDs) are typically used as first steps in postoperative pain control after otologic procedures and are adequate for most patients. Opioid prescriptions are commonly provided should patients find nonopioids alone to be insufficient. Qian et al.

prospectively studied opioid consumption following adult outpatient otologic surgery and discovered that their patients consumed roughly 75% of their prescribed opioids, and those with postauricular incisions used significantly more opioids than those with transcanal incisions.[9] It is important to note however, pain and analgesia have an important cultural component and in other geographical settings, opioid prescriptions are not routinely provided for otologic procedures.

A recent review of opioid stewardship in otolaryngology categorized ear surgery, including ventilation tubes, tympanoplasty, mastoidectomy, ossicular chain reconstruction, cochlear implantation, bone-anchored hearing aid implantation, and stapedectomy as typically associated with "mild pain" (Table 6.1). The study authors recommended preoperative use of 1000 mg acetaminophen and 400 mg gabapentin, intraoperative use of long-acting local anesthesia, and postoperative prescription of acetaminophen 500 mg every 6 h with the use of celecoxib 200 mg every 12 h or naproxen 500 mg every 8–12 h as needed for breakthrough pain.[10] However, for patients who had a history of chronic pain or preoperative opioid use, they also recommended a possible preoperative pain service consultation as well as continuation of previously prescribed narcotics in addition to the aforementioned regimen.[10]

Several studies have examined analgesic regimens for specific otologic surgeries. For example, adults are generally counseled to take acetaminophen and ibuprofen as needed for pain related to tympanostomy tube placement, and this procedure can be

Table 6.1 Select studies examining analgesia in otologic surgeries.

Surgery	Analgesia under study	References
Common otologic surgeries (e.g., PE tube, ossicular chain reconstruction, tympanoplasty)	Recommended 500 mg acetaminophen q6h with celecoxib 200 mg q12h or naproxen 500 mg q8-12h for breakthrough pain postoperatively	Cramer et al.[10]
Myringotomy with bilateral PE tube placement	Preoperative ketorolac, but not acetaminophen, provided postoperative pain control in children	Watcha et al.[11]
Myringotomy with bilateral PE tube placement	Preoperative ketorolac was associated with decreased pain scores postoperatively, but imparted no clinically meaningful difference on discharge analgesic requirements	Bean-Lijewski et al.[12]
Myringotomy with bilateral PE tube placement	No difference in analgesic requirements was discovered in patients receiving preoperative analgesia versus placebo	McHale et al.[14]
Children undergoing tympanomastoidectomy surgery	Great auricular nerve block may reduce postoperative opioid requirements	Suresh et al.[18]

performed under local analgesia, although in pediatric patients, general analgesia is used. Watcha et al. reported that administering oral ketorolac preoperatively provided superior postoperative pain control relative to acetaminophen in children undergoing bilateral tympanostomy tube placement and myringotomy.[11] However, Bean-Lijewski et al. found that although the use of preoperative ketorolac was associated with decreased pain scores at five and 10 min postoperatively, there was no difference in discharge analgesic requirements, therefore bringing into question whether ketorolac use results in a clinically meaningful difference in pain control.[12] The transient improvement in postoperative pain must be balanced with the risks of ketorolac, especially since in the pediatric population, tympanostomy tube placement may be performed in conjunction with adenotonsillectomy, where persistent concerns exist regarding the association between ketorolac and postoperative hemorrhage.[13] A more recent double-blinded randomized controlled trial studied the use of preoperative analgesia versus placebo in patients undergoing bilateral myringotomy with tympanostomy tube placement. The study discovered no statistically significant difference in median pain scores at 90 min or need for additional analgesia, suggesting that preoperative analgesia in this population should not be routinely administered.[14] Alternatives to acetaminophen for preoperative analgesia include administration of topical 2% lidocaine ear drops, which have been shown to provide comparative analgesia postoperatively.[15] Other options include blockade of the auricular branch of the vagus nerve, which provides sensory innervation to the external auditory canal and tympanic membrane, using local bupivacaine.[16]

The pain associated with mastoid surgery is also typically categorized as mild. A recent systematic review of pain management in otology reported five randomized controlled trials studying perioperative pain management for tympanomastoid surgery.[17] Two of these studies reported the effect of block of the great auricular nerve in children, with one study finding a benefit to intraoperative blockade of the nerve 1 h before the end of the surgery with reductions in postoperative opioid requirements, while another study found no benefit.[17,18] A separate study examined the combination of bupivacaine and 100 µg fentanyl compared to bupivacaine and 50 µg fentanyl for local analgesia and found that the higher fentanyl dosing led to lower pain scores for patients undergoing modified radical mastoidectomy.[19] Lastly, a randomized controlled trial examined three interventions (acetaminophen, acetaminophen plus codeine, and ibuprofen plus midazolam) and their effect on pain control in pediatric patients undergoing tympanocentesis.[20] Results showed that children treated with acetaminophen alone had the highest peak heart rates and pain scores suggesting that acetaminophen alone may not be effective in reducing pain.[20]

Similarly, the pain associated with cochlear implantation is typically mild and lasts for less than 1 week. Persistent pain following cochlear implantation is rare, and previous studies have found this affects only 1%–3% of patients.[21,22] Mahairas et al. studied opioid prescribing patterns and usage following cochlear implant surgery and reported that hydrocodone 5 mg was the most frequently prescribed opioid, with opioids prescribed for on average 5.5 days. Furthermore, they noted that each additional tablet of hydrocodone or oxycodone beyond 8 and 5 tablets per day, respectively, increased the likelihood of becoming a recurrent user of opioids by 15% and 22.5%. They concluded that limiting the total amount of opioids prescribed per day to no more than 40 morphine milligrams equivalents may be effective in decreasing the number of recurrent opioid users postoperatively.[23]

Neurotology

Neurotologic, or lateral skull base surgeries, can cause significant postoperative pain due to the need for a craniotomy and more extensive tissue manipulation. Contrary to popular belief, pain after craniotomy can be severe in up to 90% of patients within days of surgery, with as many as 30% developing a chronic headache.[24] Pain control in these patients can be particularly challenging due to the need for reliable neurologic examinations in the postoperative period to ensure patient safety.[25] These competing demands may lead to the undertreatment of postoperative pain following intracranial surgery.[26]

Multiple approaches are used to access the cerebellopontine angle for acoustic neuroma surgery, including the retrosigmoid, translabyrinthine, and middle cranial fossa approaches. Several sources of pain following craniotomy have been described and include neck pain due to patient positioning, scalp pain, and postoperative pain due to dural irritation.[27] The diversity of approaches to the skull base warrants individualized management of pain for patients undergoing these surgeries. For example, retrosigmoid craniotomies may be associated with a higher incidence of postoperative nausea, vomiting, and headache due to manipulation of the occipital nerve extracranially, and the cerebellum and brainstem intracranially.[28,29]

A variety of approaches to pain control have been proposed for postoperative pain after intracranial surgery (Table 6.2). Patient-controlled analgesia (PCA) has

Table 6.2 Selected studies examining analgesia in neurotologic surgery.

Surgery	Analgesia under study	References
Craniotomy/ Skull base surgery	Reported use of a PCA dosing protocol of 1.5 mg morphine/dose with an 8-min lockout period such that the total dose of morphine over 4 h does not exceed 40 mg	Jellish et al.[29]
Craniotomy	Premedication with acetaminophen or gabapentin may decrease analgesic consumption after surgery	Ture et al.[30]
Craniotomy	Scalp infiltration with local anesthetic reduces the hemodynamic response to placement of surgical pins and head fixation devices	Geze et al.[31]
Craniotomy	Intraoperative dexmedetomidine may reduce postoperative opioid consumption	Peng et al.[32]

been found to improve pain and lead to lower opioid use. Jellish et al. reported a dosing protocol of 1.5 mg morphine/dose with an 8-min lockout period such that the total dose of morphine over 4 h does not exceed 40 mg following skull base surgery.[29] Nausea and vomiting should also be managed vigilantly as they can lead to increased intracranial pressures and other complications. Ondansetron may be used in combination with patient-controlled morphine for postoperative pain and emesis. However, studies have shown that patient control of ondansetron administration in addition to patient-controlled morphine increased the cost of the PCA almost tenfold with no statistically significant difference in nausea or vomiting for patients undergoing infratentorial skull base resections.[29]

PCA should be used in combination with perioperative multimodal analgesia for pain in neurotologic surgery. Preoperatively, patients may receive acetaminophen or gabapentin, which has been shown to decrease analgesic consumption after surgery but is also associated with delays in extubation and increased sedation.[30] Intraoperatively, remifentanil may be used; however, it may lead to amplification of postoperative pain, opioid tolerance, and opioid-induced hyperalgesia, though these effects may be mitigated by limiting its dosing.[24] Local analgesia in the form of infiltration of the scalp with local anesthetic and epinephrine is used to not only control pain but to also induce local vasoconstriction, increasing the effects of the analgesia and reducing local bleeding. Studies have shown that scalp infiltration also reduces the hemodynamic response to placement of surgical pins and head fixation devices during neurosurgery.[31] Other therapies, including dexmedetomidine, ketamine, and corticosteroids may be administered perioperatively. Dexmedetomidine has been shown to have an opioid-sparing effect and may also mitigate postcraniotomy pain, nausea, and vomiting.[24,32]

While some studies have shown that the use of NSAIDs such as ketorolac is not associated with increased postoperative bleeding risk, in practice, the potentially catastrophic consequences of intracranial bleeding render NSAIDs seldom used in practice.[24,33] At our institution, patients who have undergone an open intracranial procedure are provided with a regimen of acetaminophen and opioid narcotic in the immediate postoperative period and on discharge, with instruction to supplement with over-the-counter NSAIDs (e.g., ibuprofen) starting 7 days postoperatively. For patients who underwent smaller craniotomies (e.g., middle fossa approach for superior canal dehiscence repair) that may require less-intensive postoperative neurologic monitoring, a PCA pump is used which can be transitioned to a precise oral dose based on recorded usage.

Approaches to reduce opioid prescription

Aside from an improved understanding of the uses of nonopioid analgesia, system-level initiatives should also be considered in the effort to reduce opioid prescription. Firstly, preoperative discussions about pain control and patient expectations should be routine. A shared decision-making model may be used during this stage so patients can be more active in their pain control choices. These discussions may enhance patient education, and oftentimes patients may decline a prescription following this discussion. One study showed that after undergoing preoperative pain control education 2 weeks before surgery, 90% of patients declined hydrocodone prescriptions and chose nonopioid alternatives.[34]

Furthermore, ERAS pathways may combine opioid and nonopioid medications for use postoperatively. Thuener et al. studied a perioperative pain management protocol and discovered a reduction in the number of oxycodone prescriptions (83%–26%) and number of pills per prescription (35–25) following implementation of a protocol for patients undergoing otolaryngologic surgery.[35] A high satisfaction with pain management was reported by 90% of patients, highlighting that comprehensive pain management protocols can reduce the amount and potency of opioids prescribed following head and neck surgery.[35] The study authors emphasized the importance of educating all team members involved in patient care to ensure adherence to protocols; however, in their study, 93% of discharge pain prescriptions were written by a resident or nurse practitioner.[35] Other ERAS pathways for free tissue transfer in otolaryngology have been published and emphasize the use of multimodal analgesia, opioid-sparing approaches, and use of NSAIDs and selective cyclo-oxygenase inhibitors.[36] ERAS protocols have been shown to lead to high levels of patient satisfaction with pain control and less opioid consumption, and Cramer et al. published a framework based on ERAS protocols for perioperative pain management in head and neck surgery.[10] They emphasized preoperative patient education and risk stratification for warning signs of chronic pain or opioid use disorder and preoperative use of acetaminophen, celecoxib, and gabapentin. Intraoperatively they recommended the use of a long-acting local anesthetic before incision. Postoperatively, they proposed the use of acetaminophen and celecoxib/NSAIDs, as well as gabapentin or tramadol in the event of more severe pain. Upon discharge, if opioids are required, they proposed using institutional guidelines for the quantity and duration of the dose, monitoring for signs of opioid misuse using prescription drug monitoring programs, and referral to pain specialists if concerned for the development of abuse.[10]

Other system-wide pain management efforts may be applied to the field of otology and neurotology. Frazee et al. studied an intervention at a regional healthcare system in which a series of pain management and opioid stewardship conferences were held along with the simultaneous implementation of ERAS protocols.[37] They also implemented a quality metric linked to surgeon compensation that rewarded surgeons for limiting postoperative discharge opioid prescriptions. These initiatives significantly reduced opioid discharge prescriptions that extended more than 5 days.[37] A different resident-led initiative at a tertiary care academic otolaryngology department standardized postoperative analgesia regimes and led to a 26% reduction in total prescriptions and morphine milligram equivalents. The study authors noted that surgical residents and interns are most frequently responsible for managing postoperative analgesia yet have the most variability in prescribing practices.[38] Taken together, these programs suggest that greater trainee education and standardization of postoperative pain protocols may be beneficial in implementing safer pain management.

Conclusion

The fields of otology and neurotology encompass a breadth of patients and procedures, which required pain management customized to each patient and procedure, but also provide opportunities for the application of opioid-sparing pain management principles. The pain associated with otologic surgery is typically mild and can be managed with acetaminophen and NSAIDs, and the use of adjunct therapies such as preoperative medication, surgical site infiltration with a local anesthetic, and nerve blocks may allow for superior pain control. Neurotologic surgery often requires a higher level of analgesia and can be managed with premedication before surgery, local anesthesia, nerve blocks, and patient-controlled analgesia. Hospital system-level initiatives such as ERAS protocols should be developed specific to the field of neurotology to allow for standardization of opioid-sparing approaches to pain management and have already been successfully implemented in other fields within otolaryngology.

References

1. Levy B, Paulozzi L, Mack KA, Jones CM. Trends in opioid analgesic—prescribing rates by specialty, U.S., 2007—2012. *Am J Prev Med.* 2015;49(3):409—413. https://doi.org/10.1016/j.amepre.2015.02.020.
2. Dang S, Duffy A, Li JC, et al. Postoperative opioid-prescribing practices in otolaryngology: a multiphasic study. *Laryngoscope.* 2020;130(3):659—665. https://doi.org/10.1002/lary.28101.
3. Gerbershagen HJ, Aduckathil S, van Wijck AJM, Peelen LM, Kalkman CJ, Meissner W. Pain intensity on the first day after surgery. *Anesthesiology.* 2013;118(4):934—944. https://doi.org/10.1097/aln.0b013e31828866b3.
4. Mohan S, Bhattacharyya N. Opioids and the otolaryngologist: an ambulatory assessment. *Otolaryngol Head Neck Surg.* 2018;159(1):29—34. https://doi.org/10.1177/0194599818765125.
5. Murphey AW, Munawar S, Nguyen SA, Meyer TA, O'Rourke AK. Opioid prescribing patterns within otolaryngology. *World J Otorhinolaryngol Head Neck Surg.* 2019;5(2):112—116. https://doi.org/10.1016/j.wjorl.2019.03.004.
6. Klimczak J, Badhey A, Wong A, Colley P, Teng M. Pain management and prescribing practices in otolaryngology residency programs. *Am J Otolaryngol Head Neck Med Surg.* 2020;41(1):102265. https://doi.org/10.1016/j.amjoto.2019.07.009.
7. Pruitt LCC, Casazza GC, Newberry CI, et al. Opioid prescribing and use in ambulatory otolaryngology. *Laryngoscope.* 2020;130(8):1913—1921. https://doi.org/10.1002/lary.28359.
8. Bonnafous S, Hermann R, Zaouche S, Tringali S, Fieux M. Evolution and safety of day-case major ear surgery. *Eur Ann Otorhinolaryngol Head Neck Dis.* 2020. (xxxx). https://doi.org/10.1016/j.anorl.2020.09.006.

9. Qian ZJ, Alyono JC, Woods OD, Ali N, Blevins NH. A prospective evaluation of post-operative opioid use in otologic surgery. *Otol Neurotol.* 2019;40(9):1194−1198. https://doi.org/10.1097/MAO.0000000000002364.

10. Cramer JD, Wisler B, Gouveia CJ. Opioid stewardship in otolaryngology: state of the art review. *Otolaryngol Head Neck Surg.* 2018;158(5):817−827. https://doi.org/10.1177/0194599818757999.

11. Watcha MF, Ramirez-Ruiz M, White PF, Jones MB, Lagueruela RG, Terkonda RP. Perioperative effects of oral ketorolac and acetaminophen in children undergoing bilateral myringotomy. *Can J Anaesth.* 1992;39(7):649−654. https://doi.org/10.1007/BF03008224.

12. Bean-Lijewski JD, Stinson JC. Acetaminophen or ketorolac for post myringotomy pain in children? A prospective, double-blinded comparison. *Paediatr Anaesth.* 1997;7(2):131−137. https://doi.org/10.1046/j.1460-9592.1997.d01-47.x.

13. Monfort R, Hill R, Sipp J. Perioperative ketorolac analgesia for patients undergoing adenoidectomy: a retrospective analysis. *Int J Pediatr Otorhinolaryngol.* 2021;140(January 2014):110522. https://doi.org/10.1016/j.ijporl.2020.110522.

14. McHale B, Badenhorst CD, Low C, Blundell D. Do children undergoing bilateral myringotomy with placement of ventilating tubes benefit from pre-operative analgesia? A double-blinded, randomised, placebo-controlled trial. *J Laryngol Otol.* 2018;132(8):685−692. https://doi.org/10.1017/S0022215118001111.

15. Bhananker SM, Azavedo L, MacCormick J, Splinter W. Topical lidocaine and oral acetaminophen provide similar analgesia for myringotomy and tube placement in children. *Can J Anaesth.* 2006;53(11):1111−1116. https://doi.org/10.1007/BF03022879.

16. Voronov P, Tobin MJ, Billings K, Coté CJ, Iyer A, Suresh S. Postoperative pain relief in infants undergoing myringotomy and tube placement: comparison of a novel regional anesthetic block to intranasal fentanyl - a pilot analysis. *Paediatr Anaesth.* 2008;18(12):1196−1201. https://doi.org/10.1111/j.1460-9592.2008.02789.x.

17. Campbell HT, Yuhan BT, Smith B, et al. Perioperative analgesia for patients undergoing otologic surgery: an evidence-based review. *Laryngoscope.* 2020;130(1):190−199. https://doi.org/10.1002/lary.27872.

18. Suresh S, Barcelona SL, Young NM, Seligman I, Heffner CL, Coté CJ. Postoperative pain relief in children undergoing tympanomastoid surgery: is a regional block better than opioids? *Anesth Analg.* 2002;94(4):859−862. https://doi.org/10.1097/00000539-200204000-00015.

19. Bhandari G, Shahi K, Parmar N, Asad M, Joshi H, Bhakuni R. Evaluation of analgesic effect of two different doses of fentanyl in combination with bupivacaine for surgical site infiltration in cases of modified radical mastoidectomy: a double blind randomized study. *Anesth Essays Res.* 2013;7(2):243. https://doi.org/10.4103/0259-1162.118979.

20. Shaikh N, Hoberman A, Kurs-Lasky M, et al. Pain management in young children undergoing diagnostic tympanocentesis. *Clin Pediatr.* 2011;50(3):231−236. https://doi.org/10.1177/0009922810385677.

21. Noblitt B, Alfonso KP, Adkins M, Bush ML. Barriers to rehabilitation care in pediatric cochlear implant recipients. *Otol Neurotol.* 2018;39(5):e307−e313. https://doi.org/10.1097/MAO.0000000000001777.

22. Celerier C, Rouillon I, Blanchard M, Parodi M, Denoyelle F, Loundon N. Pain after cochlear implantation: an unusual complication? *Otol Neurotol.* 2017;38(7):956−961. https://doi.org/10.1097/MAO.0000000000001451.

23. Mahairas AD, Neff R, Craker N, McNulty BN, Shinn JB, Bush ML. Opioid prescribing patterns and usage following cochlear implantation. *Otol Neurotol.* 2020;41(7): 922–928. https://doi.org/10.1097/MAO.0000000000002674.

24. Vacas S, Van de Wiele B. Designing a pain management protocol for craniotomy: a narrative review and consideration of promising practices. *Surg Neurol Int.* 2017;8(1): 291. https://doi.org/10.4103/sni.sni_301_17.

25. Vadivelu N, Kai AM, Tran D, Kodumudi G, Legler A, Ayrian E. Options for perioperative pain management in neurosurgery. *J Pain Res.* 2016;9:37–47. https://doi.org/10.2147/JPR.S85782.

26. Nemergut EC, Durieux ME, Missaghi NB, Himmelseher S. Pain management after craniotomy. *Best Pract Res Clin Anaesthesiol.* 2007;21(4):557–573. https://doi.org/10.1016/j.bpa.2007.06.005.

27. Chowdhury T, Garg R, Sheshadri V, et al. Perioperative factors contributing the postcraniotomy pain: a synthesis of concepts. *Front Med.* 2017;4(MAR):1–5. https://doi.org/10.3389/fmed.2017.00023.

28. Levo H, Pyykkö I, Blomstedt G. Postoperative headache after surgery for vestibular schwannoma. *Ann Otol Rhinol Laryngol.* 2000;109(9):853–858. https://doi.org/10.1177/000348940010900913.

29. Jellish WS, Murdoch J, Leonetti JP. Perioperative management of complex skull base surgery: the anesthesiologist's point of view. *Neurosurg Focus.* 2002;12(5):1–7. https://doi.org/10.3171/foc.2002.12.5.6.

30. Türe H, Sayin M, Karlikaya G, Bingol CA, Aykac B, Türe U. The analgesic effect of gabapentin as a prophylactic anticonvulsant drug on postcraniotomy pain: a prospective randomized study. *Anesth Analg.* 2009;109(5):1625–1631. https://doi.org/10.1213/ane.0b013e3181b0f18b.

31. Geze S, Yilmaz AA, Tuzuner F. The effect of scalp block and local infiltration on the haemodynamic and stress response to skull-pin placement for craniotomy. *Eur J Anaesthesiol.* 2009;26(4):298–303. https://doi.org/10.1097/EJA.0b013e32831aedb2.

32. Peng K, Jin XH, Liu SL, Ji FH. Effect of intraoperative dexmedetomidine on postcraniotomy pain. *Clin Therapeut.* 2015;37(5):1114–1121.e1. https://doi.org/10.1016/j.clinthera.2015.02.011.

33. Magni G, La Rosa I, Melillo G, Abeni D, Hernandez H, Rosa G. Intracranial hemorrhage requiring surgery in neurosurgical patients given ketorolac: a case-control study within a cohort (2001-2010). *Anesth Analg.* 2013;116(2):443–447. https://doi.org/10.1213/ANE.0b013e3182746eda.

34. Sugai DY, Deptula PL, Parsa AA, Don Parsa F. The importance of communication in the management of postoperative pain. *Hawaii J Med Public Health.* 2013;72(6):180–184.

35. Thuener JE, Clancy K, Scher M, et al. Impact of perioperative pain management protocol on opioid prescribing patterns. *Laryngoscope.* 2020;130(5):1180–1185. https://doi.org/10.1002/lary.28133.

36. Dort JC, Farwell DG, Findlay M, et al. Optimal perioperative care in major head and neck cancer surgery with free flap reconstruction: a consensus review and recommendations from the enhanced recovery after surgery society. *JAMA Otolaryngol Head Neck Surg.* 2017;143(3):292–303. https://doi.org/10.1001/jamaoto.2016.2981.

37. Frazee R, Garmon E, Isbell C, Bird E, Papaconstantinou H. Postoperative opioid prescription reduction strategy in a regional healthcare system. *J Am Coll Surg.* 2020; 230(4):631–635. https://doi.org/10.1016/j.jamcollsurg.2019.12.023.

38. Meyer C, Winters J, Brady RG, Riddick JB, Folsom C, Jardine D. Postoperative analgesia protocol: a resident-led effort to standardize opioid prescribing patterns. *Laryngoscope.* 2020. https://doi.org/10.1002/lary.29087.

Pain management in head and neck cancer

Cymon Kersch, MD, PhD [1], Ryan Li, MD [2], Ravi A. Chandra, MD, PhD [3]

[1]*Providence Portland Medical Center, Department of Internal Medicine, Medical Education, Portland, OR, United States;* [2]*Oregon Health & Science University, Department of Otolaryngology-Head and Neck Surgery, Portland, OR, United States;* [3]*Oregon Health & Science University, Department of Radiation Medicine, Portland, OR, United States*

List of abbreviations

AAO/HNSF	American Academy of Otolaryngology-Head and Neck Surgery Foundation
APCD	advanced pneumatic compression devices
CI	confidence interval
CNS	central nervous system
COX	cyclooxygenase
ERAS	enhanced recovery after surgery
FDA	Food and Drug Administration
GFR	glomerular filtration rate
HNC	head and neck cancers
IM	intramuscular
IV	intravenous
MME	morphine milligram equivalents
NCCN	National Comprehensive Cancer Network
NSAIDs	nonsteroidal antiinflammatory drugs
OM	oral mucositis
OUD	opioid use disorder
PCA	patient controlled analgesia
PNS	peripheral nervous system
PO	per os (by mouth)
POD	postoperative day
QOL	quality of life
RCT	randomized clinical trial
SC	subcutaneous
SCC	squamous cell carcinoma
SEER	surveillance, epidemiology, and end results
SNRI	serotonin-norepinephrine reuptake inhibitors
TCA	tricyclic antidepressant
VA	veterans affairs
WHO	World Health Organization

Opioid Use, Overuse, and Abuse in Otolaryngology. https://doi.org/10.1016/B978-0-323-79016-1.00011-8

Introduction: head and neck cancer-associated morbidity and pain

Head and neck cancers (HNCs) account for ~5% of cancers globally (excluding nonmelanoma skin cancers) and are associated with significant morbidity including pain.[1] HNCs primarily include malignancies of the oral cavity, oropharynx, nasopharynx, sinonasal cavities, hypopharynx, larynx, skin, and salivary glands. Prognoses for this group of cancers have only modestly improved with advances in surgical techniques, therapeutic radiation methodology, and novel targeted and immune-modulating systemic agents. There is a rise in HNC incidence rates from 2000 to 2018 according to the surveillance, epidemiology, and end results database with increased survivorship in large part related to the rising incidence of HPV-associated oropharyngeal cancers.[2] The improved survivorship necessitates concomitant progress in managing the negative sequelae of these malignancies and their treatments, such as pain syndromes commonly associated with HNC. Acute pain syndromes are experienced by up to 80% of patients with HNC, with chronic pain in up to 60% of cases.[3,4]

HNC and its treatments negatively impact patient quality of life (QOL) by causing pain, difficulties with swallowing, eating, phonation, and speech, and worsening psychosocial health that can manifest as depression, anxiety, and suicidal ideation. Importantly, these HNC-related morbidities do not exist in isolation, but intimately influence one another. Thus, understanding and alleviating pain has the capacity to improve not only the physical discomfort, but multiple aspects of QOL. For instance, greater pain is associated with an increased risk of suicide in advanced cancers.[5,6] Survivors of HNC compared to all other cancers combined were twice as likely to die from suicide, and the incidence of suicide in patients with HNC is worsening with an increase of 27% during the period from 2010 to 2014 compared to 2000–04.[5] Benefits of pain control extend beyond improving other elements of patient QOL and are also associated with improved surgical outcomes and reduced overall healthcare system burden.[7]

Pain control methods in HNC include multimodal therapeutic approaches involving opioid and nonopioid analgesics for a variety of malignancy and treatment-associated pain syndromes. Guidelines for optimal pain control in HNC are shifting with increasing knowledge of the efficacy and risks of analgesic interventions. The World Health Organization's (WHO) three-tiered cancer pain treatment ladder, beginning with nonopioid analgesics for less severe pain and increasing to stronger opioids for more severe and refractory pain, has been a widely used general guideline for treatment escalation (Fig. 7.1). Recent guideline updates from both national and international groups support the use of multimodal pain control regimens that expand treatment options and emphasize opioid stewardship. Collectively, these guidelines highlight that high-quality pain management should be an integral part of cancer care, with pain management screening at each patient contact, and a personalized plan for each individual with strong consideration of the

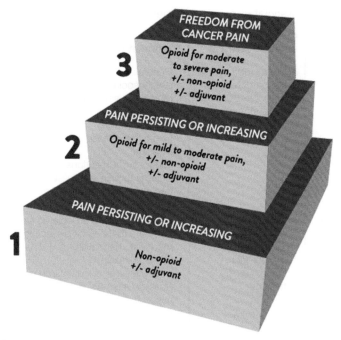

FIGURE 7.1

The WHO's three-step analgesic ladder for treatment of cancer pain.

Reprinted with permission from World Health Organization. WHO Guidelines for the pharmacological and radiotherapeutic management of cancer pain in adults and adolescents. In. Geneva, *2018*.

risks associated with specific interventions in each case. Overall guiding principles of cancer pain management recommend that when possible treatment be given by mouth, on a scheduled basis, with upfront patient education regarding a plan. Herein, we review opioid and nonopioid analgesic therapies for HNC-associated pain.

HNC-associated pain syndromes and neurobiological mechanisms

HNC-associated pain is often heterogenous in its neurobiological mechanisms, with a mixed etiologies due to the disease itself as well as treatment side-effects. Within this complex pain picture, common pain syndromes have been described that are associated with specific disease statuses and/or anticancer treatment sequelae (Table 7.1). These syndromes include acute and chronic pain from head and neck surgery, neuropathic pain, postradiation pain, myofascial pain, mucositis, dermatitis, symptomatic lymphedema, and skeletal pain, among others. The neurobiological etiology of the pain experienced in these syndromes should be addressed by

Table 7.1 HNC-associated pain syndromes.

Pain syndrome	Relation to disease and/or treatment	Treatment options overview
Surgery-associated acute and chronic pain[a]	Acute disruption of local soft tissue and/or nerves and chronic fibrosis, structural tissue changes, irreversible nerve injury	• General: nonopioid analgesics and psychosocial and behavioral support • Moderate—severe pain: add opioids • Physical therapy for stretching and improving range of motion • Myofascial release and/or soft tissue massage • Trigger point injections • Referral to pain specialist, physical therapy, integrative services, and/or physical medicine and rehabilitation
Postradiation pain[a]	Acute dermatologic and/or mucosal disruption and nerve injury, chronic scarring, fibrosis, or adhesions	• Treat the specific associated pain syndrome (if related to the neck dissection, neuropathic, mucositis, dermatitis, etc.) • Physical therapy • Possible surgical lysis of adhesions if extreme • Possible referrals, as above in surgery-associated pain.
Neuropathic pain[a]	Damage from invasive diagnostic (biopsy) or treatment procedures/radiation, local tumor invasion. Distinguished from nociceptive pain from end-organ pain stimuli	• Nonopioid analgesics including SNRIs, gabapentinoids, TCAs • CBT and psychosocial support • Local therapies including topical pharmacologic patches, compound creams and gels (ex: lidoderm, capsaicin, lidocaine, and diclofenac) and nonpharmacologic heat, ice, acupuncture, and nerve stimulation • Moderate—severe pain: opioids or dual-action opioid compounds
Myofascial pain	Severely sensitive muscle injury due to tumor or treatments	• Nonpharmacologic: physical therapy, range of motion exercises, soft tissue/myofascial release massage, ultrasonic stimulation, and/or acupuncture. • Pharmacologic: topic ointments (ketamine), patches (lidocaine), acetaminophen, NSAIDs, COX-2 inhibitors, anticonvulsant drugs, SNRIs, muscle relaxants
Mucositis[a]	Acute effect of radiation and/or chemotherapy	• Topical mouthwashes of single or multiple agents including opioids, antiinflammatory agents, growth factors or cytokines, local anesthetics (lidocaine), antihistamines with anticholinergic properties (diphenhydramine), anticonvulsants and antidepressants, antimicrobials (including antifungals), mucosal coating agents (including sucralfate), saline • Cryotherapy, laser or light therapy • Oral hygiene

Table 7.1 HNC-associated pain syndromes.—*cont'd*

Pain syndrome	Relation to disease and/or treatment	Treatment options overview
Dermatitis[a]	Acute effect of radiation and/or chemotherapy	• Hygiene practices: washing with mild soap and lukewarm water • Dressings: silver sulfadiazine, gentle moisturizers, topical corticosteroids, doxepin, • Photobiomodulation (laser therapy)
Symptomatic lymphedema[a]	Damage to lymphatics due to tumor or invasive treatments	• Patient education • Referral to certified lymphedema therapist, if available • Compression garments • Manual lymphatic drainage
Skeletal pain	Acute pain of local tumor destruction or treatment-induced osteonecrosis	• Referral to oral surgeon • Anticonvulsants or SNRIs • Opioids

[a] *Treatment is further discussed in Section "Management updates for common HNC-associated pain situations and syndromes".*
Adapted from the NCCN Survivorship Guidelines.

analgesic treatment paradigms when possible. Ideally, optimal pain control strategies are individualized to target the characteristics of each patient's pain patterns.

Further distinction of the acute or chronic nature of the pain can help establish the pain syndrome and influence treatment choice. Two time points wherein acute pain is common include malignancy-induced pain seen at initial patient presentation and in the course of treatment including surgery, chemotherapy, and/or radiotherapy. Treatments can cause disruption of tissue in and around the tumor bed, with localized inflammation and edema causing nerve compression, mucositis, and dermatitis. Chronic HNC-associated pain can be defined as pain lasting longer than 3—6 months or that extends beyond the period of "normal" healing time. In HNC this is often ongoing pain directly related to persistent malignancy or longer-term sequelae of the anticancer therapies but frequently has unclear and mixed etiologies. Multiple studies in the late 1990s and early 2000s assessed the prevalence of chronic pain in cancer patients and within the subpopulation of patients with HNCs. A meta-analysis of 52 studies spanning clinical data over 40 years found that 33% of cancer patients continued to experience pain after curative treatment and that patients with HNC had the highest prevalence of pain in a subgroup analysis of pooled data including all disease severities and treatment outcomes (70% in HNC with vs. 50% in all cancer types).[9] Similarly, a prospective study evaluating the longitudinal prevalence of pain in patients with HNC found that 26% of patients in their cohort ($n = 93$) continued to experience pain 24 months after completing curative treatment.[10] However, this study found that the prevalence of "severe" pain decreased posttreatment, with 8% of patient reporting severe pain at their first encounter and 4% at 24 months posttreatment. Recently, an analysis of 296 5-year HNC survivors in France revealed that nearly two-thirds of patients continued to experience pain up to 5 years after treatment.[4] Multivariate analysis of this dataset identified decreased levels of physical activity, oropharyngeal original primary tumor site, and a lower level of education as significant risk factors for chronic pain. Importantly, in patients with HNC who have received curative treatment, it is essential to evaluate for possible cancer progression or recurrence if new pain arises or chronic pain worsens. It is also important to acknowledge many HNC patients have comorbid conditions that can contribute to chronic pain.

Mechanistically, HNC-associated pain is classified into nociceptive and neuropathic pain (Table 7.2).[11-16]

Nociceptive pain is caused by the activation of normal nerve endings of C and Aδ fibers, often from noxious stimuli and damage to nonneuronal tissue.[15] In HNC, nociceptive pain can be caused by the destruction of local tissue by the tumor itself, invasive diagnostic and therapeutic interventions including surgery, or by effects of radiation and chemotherapy such as mucositis, dermatitis, and local injury in the tumor treatment field.[12,15,16] Nociceptive pain is subcategorized as somatic and visceral based on location and quality. Somatic pain is perceived as well-localized often sharp and/or stabbing pain, while visceral pain, mediated by the sympathetic nervous system, is more diffuse, can be referred from another area, and has a dull or achy quality. Treatments helpful in nociceptive pain include agents that inhibit inflammatory signaling and central and peripheral neurotransmission pathways.

Neuropathic pain is caused by damage to the nerve itself resulting in increased, abnormal activation patterns.[15] Frequently, this is perceived as a burning and/or

Table 7.2 Cancer pain neurobiological mechanisms.

	Type	Neural mechanism	HNC example
Nociceptive	Visceral	Stimulation of pain receptors on normal sensory nerve endings	Lung metastases
	Somatic		Mucosal tumors; bone invasion
Neuropathic	Nerve compression	Stimulation of *nervi nervorum*	Mass effect on cranial nerves of spinal rootlets
	Nerve injury	1. Lowered firing threshold in PNS sensory nerves 2. Injury to the CNS 3. Mixed PNS + CNS injury	Tumor invasion of cranial nerves or the skull base
	Sympathetically maintained	Sympathetic nervous system dysfunction	First-bite syndrome and parapharyngeal surgery

CNS, *central nervous system;* PNS, *peripheral nervous system.*
Modified from World Health Organization. WHO Guidelines for the Pharmacological and Radiotherapeutic Management of Cancer Pain in Adults and Adolescents. In. Geneva, 2018; Blasco MA, Cordero J, Dundar Y. Chronic pain management in head and neck Oncology. Otolaryngol Clin. 2020; 53:865–875; Epstein JB, Wilkie DJ, Fischer DJ, Kim YO, Villines D. Neuropathic and nociceptive pain in head and neck cancer patients receiving radiation therapy. Head Neck Oncol. 2009;1:26.

tingling sensation. In HNC, neuropathic pain can be caused by tumor invasion or compression of nerves in either or both the peripheral nervous system or central nervous system (CNS).[15,16] Analgesics that can be utilized in neuropathic pain include more centrally acting neuromodulating therapeutics that are historically utilized in the treatment of general neurologic and psychiatric disorders.

Despite these distinctive neurologic causes of pain, the experience of pain in HNC is complex. Potter and colleagues found that in HNC patients who had pain present at the time of diagnosis, 93% had mixed nociceptive and neuropathic pain.[17] Additionally, the intricate anatomy of the head and neck and the invasive patterns of primary cancers in this region contribute to the variability of pain across different types of HNCs. For instance, it has been proposed that the higher density of nerve endings in the oral cavity coupled with the higher propensity of oral cavity cancer to invade bone contribute to higher reported pain in oral cavity cancers compared to those within the larynx and pharynx, in some studies.[10,11,18] Moreover, in their most recent update, the International Association for the Study of Pain now defines pain as "an unpleasant sensory and emotional experience associated with, or resembling that associated with, actual or potential tissue damage," incorporating the psychological aspects of pain.[19]

Treatment overview for HNC-associated pain
Overview of analgesics and pain management in HNC

Given the heterogeneity of HNC-associated pain, multiple pain modifying pharmacologic and nonpharmacologic strategies exist. Analgesics refer to any intervention that modifies pain. Analgesics can be categorized into opioid, nonopioid, and other treatments (Table 7.3).

Opioids include a range of naturally occurring, semisynthetic, and synthetic compounds that modulate opioid receptors in the CNS and peripheral tissues through a variety of mechanisms. Opioids are available with different strengths, routes of administration, and length of their analgesic effects that can be tailored to the pain level and lifestyle of each patient. The potencies of different opioids and routes of administration can be approximated relative to morphine utilizing established and widely available conversion tables.

Nonopioid analgesics include pharmacologic and nonpharmacologic techniques with varying mechanisms of actions, many of which are being actively studied for their role in cancer pain modulation (Table 7.4). Annex six in the WHO Cancer Pain Guidelines provides detailed resources for drug profiles and important prescribing information of many of these medications including acetylsalicylic acid, codeine, fentanyl, hydromorphone, ibuprofen, methadone, morphine, naloxone, oxycodone, paracetamol.[8] Nonpharmacologic analgesic treatments include physical therapy, compression devices, nerve stimulation, acupuncture, and mind—body techniques.

Table 7.3 Analgesics used in HNC-associated pain.

Analgesic category	Example agents/techniques
Common opioid pharmacologic agents	• Codeine • Oxycodone • Methadone • Hydromorphone • Morphine • Fentanyl
Nonopioid pharmacologic agents	• Acetaminophen/paracetamol • NSAIDs (including COX-1 and COX-2 inhibitors) • Anticonvulsants (including gabapentinoids) • Antidepressants (including TCAs, SNRIs) • Steroids

Nonpharmacologic pain-modifying interventions	• Neurolysis, nerve blocks
	• Nerve stimulation
	• Physical therapy
	• Therapeutic compression
	• Integrative therapies
	  o Vitamin, supplements
	  o Chiropractic manipulation
	  o Acupuncture
	  o Mind—body techniques (yoga, meditation)

COX, *cyclooxygenase;* NSAIDs, *nonsteroidal antiinflammatory drugs;* SNRI, *serotonin-norepinephrine reuptake inhibitors;* TCA, *tricyclic antidepressant.*

    Treatment of HNC-associated pain is a multistep process. First, a thorough assessment of the pain's location and severity, its impact on QOL, and patient's goals of care is done. Multiple tools exist for the initial evaluation including the Brief Pain Inventory form, Pain Observation Tool, Comprehensive Pain Assessment, Pain Assessment with Advanced Dementia, and Integrated Palliative Care Outcome Scales.[8,20] Pain-related health consequences should also be assessed including depression, anxiety, and suicidal ideation. If these are identified they should be treated expeditiously as part of the overall cancer care plan.

Table 7.4 Nonopioid analgesics often utilized for HNC-associated pain.

Class	Example medications
Acetaminophen	Acetaminophen, Paracetamol
NSAIDS	Ibuprofen, ketorolac, celecoxib, acetylsalicylic acid
Steroids	Dexamethasone, methylprednisolone, prednisolone
Antidepressants	Amitriptyline, venlafaxine
Anticonvulsants	Carbamazepine, gabapentin, Pregabalin

In the pain management plan, treatment should then be selected based on the results of pain evaluation in the context of the individual's goals of care, medical comorbidities, lifestyle, and personal beliefs. HNC-associated safety risks should be considered. Direct tumor and treatment effects on the upper airway make some analgesic side effects such as nausea, vomiting, and respiratory depression uniquely dangerous.[21] Additional considerations include an increased risk of opioid dependence in this population and growing evidence of the superior therapeutic efficacy of multimodal opioid-free analgesic treatments, as described in the following subsections.[21-24] Collectively, recent society guidelines support the use of opioid-sparing regimens, often with acetaminophen or nonsteroidal antiinflammatory drugs (NSAIDs), for mild-to-moderate pain, addition of longer-acting opioids when pain is severe and/or insufficiently controlled with other multimodal techniques, and rapid-acting analgesics available for breakthrough pain.[8,11] Some nonopioid analgesics such as NSAIDs continue to be used cautiously in perioperative settings because of their perceived bleeding risk, although data on actual bleeding risk are conflicted.[21] Again whenever possible, medications should be given enterally on a scheduled basis.

Ideally pain management includes both psychosocial care and pharmacologic treatments. It is important to recognize that the experience of pain is multifactorial and includes both neurological physiology described above and psychological, social, cultural, and spiritual contexts.

Special considerations for opioid use in HNC

Opioids are often used to treat general pain and pain syndromes associated with HNC in the acute and chronic settings. However, due to their risks and emerging evidence for opioid-sparing analgesia, there is strong support to increase usage of nonopioid therapies. Nonetheless, opioids remain a staple for alleviating acute and chronic, moderate-to-severe pain (4—10 of 10 on the pain scale) in HNC. Guidelines from the WHO and National Comprehensive Cancer Network (NCCN) provide detailed recommendations for their use in adult cancer pain.[8,20,25]

Selection of the specific opioid, dose, and route of administration are done on an individualized basis. Commonly, pure agonists such as morphine, oxycodone, and fentanyl are used for cancer pain. Morphine is often one of the preferred first-line agents for opioid-naïve patients, with a starting dose of 5—15 mg PO for moderate pain or 2—5 mg IV for severe pain.[20,26,27] Of note, active morphine metabolites can accumulate in patients with renal disease; extra caution should be taken in these cases.[28-30] When possible, the WHO recommends an oral route of administration; however, this can be complicated in HNC where tumor and treatments can affect swallowing, medication safety, and where certain topical formulations may help with localized symptom management while limiting systemic side effects. When prescribing opioids, clinicians should utilize the lowest effective dose for the shortest duration to limit the risk of developing opioid dependence. Effective dosing often varies patient-to-patient due to individual opioid tolerance and metabolism. For instance, genetically derived variations in CYP3A4 enzymatic activity results in inconsistent codeine metabolism to its active metabolite, leading to variable pain control and increased toxicity risks.[31] Prescribing pain medications individually rather than in combined formulations enable dose titration of each analgesic independently. Short half-life agents such as oxycodone and morphine also assist with dose titration.

Since the late 1980s, multiple clinical studies have compared the efficacy of opioids at alleviating acute and chronic pain in cancer patients.[32−41] Collectively, no consistent advantage has been attributed to a specific choice of opioid for time to pain relief, durability of the analgesic effect, overall QOL benefit, and tolerance of adverse effects. Bandieri and colleagues recently completed a multicenter, randomized clinical trial (RCT) comparing the efficacy of low-dose morphine and weak opioids in moderate cancer pain in patients with a variety of solid and hematologic cancers.[32] In this study of 240 patients, low-dose morphine (up to 30 mg daily) was associated with a higher percentage of patients achieving at least a 20% reduction in their pain compared to weak opioids; both groups had comparable tolerance of adverse effects. Similarly, two recent RCTs comparing morphine and oxycodone for the treatment of cancer pain found no difference in adverse effects or pain relief efficacy between the agents.[34,35] Another recent four-arm multicenter, RCT (NCT01809106) compared PO morphine, PO oxycodone, TD fentanyl, or buprenorphine for 28 days.[33] As in the other studies, no significant difference was found in the tolerability or efficacy of the different opioid treatment arms. Thus, the specific opioid selection is a collective decision between patient and provider, accounting for an individual analgesic response, medical comorbidities, side effect tolerability, analgesia and QOL goals, and ability to adhere to the dosage schedule.

Breakthrough pain, an acute flare in pain in the setting of chronic pain management, remains a common issue in HNC patients. A rapid-acting opioid medication, such as immediate-release morphine, can be effective to treat acute pain crises.[20] The initial dosing will vary for opioid-naïve patients compared to patients with a history of opioid use. For opioid-naïve patients, an oral dose of 5−15 mg or an IV dose of 2−5 mg morphine sulfate is reasonable, again with the choice of other rapid-acting opioids. For patients chronically utilizing opioid medications, a dose of 10%−20% of their total opioid dose taken in the prior 24 h is recommended. Dosing should then be individually titrated based on patient assessments every 60 min for enteral formulations, and every 15 min for IV formulations (Table 7.5).

When prescribing opioids for acute or chronic pain, the risk of opioid dependence, adverse effects of long-term use, and discontinuation plans to prevent possible withdrawal should always be considered and discussed with patients. A large number of HNC patients who are started on opioid pain medications for acute pain utilize narcotics long-term.[42−45] One report found that ∼1/3 of HNC patients undergoing surgical treatment and prescribed perioperative opioid analgesics continued to fill opioid prescriptions more than 90 days postsurgery.[44] Similarly, a retrospective review of 7484 patients with laryngeal cancer who were prescribed opioids for pain control during treatment found that 17.2% continued to fill opioid prescriptions more than 90 days after treatment ended.[42] In this cohort, early opioid use in treatment, tobacco use, radiation therapy alone, and higher median morphine milligram equivalents (MMEs) were all associated with chronic opioid use. Similar risk factors for long-term opioid use were identified in a retrospective cohort study

Table 7.5 Opioid titration during acute cancer pain crisis management.

Pain score at time of reassessment	Opioid dose/route change
Unchanged or increased after 1 assessment	Increase rescue dose by 50%–100%
Reduced, but inadequately controlled, and 1 assessment	Repeat initial dose and reassess again after 60 min (for oral) or 15 min (for IV)
Moderate-to-severe and unchanged after 2–3 cycles of the opioid	Change from PO to IV route, or consider alternative intervention
Decreased to mild pain (score of 0–3/10 on pain scale)	Continue current dose as needed for 24 h then reevaluate for continued pain control

Based on NCCN Guidelines. National comprehensive cancer network adult pain guidelines. J Pain Palliat Care Pharmacother. 2006;20:94.

($n = 73$) evaluating chronic opioid use after treatment of newly diagnosed laryngeal cancer in the VA population.[43] Here, prior opioid use (more than 30 days before cancer treatment initiation) and higher MME were associated with the development of chronic use. Patients who had prior opioid use were eight times more likely to develop chronic opioid use, defined as continued use at 360 days after their cancer treatment was completed. Thus, chronic use risk factors should be considered when prescribing opioid medications and while counseling patients. The American Academy of Otolaryngology-Head and Neck Surgery Foundation recently published the Clinical Practice Guidelines: Opioid Prescribing for Analgesia after Common Otolaryngology Operations. Emphasis was placed on discussing risk factors for opioid use disorder (OUD) with patients before any surgical operation (Table 7.6).[46] In light of the risks of developing OUD and its consequences, the

Table 7.6 Risk factors for OUD in HNC patients.

• Opioid use >30 days before oncologic treatment	• Early opioid use in cancer treatment
• Personal history of alcohol or drug abuse or tobacco use	• Has prescription for anxiolytic or antipsychotic
• Family history of alcohol or drug abuse	• HNC treated with radiation therapy alone, particularly with oropharyngeal primary site
• Psychiatric disorder diagnosis including:	• For surgical patients: presence of preoperative pain, procedure intensity, and postoperative length of hospital stay
• Anxiety	• Higher MME during acute pain treatment
• Depression	• Age 16–45 years
• Personality disorder	• Lower socioeconomic status

Adapted from Zayed S, Lin C, Boldt RG, et al. Risk of chronic opioid use after radiation for head and neck cancer: a systematic review and meta-analysis. Adv Radiat Oncol. 2021;6:100583; Anne S, Mims JW, Tunkel DE, et al. Clinical practice guideline: opioid prescribing for analgesia after common otolaryngology operations. Otolaryngol Head Neck Surg. 2021;164:S1–S42.

WHO cancer pain management guidelines along with pain guidelines from multiple national and international societies including the NCCN include vigilant opioid stewardship.[8,20,46–49]

Management updates for common HNC-associated pain situations and syndromes
Acute and chronic surgery-associated pain

In recent years, there has been a strong effort to shift toward developing nonopioid multimodal analgesic regimens to use in pain management for patients undergoing surgical intervention. Collectively, guidelines support that nonopioid analgesics should be started for all patients in the perioperative setting who do not have contraindications. Nonopioid analgesics include acetaminophen, NSAIDs, anticonvulsants, antidepressants, steroids, and multimodal therapy comprised of a combination of therapeutic agents. A brief overview of common nonopioid medications used in this setting follows. Patient-specific contraindications should guide drug selection, and multimodal treatments that do not include opioids may be superior to opioids in specific scenarios.[23,24] The 2017 Enhanced Recovery After Surgery Society guidelines on perioperative care for HNC surgery recommend a multimodal, opioid-sparing pain control regimen.[49] The WHO recommends that a nonopioid monotherapy strategy is appropriate for mild pain, but suggests that these should be combined with the opioids for moderate-to-severe pain.[8]

Acetaminophen (or paracetamol) is commonly used for pain control in HNC. In surgical HNC patients, this can be used pre-, intra-, and postoperatively. Pre- and postoperatively, a single (650–1000 mg) or scheduled (650 mg every 6 h; 950 mg every 8 h) oral dosing can be used depending on the expected severity and duration of pain.[21] Intraoperatively, IV delivery is an option of great research.[21] A recent prospective single-center study evaluated the role of IV acetaminophen in postoperative pain control in patients with HNC.[50] In this study, 48 patients were treated with postoperative scheduled IV acetaminophen (1 g every 6 h for a total of four doses) in addition to a standard opioid PCA and breakthrough narcotics. This cohort used significantly less narcotics in the first 8 h after surgery and had a decreased length of stay compared to a similar retrospective cohort; the two groups had similar levels of pain control. For high dose and/or longer-term use of acetaminophen, hepatic function is important to consider. This is particularly important in patients with HNC as alcohol consumption is a risk factor for both HNC and impaired liver function.[21,51] In these cases, acetaminophen may be contraindicated or require hepatic dosing.

NSAIDs help provide pain control by inhibiting cyclooxygenase (COX) enzymes, which in turn suppresses prostaglandin production resulting in reduced inflammation. Similar to acetaminophen, NSAIDs can be used in both the pre- and postoperative settings for patients with HNC. When doing so, caution must be taken in drug selection to reduce the risk of bleeding and renal injury. Their use may be contraindicated in patients with chronic kidney disease, severely reduced glomerular filtration rate, or those undergoing treatment with nephrotoxic chemotherapy agents. Selective COX-2 inhibition by celecoxib may decrease the risk of platelet dysfunction and associated risk of postoperative hemorrhage. In patients with HNC undergoing tumor resection with free flap reconstruction, retrospective studies found no increased risk of bleeding with the use of perioperative celecoxib and/or ketorolac.[24,52,53] Importantly, these studies reported no impact on free flap healing. However, their efficacy in reducing perioperative pain remains unclear as studies have shown mixed results.[52,53] A recent retrospective matched-cohort study of 147 patients who underwent surgery for the treatment of HNC with free tissue reconstruction found that the cohort receiving postoperative celecoxib for pain utilized less total opioids without increased flap-related complications.[53] These results suggest that celecoxib may help decrease opioid use in HNC patients in the acute postoperative setting. Notably, in this study, the observed decrease in opioid utilization in the celecoxib cohort from 55.5 to 26.9 MME per day is clinically significant, as opioid dosages greater than 50 MME double the risk of opioid dependence and opioid-related complications.

Corticosteroids can also be used in the treatment of acute cancer pain while also reducing edema and nausea.[8,21] Evidence for their benefit is mixed in the perioperative setting. A recent prospective double-blind randomized controlled trial of 93 patients who underwent reconstructive HNC surgery calls into question the safety of dexamethasone in this setting.[54,55] In the dexamethasone treatment group ($n = 51$; 60 mg total dexamethasone administered in 10 mg doses every 8–12 h over 3 days pre- and postoperatively), no significant benefits were identified, and this group experienced increased major complications, including infections resulting in additional surgeries within 3 weeks. However, other studies have demonstrated the safe use of these agents with pain reduction benefits. A recent, double-blind, placebo-controlled RCT evaluated the use of corticosteroids to reduce postoperative pain in HNC patients being treated with transoral robotic surgery.[56] In this study, all patients received 10 mg dexamethasone intraoperatively and then were randomized to receive 8 mg dexamethasone or placebo every 8 h after surgery up to 4 days. While there were minimal differences in the postoperative pain control between the two groups, the extended corticosteroid arm had a trend toward earlier improvement in diet consistency, decreased length of hospital stay, and importantly no difference in complications. The WHO cancer pain treatment guidelines recommend that steroids should always be (1) prescribed for the shortest possible period of time and (2) dosed based on the cancer stage, goals of care, and with consideration of additional medical comorbidities such as diabetes mellitus.[8] When being used for cancer pain due at least in part to peritumoral edema, a steroid with the least mineralocorticoid effect should be selected.[8] When being used, their potential side effect profile includes hypertriglyceridemia, hyperglycemia, electrolyte imbalance, bone loss, psychosis, risk of infection, and impaired wound healing. These are critical to consider for patients undergoing HNC treatments such as complex surgical procedures and chemoradiotherapy.

Locoregional analgesia is also being explored for use in perioperative pain management for HNC patients. Intra- and postoperative continuous wound infusion (CWI) with local anesthetics can reduce acute pain in the postoperative period for HNC patients undergoing neck dissection. In a newly published nonrandomized clinical trial, Gostian and colleagues found that intra- and postoperative CWI with ropivacaine (0.2%, 3 mL/h) for 72 h after surgery was associated with reduced pain and analgesic use compared to a standard escalating oral regimen including ibuprofen, metamizole, and opioids.[57] Recent work also supports that preoperative local anesthesia can improve postoperative pain. For instance, one study randomized 74 patients undergoing thyroid surgery to preoperative ultrasound-guided bilateral superficial cervical plexus block with 10 mL of ropivacaine 0.5% or to similarly administered normal saline. The treatment group experienced significantly reduced postoperative pain in addition to improved overall satisfaction and decreased length of stay in the postanesthesia care unit.[58]

Multimodal analgesia (MMA) refers to combination treatments that target multiple, different pain mechanisms, with the goal of increasing pain control and decrease narcotic use. Clinical trials are exploring the efficacy of MMA regimens with and without narcotics in HNC. In a retrospective cohort study assessing pain control after head and neck free flap reconstructive surgery, the use of MMA ($n = 28$ patients) was associated with lower MME doses in the postoperative period and at the time of hospital discharge as well as lower pain scores compared to a control group ($n = 37$) treated with standard narcotic-based analgesia.[24] Perioperative MMA in this study included the use of scheduled and as-needed neuromodulating and antiinflammatory agents including acetaminophen, gabapentin, celecoxib, and ketorolac with IV fentanyl for breakthrough pain and PCA for the first 24 h after surgery, while the control narcotic-based cohort was treated with traditional acetaminophen, hydrocodone-acetaminophen, and IV morphine as needed. Similarly, a retrospective study evaluating the efficacy of MMA in HNC patients ($n = 138$) who underwent extensive head and neck surgery with free flap reconstruction also found that MMA was associated with improved pain control and reduced opioid use.[59] Their MMA regimen was implemented as an electronic order set and developed based on a consensus-based protocol.[49] An additional study involving 528 adults who underwent thyroid and parathyroid surgery at a single institution found that over several years of implementing an MMA protocol, the prescription frequency of opioids at discharge significantly decreased (Fig. 7.2).[59a] The use and efficacy of MMA versus opioid therapy for treating radiation-induced oral mucositis (OM) pain in HNC patients is an area of ongoing research with at least one active RCT (NCT04221165).[60] While implementing organized, multimodal pain regimens are challenging, recent investigation supports their feasibility even at high-volume cancer care centers.[59a,61]

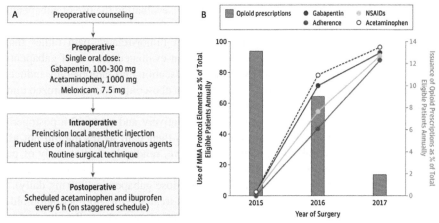

FIGURE 7.2 Association of the development of a multimodal analgesia (MMA) protocol with discharge opioid prescription patterns.

(A) MMA protocol. (B) The annual frequency of MMA adherence, use of individual MMA components, and opioids prescriptions at discharge at a single institution cohort of 528 adults who underwent thyroid and parathyroid surgery, demonstrating a progressive increase in MMA adherence with reduction in the frequency of opioid prescription at discharge.

Reprinted with permission from Hinther A, Nakoneshny SC, Chandarana SP, et al. Efficacy of multimodal analgesia for postoperative pain management in head and neck cancer patients. Cancers. 2021;13.

Postradiation pain

Acute and chronic pain can occur following radiation therapy treatment due to skin, oral mucosa, nerve, soft tissue, and bone damage. Acute pain often includes oral mucositis and dermatitis, which are discussed separately below. Longer-term pain can occur weeks to months following completion of radiation therapy and include neuropathic pain (most common), myofascial pain, and lymphedema[62]; these are discussed in the following subsections with specific treatment considerations. Importantly, with chronic postradiation pain it is essential to evaluate for possible tumor recurrence. One retrospective data review of 86 patients with HNC treated with radiotherapy who continued to have pain 6 weeks after completion of their treatment found that those whose pain resolved at 3 months ($n = 39$) had greater disease-free survival than those persistent pain beyond 3 months ($n = 47$).[63]

Neuropathic pain

Neuropathic pain can occur in the acute and chronic setting in patients with HNC due to both the malignancy itself and complications of the anticancer treatments. Anticonvulsants and antidepressants can be used to modulate these pain pathways. Of these pharmacologic classes, gabapentinoid anticonvulsants (e.g., gabapentin and pregabalin) and tricyclic antidepressants (TCAs) are frequently used for treating neuropathic pain.[8,11,64,65] In particular, gabapentin has been widely studied and extensively used for neuropathic pain. Recent and ongoing studies are seeking to better define its utility.[66,67]

A recent review of 13 randomized clinical trials evaluating the use of gabapentin and pregabalin for pain control in cancer patients found that the pain modulating benefit of the gabapentinoid may be greater in tumor-related pain rather than treatment-related pain. However, recent RTCs that evaluated the use of gabapentinoids in acute settings related to HNC surgical resection and radiotherapy-induced pain have shown benefits. In a double-blinded, placebo-controlled, randomized clinical trial of 110 patients undergoing head and neck mucosal surgery, patients who received gabapentin (300 mg twice daily preoperatively and up to 72 h postoperatively) reported clinically important reductions in their pain scores but did not use fewer narcotics.[68] Alternately, a recent prospective, randomized pilot study of patients with HNC undergoing chemoradiation evaluated the safety and efficacy of prophylactic high (2700 mg daily) compared to low dose gabapentin (900 mg daily).[64] For significant pain, patients in group 1 were then treated with short-acting opioids, while those in group 2 were treated with longer-acting methadone. Results demonstrated no difference in pain between the two arms. However, the study did find that more patients in the high-dose arm required no opioid during treatment (42% vs. 7%), but that those in group 2 reported high QOL suggesting that higher dose gabapentin may reduce the need for opioids, but in patients requiring opioids use of methadone rather than standard shorter-acting opioids may be beneficial. Pregabalin has also been evaluated for use with radiotherapy-related pain in patients with HNC.[69] In a randomized, double-blind, placebo-controlled trial of 128 patients, 59.4% patients in the pregabalin arm experienced at least a 30% reduction in their reported pain, compared to 32.8% in the placebo group. Overall, the pregabalin arm had improved pain control, mood, and QOL.

Oral mucositis

A common cause of acute pain during and after chemotherapy and radiation treatment for HNC is OM. In addition to the direct discomfort, mucositis, and mucositis-related pain can lead to decreased nutritional intake, dehydration, weight loss, declining performance status, and increased risk of infection requiring hospitalization, which negatively impacts patient QOL and mortality.[70] Many treatments and treatment guidelines for the prevention and treatment of OM exist, which include topical opioid and nonopioid therapies as well as general hygiene recommendations, all described later.

Topical opioids can be used to help relieve OM-related pain. Following a systemic review, the Mucositis Study Group of the Multinational Association of Supportive Care in Cancer/International Society of Oral Oncology (MASCC/ISOO) added a new suggestion to their 2014 practice guidelines (which is maintained in their updated 2020 guidelines) to include the use of topical 0.2% morphine mouthwash for the treatment of OM-associated pain in HNC cancer being treated with combination chemoradiotherapy.[70–72] Several randomized clinical trials have compared the efficacy of morphine-containing mouthwashes to commonly used nonopioid multiagent mouthwashes that include lidocaine, diphenhydramine, and magnesium-aluminum chloride (so-called "Magic Mouthwash"). While results were mixed across the trials, patients being treated with the morphine-containing mouthwash showed a probable improvement in their pain control.[73–75] Transdermal and intranasally administered fentanyl has also been studied in at least eight clinical trials; however, due to mixed efficacy results and varied trial structures, no clear guidelines arose from these data.[71] Notably, topical opioid analgesics have the benefit of diminished central nervous system side effects compared to systemic administration.

Nonopioid OM interventions include oral hygiene care, antiinflammatory agents, growth factors or cytokines, local anesthetics (e.g., lidocaine), antihistamines with anticholinergic properties (e.g., diphenhydramine), anticonvulsants and antidepressants, antimicrobials (including antifungals), mucosal coating agents (including sucralfate), cryotherapy, laser or light therapy, and natural products such as honey.[71,72,76,77] Expert recommendations on the use of these agents have been published elsewhere and are reviewed here in brief.[70–72]

As oral hygiene and periodontal diseases are risk factors for developing or worsening OM, basic oral care to both prevent and treat OM is recommended.[76] These include tooth brushing, flossing, and possible use of salt and sodium bicarbonate mouthwashes. As of the 2016 Italian consensus review, there was no consistent, clear benefit of any mouthwash over saline or bicarbonate oral rinses.[76]

Multiple antiinflammatory agents show utility in relieving pain from OM and have been systematically reviewed.[78,79] Of these, benzydamine—an NSAID—in a mouthwash formulation has been recommended for patients receiving radiation therapy doses up to 50 Gy.[70,72] The 2014 and 2020 MASCC/ISOO reports did not provide guidelines for the use of celecoxib, misoprostol, indomethacine, and other agents that have been tested in this setting, as evidence for analgesic efficacy is mixed. Amifostine is costly, and commonly can cause nausea and vomiting, and more rarely anaphylactoid reactions.[72,76] A recent double-blind, placebo-controlled trial (JORTC-PAL04) evaluating the efficacy of an oral indomethacin spray to treat OM pain in 60 patients with HNC being treated with chemoradiation found that the spray was associated with improved pain control for up to 180 min and improved ability to drink liquids and converse.[80] Multiple growth factors and cytokines have been explored for their ability to treat OM. One growth factor has been approved by the FDA for use in OM, palifermin (keratinocyte growth factor-1). Palifermin was recommended for use in 2014 MASCC/ISOO guidelines for patients with hematologic malignancies but has not been recommended for routine use in HNCs.[72,76]

Local anesthetics and diphenhydramine are commonly used to treat OM alone and in combination mouthwash products—as referred to above, "Magic Mouthwash." The exact composition of these formulations can vary, including proportions of diphenhydramine, a local anesthetic such as lidocaine, and an antacid, sometimes with the addition of an antimicrobial, opioid, and/or steroid agent. The Alliance A221304 RCT evaluated the effects of a diphenhydramine-lidocaine-antacid mouthwash compared to a doxepin mouthwash or a placebo mouthwash to alleviate radiation-induced OM pain.[81] Results demonstrated a significant effect of both preparations on reducing pain compared to the control group. The MASCC/ISOO guidelines recommend the use of multiagent combination care protocols for HCN patients receiving either or both RT and chemotherapy but reviews of mixed agent preparation were not analyzed given their variable ingredients; mixed agent mouthwashes continue to be the subject of ongoing studies.[70,82]

The use of gabapentinoids and TCAs are being explored for utility in OM, but do not have recommendations for or against their use yet. Retrospective evaluation of 30 patients who received radiation therapy for HNC found that using a median dose of 2700 mg/day of gabapentin reduced the use of narcotic pain medication for OM throughout radiation therapy.[83] In this study, grade 2 or higher OM was present in 80% of patients during the last weeks of radiation; however, only 35% of patients used narcotics during that time. Antidepressants may also have utility in this setting. Doxepin is a TCA that has topical analgesic and anesthetic properties. A phase II, randomized, double-blinded, placebo-controlled trial assessing the efficacy of a doxepin rinse for reducing radiotherapy-induced OM-related pain found that the doxepin rinse was associated with reduced mouth and throat pain and increased patient desire to continue treatment.[84]

Phototherapy, also termed photobiomodulation, may also be a useful adjunct to treat chemoradiation-induced OM, as has been recently reviewed.[85] Of note, while there are no anecdotal reports of tumorigenic properties of phototherapy, based on its mechanisms of action future studies confirming its safety profile are important. The most recent MASCC/ISOO 2020 guidelines recommend the use of intraoral photobiomodulation with a low-level laser to help prevent OM in adults receiving RT along or RT-CT, though with extra safety considerations for oral cancer.[70]

Recommendations for or against the use of other agents to treat OM associated with HNC are mixed based on the specific patient risk factors and use of chemotherapy and/or radiation therapy and should be reviewed before treatment.[70–72,76] Of note, recently guidelines also now suggest the use of honey in preventing OM in HNC patients undergoing treatment with RT alone or with chemotherapy.[70]

Acute and chronic radiation dermatitis

Radiation-induced dermatitis is a common sequelae of radiation therapy that causes significant pain. Up to 95% of patients undergoing radiation treatments can experience moderate-to-severe dermatitis, which can be associated with ulceration, burning, itching, and barrier breakdown increasing the risk of opportunistic infections.[86,87] Grade 1 dermatitis is common in the first few weeks of radiation therapy and is defined as a mild, transient erythema. Grade 2 dermatitis often occurs in weeks 2–4 of radiation therapy and is defined by dry desquamation with hyperpigmentation. Grade 3 dermatitis can occur weeks to months into and following radiation therapy and is severely painful with moist desquamation.

The mainstay of treatments for radiation dermatitis includes hygiene practices and topical dressings/treatments. Clinical practice guidelines have been established by the MASCC Skin Toxicity Study Group.[88] Hygiene practices have been studied in RCTs to evaluate their benefit in alleviating symptoms of radiation dermatitis and support washing with mild soap and lukewarm water to reduce the severity of dermatitis and associated pruritus in patients with breast cancer undergoing radiation therapy.[89,90] Multiple RCTs have evaluated the efficacy of topical agents in allevi-ating dermatitis in patients with HNC. Agents evaluated include silver sulfadiazine, moisturizers, topical corticosteroids, and natural agents including aloe vera, doxe-pin, and topical atorvastatin among others, many of which show evidence of decreasing pain or severity of the radiation dermatitis.[87] For patients experiencing desquamation, the use of at least a hydrophilic moisturizer is often recommended. Topical steroids that are medium potency can be beneficial in relieving pain and itch associated with dermatitis. A recent RCT evaluated the use of topical steroids in radiation dermatitis for patients with HNC.[91] In this study, patients were random-ized to either receive topical steroids or a placebo when they experienced either grade 1 dermatitis or reached 30 Gy cumulative radiation dosage. The steroid group experienced significantly reduced frequency of grade 3 or higher dermatitis (13.9% vs. 25.5%). There was no difference in grade 2 dermatitis. Thus, topical steroids may reduce dermatitis severity in patients with HNC undergoing radiation therapy.

Symptomatic lymphedema

A frequent cause of pain in cancer patients is tumor- and treatment-induced lymphe-dema, which can involve the face and neck as well as internal structures including the pharynx and larynx.[92] Up to 90% of HNC patients can experience lymphedema at some point over the course of their cancer treatment and posttreatment period.[93]

Standard treatment includes manual lymphatic drainage, compression, exercise, and skincare. Challenges for these treatments include variable efficacy across pa-tients, access to and affordability of therapy, and few trained lymphedema therapists. Investigators have also explored the use of selenium, liposuction, and lymphaticove-nular anastomoses to relieve symptomatic lymphedema.[94] Of these, manual drainage has been the most robustly studied to date, but liposuction and surgical in-terventions show efficacy in smaller studies. Newer strategies aimed at mitigating obstacles in lymphedema treatment such as cost and access to treatment are active areas of research. Advanced pneumatic compression devices (APCD), which have the advantage of use at home, have received premarket clearance from the FDA. In a randomized, wait-list controlled clinical trial of APCD for HNC-associated lymphedema, preliminary data suggest efficacy for improving lymphedema and visible external swelling.[92]

Additional therapies being explored for HNC-associated pain management

Targeted chronic pain management for head and neck pain include direct inhibition of sensory nerves via neurolysis and local anesthetic blocks, both of which function by disrupting the transmission of pain signals to the CNS. Nerves that may be amenable to anesthetic block in HNC include the trigeminal ganglion and branches, gasserian ganglion, sphenopalatine ganglion, occipital nerve, superior laryngeal nerve, and the glossopharyngeal nerve.[11] This is an active area of research for alle-viating pain associated with HNC and its treatments.

Integrative therapies provide additional multimodal techniques to alleviate acute and chronic pain. A combination of these methods is used by up to half of the cancer patients.[95–97] Integrative therapies include the use of natural products such as herbs and vitamin, mind-body techniques including yoga and meditation, homeopathy, chiropractic manipulation, therapeutic compression devices, and acupuncture. Of these, the most robust studies to date have been conducted on the adjuvant use of acupuncture, where benefits have been shown in both the acute and chronic setting.[98–102]

A recent prospective randomized open-label trial of 60 HNC patients undergoing curative and adjuvant chemoradiotherapy assessed the impact of acupuncture throughout standard anticancer treatment on pain severity and analgesic consumption.[98] Results demonstrated that the acupuncture cohort ($n = 30$) had significantly lower average pain, improved rating of the worst pain of the day, and decreased analgesic use during and 3 months after radiotherapy.

In the chronic setting, acupuncture has been found to reduce both pain and xerostomia, a common side effect of HNC treatment.[101,102] A prospective, open-label, RCT assessed the role of acupuncture in patients with pain at least 3 months after undergoing neck dissection and radiation at Memorial Sloan Kettering Cancer Center.[102] Patients were randomized to receive weekly acupuncture or standard care (physical therapy, analgesia, and/or antiinflammatory drugs). Both the Constant-Murley score, a composite measure of pain, activities of daily living, and function, and reported xerostomia had greater improvement in the acupuncture arm. Supporting this, a large 2-center, phase 3 randomized clinical trial evaluated standard of care with true acupuncture and sham acupuncture in 399 patients experiencing xerostomia who were treated for HNC.[101] Results suggested that true acupuncture may reduce and decrease the severity of xerostomia 1 year after treatment. However, post hoc analyses identified differences in treatment effects at the two centers with the true acupuncture only being beneficial at the Fudan University Cancer Center in Shanghai, China study site, and not at the University of Texas MD Anderson Cancer Center in Houston, Texas site.

Conclusion and summary for pain management in HNC

The treatment of acute and chronic pain in HNC patients is a critical element of oncologic care. Similar to the evolution of the anticancer treatments these patients receive—that is shifting toward a personalized medicine paradigm targeting unique attributes of each patient's cancer—pain management strategies are similarly becoming more personalized. Multiple tools exist for developing these treatment plans including opioid and nonopioid pharmacologic and nonpharmacologic interventions. In recent years, there has been a growing emphasis on opioid stewardship with newer multimodal, opioid-sparing pain regimens showing promise in both feasibility and efficacy. Future work aims to improve methods to prevent and treat pain while limiting adverse side effects of analgesics. The evolution of pain management aims to improve the overall well-being and QOL of patients with HNC.

References

1. Auperin A. Epidemiology of head and neck cancers: an update. *Curr Opin Oncol.* 2020; 32:178−186.
2. Howlader NNA, Krapcho M, Miller D, et al. *SEER Cancer Statistics Review, 1975-2018, National Cancer Institute.* Bethesda, MD. 2021. based on November 2020 SEER data submission, posted to the SEER web site, April 2021.
3. Bossi P, Giusti R, Tarsitano A, et al. The point of pain in head and neck cancer. *Crit Rev Oncol Hematol.* 2019;138:51−59.
4. Dugue J, Humbert M, Bendiane MK, Bouhnik AD, Babin E, Licaj I. Head and neck cancer survivors' pain in France: the VICAN study. *J Cancer Surviv.* 2021. https://doi.org/10.1007/s11764-021-01010-0.
5. Osazuwa-Peters N, Simpson MC, Zhao L, et al. Suicide risk among cancer survivors: head and neck versus other cancers. *Cancer.* 2018;124:4072−4079.
6. Park SA, Chung SH, Lee Y. Factors associated with suicide risk in advanced cancer patients: a cross-sectional study. *Asian Pac J Cancer Prev.* 2016;17:4831−4836.
7. Noel CW, Sutradhar R, Zhao H, et al. Patient-reported symptom burden as a predictor of emergency department use and unplanned hospitalization in head and neck cancer: a longitudinal population-based study. *J Clin Oncol.* 2021;39:675−684.
8. World Health Organization. *WHO Guidelines for the Pharmacological and Radiotherapeutic Management of Cancer Pain in Adults and Adolescents. In. Geneva.* 2018.
9. van den Beuken-van Everdingen MHJ, de Rijke JM, Kessels AG, Schouten HC, van Kleef M, Patijn J. High prevalence of pain in patients with cancer in a large population-based study in The Netherlands. *Pain.* 2007;132:312−320.
10. Chaplin JM, Morton RP. A prospective, longitudinal study of pain in head and neck cancer patients. *Head Neck.* 1999;21:531−537.
11. Blasco MA, Cordero J, Dundar Y. Chronic pain management in head and neck Oncology. *Otolaryngol Clin.* 2020;53:865−875.
12. Epstein JB, Wilkie DJ, Fischer DJ, Kim YO, Villines D. Neuropathic and nociceptive pain in head and neck cancer patients receiving radiation therapy. *Head Neck Oncol.* 2009;1:26.
13. McMenamin EM, Grant M. Pain prevention using head and neck cancer as a model. *J Adv Pract Oncol.* 2015;6:44−49.
14. Classification of chronic pain. Descriptions of chronic pain syndromes and definitions of pain terms. Prepared by the International Association for the Study of Pain, Subcommittee on Taxonomy. *Pain Suppl.* 1986;3:S1−S226.
15. Ing JW. Head and neck cancer pain. *Otolaryngol Clin.* 2017;50:793−806.
16. Chua KS, Reddy SK, Lee MC, Patt RB. Pain and loss of function in head and neck cancer survivors. *J Pain Symptom Manag.* 1999;18:193−202.
17. Potter J, Higginson IJ, Scadding JW, Quigley C. Identifying neuropathic pain in patients with head and neck cancer: use of the Leeds Assessment of Neuropathic Symptoms and Signs Scale. *J R Soc Med.* 2003;96:379−383.
18. Mu L, Chen J, Li J, et al. Sensory innervation of the human soft palate. *Anat Rec.* 2018; 301:1861−1870.
19. Raja SN, Carr DB, Cohen M, et al. The revised International Association for the Study of Pain definition of pain: concepts, challenges, and compromises. *Pain.* 2020;161: 1976−1982.

20. National Comprehensive Cancer network adult pain guidelines. *J Pain Palliat Care Pharmacother.* 2006;20:94.

21. Bobian M, Gupta A, Graboyes EM. Acute pain management following head and neck surgery. *Otolaryngol Clin.* 2020;53:753−764.

22. McDermott JD, Eguchi M, Stokes WA, et al. Short- and long-term opioid use in patients with oral and oropharynx cancer. *Otolaryngol Head Neck Surg.* 2019;160:409−419.

23. Du E, Farzal Z, Stephenson E, et al. Multimodal analgesia protocol after head and neck surgery: effect on opioid use and pain control. *Otolaryngol Head Neck Surg.* 2019;161: 424−430.

24. Eggerstedt M, Stenson KM, Ramirez EA, et al. Association of perioperative opioid-sparing multimodal analgesia with narcotic use and pain control after head and neck free flap reconstruction. *JAMA Facial Plast Surg.* 2019;21:446−451.

25. Swarm RA, Abernethy AP, Anghelescu DL, et al. Adult cancer pain. *J Natl Compr Cancer Netw.* 2013;11:992−1022.

26. Klepstad P, Kaasa S, Borchgrevink PC. Start of oral morphine to cancer patients: effective serum morphine concentrations and contribution from morphine-6-glucuronide to the analgesia produced by morphine. *Eur J Clin Pharmacol.* 2000;55:713−719.

27. Klepstad P, Kaasa S, Skauge M, Borchgrevink PC. Pain intensity and side effects during titration of morphine to cancer patients using a fixed schedule dose escalation. *Acta Anaesthesiol Scand.* 2000;44:656−664.

28. Portenoy RK, Foley KM, Stulman J, et al. Plasma morphine and morphine-6-glucuronide during chronic morphine therapy for cancer pain: plasma profiles, steady-state concentrations and the consequences of renal failure. *Pain.* 1991;47: 13−19.

29. Portenoy RK, Khan E, Layman M, et al. Chronic morphine therapy for cancer pain: plasma and cerebrospinal fluid morphine and morphine-6-glucuronide concentrations. *Neurology.* 1991;41:1457−1461.

30. Tiseo PJ, Thaler HT, Lapin J, Inturrisi CE, Portenoy RK, Foley KM. Morphine-6-glucuronide concentrations and opioid-related side effects: a survey in cancer patients. *Pain.* 1995;61:47−54.

31. Gasche Y, Daali Y, Fathi M, et al. Codeine intoxication associated with ultrarapid CYP2D6 metabolism. *N Engl J Med.* 2004;351:2827−2831.

32. Bandieri E, Romero M, Ripamonti CI, et al. Randomized trial of low-dose morphine versus weak opioids in moderate cancer pain. *J Clin Oncol.* 2016;34:436−442.

33. Corli O, Floriani I, Roberto A, et al. Are strong opioids equally effective and safe in the treatment of chronic cancer pain? A multicenter randomized phase IV 'real life' trial on the variability of response to opioids. *Ann Oncol.* 2016;27:1107−1115.

34. Zecca E, Brunelli C, Bracchi P, et al. Comparison of the tolerability profile of controlled-release oral morphine and oxycodone for cancer pain treatment. An open-label randomized controlled trial. *J Pain Symptom Manag.* 2016;52:783−794 e786.

35. Riley J, Branford R, Droney J, et al. Morphine or oxycodone for cancer-related pain? A randomized, open-label, controlled trial. *J Pain Symptom Manag.* 2015;49:161−172.

36. Arkinstall WW, Goughnour BR, White JA, Stewart JH. Control of severe pain with sustained-release morphine tablets v. oral morphine solution. *Cancer Med Assoc J.* 1989;140:653−657, 661.

37. Goughnour BR, Arkinstall WW, Stewart JH. Analgesic response to single and multiple doses of controlled-release morphine tablets and morphine oral solution in cancer patients. *Cancer.* 1989;63:2294−2297.

38. Broomhead A, Kerr R, Tester W, et al. Comparison of a once-a-day sustained-release morphine formulation with standard oral morphine treatment for cancer pain. *J Pain Symptom Manag.* 1997;14:63–73.

39. Bruera E, Belzile M, Pituskin E, et al. Randomized, double-blind, cross-over trial comparing safety and efficacy of oral controlled-release oxycodone with controlled-release morphine in patients with cancer pain. *J Clin Oncol.* 1998;16:3222–3229.

40. Hagen NA, Babul N. Comparative clinical efficacy and safety of a novel controlled-release oxycodone formulation and controlled-release hydromorphone in the treatment of cancer pain. *Cancer.* 1997;79:1428–1437.

41. Hanna M, Thipphawong J, Study G. A randomized, double-blind comparison of OROS(R) hydromorphone and controlled-release morphine for the control of chronic cancer pain. *BMC Palliat Care.* 2008;7:17.

42. Starr N, Oyler DR, Schadler A, Aouad RK. Chronic opioid use after laryngeal cancer treatment. *Head Neck.* 2021;43:1242–1251.

43. Craker NC, Gal TJ, Wells L, Schadler A, Pruden S, Aouad RK. Chronic opioid use after laryngeal cancer treatment: a VA study. *Otolaryngol Head Neck Surg.* 2020;162: 492–497.

44. Saraswathula A, Chen MM, Mudumbai SC, Whittemore AS, Divi V. Persistent postoperative opioid use in older head and neck cancer patients. *Otolaryngol Head Neck Surg.* 2019;160:380–387.

45. Zayed S, Lin C, Boldt RG, et al. Risk of chronic opioid use after radiation for head and neck cancer: a systematic review and meta-analysis. *Adv Radiat Oncol.* 2021;6:100583.

46. Anne S, Mims JW, Tunkel DE, et al. Clinical practice guideline: opioid prescribing for analgesia after common otolaryngology operations. *Otolaryngol Head Neck Surg.* 2021; 164:S1–S42.

47. Binczak M, Navez M, Perrichon C, et al. Management of somatic pain induced by head-and-neck cancer treatment: definition and assessment. Guidelines of the French Oto-Rhino-Laryngology- Head and Neck Surgery Society (SFORL). *Eur Ann Otorhinolaryngol Head Neck Dis.* 2014;131:243–247.

48. Blanchard D, Bollet M, Dreyer C, et al. Management of somatic pain induced by head and neck cancer treatment: pain following radiation therapy and chemotherapy. Guidelines of the French Otorhinolaryngology Head and Neck Surgery Society (SFORL). *Eur Ann Otorhinolaryngol Head Neck Dis.* 2014;131:253–256.

49. Dort JC, Farwell DG, Findlay M, et al. Optimal perioperative care in major head and neck cancer surgery with free flap reconstruction: a consensus review and recommendations from the enhanced recovery after surgery society. *JAMA Otolaryngol Head Neck Surg.* 2017;143:292–303.

50. Smith E, Lange J, Moore C, Eid I, Jackson L, Monico J. The role of intravenous acetaminophen in post-operative pain control in head and neck cancer patients. *Laryngoscope Investig Otolaryngol.* 2019;4:250–254.

51. Kawakita D, Matsuo K. Alcohol and head and neck cancer. *Cancer Metastasis Rev.* 2017;36:425–434.

52. Schleiffarth JR, Bayon R, Chang KE, Van Daele DJ, Pagedar NA. Ketorolac after free tissue transfer: a comparative effectiveness study. *Ann Otolaryngol Rhinol Laryngol.* 2014;123:446–449.

53. Carpenter PS, Shepherd HM, McCrary H, et al. Association of celecoxib use with decreased opioid requirements after head and neck cancer surgery with free tissue reconstruction. *JAMA Otolaryngol Head Neck Surg.* 2018;144:988–994.

54. Kainulainen S, Lassus P, Suominen AL, et al. More harm than benefit of perioperative dexamethasone on recovery following reconstructive head and neck cancer surgery: a prospective double-blind randomized trial. *J Oral Maxillofac Surg.* 2018;76: 2425–2432.

55. Kainulainen S, Tornwall J, Koivusalo AM, Suominen AL, Lassus P. Dexamethasone in head and neck cancer patients with microvascular reconstruction: No benefit, more complications. *Oral Oncol.* 2017;65:45–50.

56. Clayburgh D, Stott W, Bolognone R, et al. A randomized controlled trial of corticosteroids for pain after transoral robotic surgery. *Laryngoscope.* 2017;127:2558–2564.

57. Gostian M, Loeser J, Albert C, et al. Postoperative pain treatment with continuous local anesthetic wound infusion in patients with head and neck cancer: a nonrandomized clinical trial. *JAMA Otolaryngol Head Neck Surg.* 2021;147(6):553–560.

58. Yao Y, Lin C, He Q, Gao H, Jin L, Zheng X. Ultrasound-guided bilateral superficial cervical plexus blocks enhance the quality of recovery in patients undergoing thyroid cancer surgery: a randomized controlled trial. *J Clin Anesth.* 2020;61:109651.

59. Hinther A, Nakoneshny SC, Chandarana SP, et al. Efficacy of multimodal analgesia for postoperative pain management in head and neck cancer patients. *Cancers.* 2021;13.

59a. Militsakh O, Lydiatt W, Lydiatt D, et al. Development of Multimodal Analgesia Pathways in Outpatient Thyroid and Parathyroid Surgery and Association With Postoperative Opioid Prescription Patterns. *JAMA Otolaryngol Head Neck Surg.* 2018;144(11): 1023–1029.

60. Zayed S, Lang P, Mendez LC, et al. Opioid therapy vs. multimodal analgesia in head and neck Cancer (OPTIMAL-HN): study protocol for a randomized clinical trial. *BMC Palliat Care.* 2021;20:45.

61. Low GMI, Kiong KL, Amaku R, et al. Feasibility of an Enhanced Recovery after Surgery (ERAS) pathway for major head and neck oncologic surgery. *Am J Otolaryngol.* 2020;41:102679.

62. Kallurkar A, Kulkarni S, Delfino K, Ferraro D, Rao K. Characteristics of chronic pain among head and neck cancer patients treated with radiation therapy: a retrospective study. *Pain Res Manag.* 2019;2019:9675654.

63. Srivastava P, Kingsley PA, Srivastava H, Sachdeva J, Kaur P. Persistent postradiotherapy pain and locoregional recurrence in head and neck cancer-is there a hidden link? *Korean J Pain.* 2015;28:116–121.

64. Hermann GM, Iovoli AJ, Platek AJ, et al. A single-institution, randomized, pilot study evaluating the efficacy of gabapentin and methadone for patients undergoing chemoradiation for head and neck squamous cell cancer. *Cancer.* 2020;126:1480–1491.

65. Lee TS, Wang LL, Yi DI, Prasanna PD, Kandl C. Opioid sparing multimodal analgesia treats pain after head and neck microvascular reconstruction. *Laryngoscope.* 2020;130: 1686–1691.

66. Vedula SS, Bero L, Scherer RW, Dickersin K. Outcome reporting in industry-sponsored trials of gabapentin for off-label use. *N Engl J Med.* 2009;361:1963–1971.

67. Vedula SS, Li T, Dickersin K. Differences in reporting of analyses in internal company documents versus published trial reports: comparisons in industry-sponsored trials in off-label uses of gabapentin. *PLoS Med.* 2013;10:e1001378.

68. Townsend M, Liou T, Kallogjeri D, et al. Effect of perioperative gabapentin use on postsurgical pain in patients undergoing head and neck mucosal surgery: a randomized clinical trial. *JAMA Otolaryngol Head Neck Surg.* 2018;144:959–966.

69. Avraham HK, Jiang S, Fu Y, Nakshatri H, Ovadia H, Avraham S. Angiopoietin-2 mediates blood-brain barrier impairment and colonization of triple-negative breast cancer cells in brain. *J Pathol*. 2014;232:369–381.

70. Elad S, Cheng KKF, Lalla RV, et al. MASCC/ISOO clinical practice guidelines for the management of mucositis secondary to cancer therapy. *Cancer*. 2020;126:4423–4431.

71. Saunders DP, Rouleau T, Cheng K, et al. Systematic review of antimicrobials, mucosal coating agents, anesthetics, and analgesics for the management of oral mucositis in cancer patients and clinical practice guidelines. *Support Care Cancer*. 2020;28:2473–2484.

72. Lalla RV, Bowen J, Barasch A, et al. MASCC/ISOO clinical practice guidelines for the management of mucositis secondary to cancer therapy. *Cancer*. 2014;120:1453–1461.

73. Cerchietti LC, Navigante AH, Bonomi MR, et al. Effect of topical morphine for mucositis-associated pain following concomitant chemoradiotherapy for head and neck carcinoma. *Cancer*. 2002;95:2230–2236.

74. Sarvizadeh M, Hemati S, Meidani M, Ashouri M, Roayaei M, Shahsanai A. Morphine mouthwash for the management of oral mucositis in patients with head and neck cancer. *Adv Biomed Res*. 2015;4:44.

75. Vayne-Bossert P, Escher M, de Vautibault CG, et al. Effect of topical morphine (mouthwash) on oral pain due to chemotherapy- and/or radiotherapy-induced mucositis: a randomized double-blinded study. *J Palliat Med*. 2010;13:125–128.

76. De Sanctis V, Bossi P, Sanguineti G, et al. Mucositis in head and neck cancer patients treated with radiotherapy and systemic therapies: literature review and consensus statements. *Crit Rev Oncol Hematol*. 2016;100:147–166.

77. Cho HK, Jeong YM, Lee HS, Lee YJ, Hwang SH. Effects of honey on oral mucositis in patients with head and neck cancer: a meta-analysis. *Laryngoscope*. 2015;125:2085–2092.

78. Nicolatou-Galitis O, Sarri T, Bowen J, et al. Systematic review of anti-inflammatory agents for the management of oral mucositis in cancer patients. *Support Care Cancer*. 2013;21:3179–3189.

79. Nicolatou-Galitis O, Sarri T, Bowen J, et al. Systematic review of amifostine for the management of oral mucositis in cancer patients. *Support Care Cancer*. 2013;21:357–364.

80. Nagaoka H, Momo K, Hamano J, et al. Effects of an indomethacin oral spray on pain due to oral mucositis in cancer patients treated with radiotherapy and chemotherapy: a double-blind, randomized, placebo-controlled trial (JORTC-PAL04). *J Pain Symptom Manag*. 2021;62(3):537–544.

81. Sio TT, Le-Rademacher JG, Leenstra JL, et al. Effect of doxepin mouthwash or diphenhydramine-lidocaine-antacid mouthwash vs placebo on radiotherapy-related oral mucositis pain: the alliance A221304 randomized clinical trial. *J Am Med Assoc*. 2019;321:1481–1490.

82. Uberoi AS, Brown TJ, Gupta A. Finding the magic in magic mouthwash-reply. *JAMA Int Med*. 2019;179:724–725.

83. Bar AV, Weinstein G, Dutta PR, et al. Gabapentin for the treatment of pain syndrome related to radiation-induced mucositis in patients with head and neck cancer treated with concurrent chemoradiotherapy. *Cancer*. 2010;116:4206–4213.

84. Leenstra JL, Miller RC, Qin R, et al. Doxepin rinse versus placebo in the treatment of acute oral mucositis pain in patients receiving head and neck radiotherapy with or without chemotherapy: a phase III, randomized, double-blind trial (NCCTG-N09C6 [Alliance]). *J Clin Oncol*. 2014;32:1571–1577.

85. Zecha JA, Raber-Durlacher JE, Nair RG, et al. Low-level laser therapy/photobiomodulation in the management of side effects of chemoradiation therapy in head and neck cancer: part 2: proposed applications and treatment protocols. *Support Care Cancer.* 2016;24:2793−2805.

86. Rosenthal A, Israilevich R, Moy R. Management of acute radiation dermatitis: a review of the literature and proposal for treatment algorithm. *J Am Acad Dermatol.* 2019;81: 558−567.

87. Iacovelli NA, Torrente Y, Ciuffreda A, et al. Topical treatment of radiation-induced dermatitis: current issues and potential solutions. *Drugs Context.* 2020;9.

88. Wong RK, Bensadoun RJ, Boers-Doets CB, et al. Clinical practice guidelines for the prevention and treatment of acute and late radiation reactions from the MASCC Skin Toxicity Study Group. *Support Care Cancer.* 2013;21:2933−2948.

89. Campbell IR, Illingworth MH. Can patients wash during radiotherapy to the breast or chest wall? A randomized controlled trial. *Clin Oncol.* 1992;4:78−82.

90. Roy I, Fortin A, Larochelle M. The impact of skin washing with water and soap during breast irradiation: a randomized study. *Radiother Oncol.* 2001;58:333−339.

91. Yokota T, Zenda S, Ota I, et al. Phase 3 randomized trial of topical steroid versus placebo for prevention of radiation dermatitis in patients with head and neck cancer receiving chemoradiation. *Int J Radiat Oncol Biol Phys.* 2021;111(3):794−803.

92. Ridner SH, Dietrich MS, Deng J, Ettema SL, Murphy B. Advanced pneumatic compression for treatment of lymphedema of the head and neck: a randomized wait-list controlled trial. *Support Care Cancer.* 2021;29:795−803.

93. Ridner SH, Dietrich MS, Niermann K, Cmelak A, Mannion K, Murphy B. A prospective study of the lymphedema and fibrosis continuum in patients with head and neck cancer. *Lymphatic Res Biol.* 2016;14:198−205.

94. Tyker A, Franco J, Massa ST, Desai SC, Walen SG. Treatment for lymphedema following head and neck cancer therapy: a systematic review. *Am J Otolaryngol.* 2019;40:761−769.

95. Asher BF, Seidman M, Snyderman C. Complementary and alternative medicine in otolaryngology. *Laryngoscope.* 2001;111:1383−1389.

96. Molassiotis A, Ozden G, Platin N, et al. Complementary and alternative medicine use in patients with head and neck cancers in Europe. *Eur J Cancer Care.* 2006;15:19−24.

97. Warrick PD, Irish JC, Morningstar M, Gilbert R, Brown D, Gullane P. Use of alternative medicine among patients with head and neck cancer. *Arch Otolaryngol Head Neck Surg.* 1999;125:573−579.

98. Dymackova R, Selingerova I, Kazda T, et al. Effect of acupuncture in pain management of head and neck cancer radiotherapy: prospective randomized unicentric study. *J Clin Med.* 2021;10.

99. Matovina C, Birkeland AC, Zick S, Shuman AG. Integrative medicine in head and neck cancer. *Otolaryngol Head Neck Surg.* 2017;156:228−237.

100. Alimi D, Rubino C, Pichard-Leandri E, Fermand-Brule S, Dubreuil-Lemaire ML, Hill C. Analgesic effect of auricular acupuncture for cancer pain: a randomized, blinded, controlled trial. *J Clin Oncol.* 2003;21:4120−4126.

101. Garcia MK, Meng Z, Rosenthal DI, et al. Effect of true and sham acupuncture on radiation-induced xerostomia among patients with head and neck cancer: a randomized clinical trial. *JAMA Netw Open.* 2019;2:e1916910.

102. Pfister DG, Cassileth BR, Deng GE, et al. Acupuncture for pain and dysfunction after neck dissection: results of a randomized controlled trial. *J Clin Oncol.* 2010;28: 2565−2570.

Nonopioid pain management in otolaryngology—head and neck surgery: the pharmacist's perspective

Rebecca Britton, PharmD, BCPS, Kylee Kastelic, PharmD, Robert Osten, PharmD, BCPS, BCGP, Renita Patel, PharmD, BCPS

Department of Pharmacy, Oregon Health and Science University, Portland, OR, United States

Introduction

With the setting of the opioid epidemic, a focus has been placed on understanding the prescribing patterns of physicians for postoperative surgery pain. A 2018 survey of 1770 members of the American Rhinologic Society was conducted regarding the prescribing patterns for pain management after endoscopic sinus surgery (ESS).[1] The overall survey response rate was low at 9.49% ($N = 168$). At least one kind of opioid was prescribed by 94.05% of respondents with an average of 27 pills. Those in private practice were less likely to prescribe oxycodone ($p = .000105$). Private practice physicians were also less likely to refer patients to pain management ($p = .0117$) and were more likely to refer patients to nontraditional forms of pain management ($p = .0164$). There was no statistical difference between prescribing of acetaminophen between the groups. Academic physicians were less likely to prescribe nonsteroidal antiinflammatories (NSAIDs) ($p = .032$). All across the country, regardless of practice setting, most providers prescribe opioids after ESS. Given this, multimodal pain strategies are essential to understand and implement perioperatively to decrease opioid use and more safely treat patients. Most data are for the (non-opioid) analgesics of acetaminophen, NSAIDs, and gabapentinoids, thus will be the focus of this chapter.

Acetaminophen

Overview

Acetaminophen (APAP) is a nonopioid analgesic that is available without a prescription and found both individually and in a wide variety of combination products (fixed dose with other analgesics, headache remedies, sleep aids, cold and flu preparations). Its full mechanism of action is not well understood. It is believed to provide analgesic effects through inhibiting descending serotonergic pathways in the central nervous system (CNS) in addition to possible interaction with other nociceptive systems.[2,3] It is commonly used for mild-to-moderate pain such as headaches and myalgia. It also provides antipyretic effects through inhibition of the hypothalamic heart-regulating center. It only weakly inhibits COX-1 and COX-2 enzymes in peripheral tissues and therefore has little antiinflammatory effects.

APAP is readily orally absorbed with an onset of action and peak effects reached within 60 min depending on gastric emptying time.[2] It is also available in intravenous (IV) form, which may provide peak effects in as little as 15 min. APAP is widely distributed throughout the body. It has a 2–3 h half-life with a 4–6 h duration of effect (antipyretic effects may last longer). It is primarily metabolized through hepatic conjugation with glucuronic acid ($\sim$60%) and sulfuric acid ($\sim$35%). See Table 8.1 for specific dosing recommendations.

Common adverse effects include the following: nausea, vomiting, dizziness, mild hepatic enzyme elevation, and difficulty sleeping.[2] At higher doses, a minor toxic metabolite (N-acetyl-p-benzoquinone or NAPQI) can accumulate when normal metabolic pathways become saturated. The accumulation of NAPQI can lead to severe hepatotoxicity and acute renal impairment. It is recommended to avoid total daily doses of APAP greater than 4000 mg or single doses greater than 1000 mg in patients with normal hepatic function to reduce the risk of toxicity. Lower dosing cutoffs should be considered in patients with mild to moderate hepatic impairment and use should be avoided in patients with severe hepatic impairment. APAP has few clinically significant drug–drug interactions.

Use in otolaryngology surgery

APAP has been utilized for surgeries as both a single analgesic and as part of a multimodal pain medication approach. There is a large controversy around whether IV APAP is superior to oral. Most of the studies involving APAP use, either preoperatively or postoperatively, include IV APAP. There are conflicting data as a whole, but the proposed benefits include lower pain scores (VAS), less narcotic use, and longer time to rescue medication, as well as less nausea and vomiting compared to other analgesics. There are many studies involving APAP use in adenoidectomies, tonsillectomies, and ESS.

Most of the evidence for APAP use in otolaryngology involves pediatric patients undergoing adenoidectomies and tonsillectomies. APAP was reviewed in three studies, two for adenotonsillectomy and one for tonsillectomy. A double-blind randomized controlled trial of a single dose of IV APAP did not reduce pain scores in pediatric patients (ages 2–8) undergoing adenotonsillectomy ($N = 239$).[4] Patients received oral midazolam, propofol, and morphine before tracheal intubation. Intraoperatively IV APAP at 15 mg/kg ($n = 118$) or saline placebo ($n = 121$) was administered. Faces, Legs, Activity, Cry, Consolability (FLACC) scores and rescue analgesics did not differ at any postoperative time point between groups. Results

Table 8.1 Nonopioid pain medication overview.[2,15]

Medication	Preoperative dose	Postoperative dose	Maximum total daily dose	Dose adjustments	Adverse effects/Precautions
Acetaminophen (IV/PO)	500–1000 mg	500–1000 mg Q6-8 H	4000 mg	Reduce dose for hepatic impairment	GI upset, risk of severe hepatic impairment with excessive use
NSAIDs					
Celecoxib (PO)	200–400 mg	100–200 mg twice daily	400 mg	Avoid use with CrCl <30 mL/min	GI upset, increased risk of CV events
Ketorolac (IV)	15–30 mg	15–30 mg Q6 H	120 mg	50% reduction for CrCl 30–50 mL/min, weight <50 kg or age >65 years; Avoid use with CrCl <30 mL/min	Increased risk of bleeding/CV events with use greater than 5 days
Ibuprofen (PO)	400–800 mg	400–800 mg Q6-8 H	3200 mg	Avoid use with CrCl <30 mL/min	GI upset, increased risk of GI bleed and renal impairment with prolonged use
Naproxen (PO)	250–500 mg	250–500 mg Q8-12 H	1500 mg	50% reduction for CrCl 30–50 mL/min; avoid use with CrCl <30 mL/min	GI upset, increased risk of GI bleed and renal impairment with prolonged use; potentially least risk of CV events
Gabapentinoids					
Gabapentin (PO)	300–900 mg	300–900 mg Q8 H	3600 mg	50% dose reduction for CrCl 30–50 mL/min; 75% dose reduction for CrCl 15–30 mL/min	Sedation, potential for abuse, potential for withdrawal with prolonged use or high dose if stopped abruptly
Pregabalin (PO)	150 mg	50–200 mg Q8-12 H	600 mg	50% reduction for CrCl 30–50 mL/min or age >65 years; 75% dose reduction and not more than Q12H interval for	Sedation, potential for abuse, potential for withdrawal with prolonged use or high dose if stopped abruptly

CV, *cardiovascular;* CrCl, *creatinine clearance,* GI, *gastrointestinal;* H, *hours;* NSAIDs, *nonsteroidal antiinflammatories;* PO, *oral;* Q, *every.*

were similar in a prospective trial of pediatric patients (ages 3—17) undergoing tonsillectomy or adenotonsillectomy ($N = 260$).[5] Patients either received IV APAP intraoperatively at 15 mg/kg ($n = 131$) or did not. There were no differences in FLACC scores between the two groups up to 24 h postoperatively, but more incidences of nausea and vomiting with IV APAP. Lastly, a retrospective cohort study of 166 pediatric patients (age 1—16 years) evaluated the use of IV APAP ($n = 74$) compared to none as the control group ($n = 92$).[6] Patients in the APAP cohort received a single dose of 15 mg/kg before anesthesia induction. Patients who received APAP received statistically significantly less morphine compared to the control cohort. Of note, this is a retrospective design compared to the prospective design of the previous two studies and they were assessing different outcomes.

APAP has also been utilized for postoperative pain control in ESS. Two double-blind, randomized controlled trials evaluated 1000 mg of IV APAP compared to placebo in adults undergoing ESS surgery.[7,8] In one study, there was a trend toward lower visual analog scores (VASs) in the APAP group at 1 h postoperatively, but also a trend toward the placebo at 12 and 24 h ($N = 62$).[7] However in the next study, significantly fewer patients in the APAP group required rescue analgesia and had less incidence of severe pain ($N = 74$).[8] The APAP dosing strategies were slightly different, with patients receiving APAP before surgery and then a second dose 4 h after versus right after completion of the surgery in the first and second studies, respectively. Another randomized, double-blind study evaluated 1000 mg of IV APAP 15 min before induction (Group I, $n = 20$) compared to at the end of surgery (Group II, $n = 19$) in adult ESS patients.[9] Postoperative VAS pain scores were statistically significantly higher in Group II up to 6 h postoperatively, and the time to first analgesic was significantly longer in Group I. With conflicting results, it is hard to determine the optimal timing of APAP. Of note, the first trial had inconclusive results within the trial, possibly making a case that APAP should be dosed before surgery and continued throughout.[7,9] Lastly, a prospective study evaluated oral APAP at 665 mg modified-release tablets as either a scheduled regimen of three times daily for 5 days ($n = 38$) versus on an as-needed basis ($n = 40$).[10] Although there was no difference between the scheduled and as-needed group in regards to recovery (average 9—10 days), there were significantly lower pain scores in the scheduled group. If using oral medication, due to the delay in absorption and peak effect, it is beneficial to schedule the medication rather than use as needed.

APAP has also been studied in combination with other analgesics. In a randomized, double-blind study, the efficacy of APAP alone was tested against the combination of APAP with codeine in pediatric patients (ages 3—12 years) undergoing outpatient tonsillectomy and adenoidectomy ($N = 51$).[11] Patients were transitioned to either APAP 15 mg/kg ($n = 31$) or APAP/codeine 1 mg/kg ($n = 20$), based on codeine dose. There was no difference in postoperative pain reported by the patients. APAP has also been reported to help with goal recovery (lower rates of severe pain) when used with remifentanil in ESS patients.[12] A meta-analysis including 23 studies of otologic surgeries (myringotomy/tympanostomy, tympanomastoid, microtia reconstruction, middle ear surgeries) concluded that combination analgesics, such as APAP and codeine provided superior analgesia, while NSAIDs and α-agonists may be monotherapy options.[13] Caution must be taken when using codeine in pediatric patients after tonsillectomy or adenoidectomy as there is now a Black Box Warning on the combination product.[14] Due to a subset of the population being ultrarapid metabolizers of codeine, from a Cytochrome P450 2D6 polymorphism, codeine is converted to morphine at higher levels. The Black Box Warning came after pediatric deaths occurred with the use of APAP/codeine after tonsillectomies and adenoidectomies.

Common misconceptions

As seen in the evidence presented in this section, there is conflict in the data about whether APAP should be given IV or orally when used perioperatively. In adult clinical practice, IV APAP has a specific place in therapy for a patient that cannot take APAP via an enteral route and there is significant rectal pathology or a history of sexual abuse or trauma where administering rectal APAP could cause a psychological disturbance for the patient. Patients that are neutropenic (absolute neutrophil count less than 500) and do not have enteral access would be another reason to use IV APAP. We have created this type of restriction criteria at our institution to help curb unnecessary use of IV APAP, especially in the historical setting of the significant increased cost compared to the oral and rectal suppository formulations.

As of April 2021, the cost of generic APAP IV (10 mg/mL, 100 mL bottle) is ~$0.45 per mL.[15] With the IV route typically dosed at 1000 mg per dose, that is almost $50 per dose, whereas an oral APAP tablet (500 mg dose per tablet) and a rectal APAP suppository (650 mg dose per suppository) are roughly the same cost as 1 mL (10 mg) of IV APAP ($0.45 per tablet or suppository). If a patient is on scheduled APAP 1000 mg every 6 h for multimodal pain management, the cost of administering this regimen via an IV route definitely adds up and can generate thousands of dollars of unnecessary yearly drug spend for a hospital.

Another question that often comes up when putting together postoperative multimodal pain regimens is how to best utilize APAP with NSAID medications in patients where both medication classes are deemed safe for use. You may have heard before that alternating timing of NSAIDs with APAP can improve the effectiveness of pain control more than taking the medications together at the same time or even alone but is there evidence to support this strategy?

A retrospective chart review described outcomes in pain relief in children who received alternating regimens of APAP and ibuprofen after tonsillectomy or adenoidectomy.[16] Out of 583 patients that were 1–18 years of age, only 56 (9.6%) reported inadequate pain control with this regimen. Overall, the incidence of postoperative bleeding and bleeding requiring surgical intervention was low at 24 patients (4.1%) and 9 patients (1.5%), respectively. Although this review was conducted in children, it is reasonable to say an alternating regimen of APAP and ibuprofen at doses appropriate for adults would also allow for improved pain control with little risk of postoperative bleeding concerns.

In contrast, a randomized controlled trial described a combined regimen of APAP 500 mg and ibuprofen 150 mg per tablet (studying the British prescription product Maxigesic), two tablets by mouth preoperatively, and then two tablets every 6 h for up to 48 h postoperatively in patients undergoing dental molar removal.[17] This was compared to monotherapy of either APAP 500 mg by mouth every 6 h or ibuprofen 150 mg by mouth every 6 h. Of general relevance was the secondary endpoint of global pain rating, a subjective patient report, with the favored group being the combined regimen (68.4% of patients reported "none" or "mild" pain scores compared to 37.5% of patients taking APAP alone and 54.3% of patients taking ibuprofen alone). To note, only the APAP group had a statistically significant difference compared to the combined regimen ($p = .008$). Also, patients on the combined therapy required less use of rescue pain medication, though this was not statistically significant. This example shows the potential of combined APAP/ibuprofen providing greater pain control compared to monotherapy with either of these agents. Although there is little evidence looking at a combined regimen versus an alternating regimen of these two medications, from a patient adherence standpoint a combined regimen, either in a combined tablet (not available in the United States as of May 2021) or taking these medications at the same time with equal frequency, will allow for better patient medication adherence and less confusion in trying to stagger medications and higher risk of potentially exceeding recommended maximum daily doses.

Nonsteroidal antiinflammatory drugs
Overview

NSAIDs are a large class of nonopioid analgesics. NSAIDs as a whole have analgesic, antiinflammatory, and antipyretic effects through both nonselective COX inhibition and selective COX-2 inhibition depending on the agent. They are particularly effective at treating pain when inflammation is involved in triggering pain perception.[2,3] Many NSAIDs are available without a prescription and can commonly be found as individual agents and in multiple combination products similar to APAP. A few NSAIDS are available in formulations other than oral (i.e., topical diclofenac gel; IV and ophthalmic ketorolac).

Most NSAIDs have rapid absorption after oral intake with the onset of action within 30–60 min and peak effects generally in 1–3 h.[2,3] They are widely distributed throughout the body including relatively high concentrations in the CNS providing central analgesic effects. They are primarily metabolized through hepatic pathways and renally excreted. Half-life and duration of effect can vary greatly depending on the specific agent used. See Table 8.1 for specific dosing recommendations.

Common adverse effects include the following: abdominal pain and cramping, nausea, vomiting, dizziness, headache, and fluid retention.[2,3] More serious adverse effects include the following: severe gastrointestinal events (including inflammation, ulceration, and bleeding), rash (including Stevens-Johnson Syndrome and toxic epidermal necrosis), bleeding (through inhibition of platelet adhesion and aggregation), hepatic and renal impairment, and cardiovascular events (including myocardial infarction and stroke). The risk of gastrointestinal adverse effects increases significantly when NSAIDs are taken in combination with aspirin or other antiplatelet agents, anticoagulants, selective serotonin reuptake inhibitors, or prolonged use of corticosteroids. The risk of renal impairment is significantly increased when NSAIDs are taken in combination with ACE inhibitors. NSAIDs are also highly protein bound and may displace other protein-bound medications increasing the risk of toxicity of these agents (such as methotrexate or warfarin).

Use in otolaryngology surgery

NSAIDs are a cornerstone for opioid-sparing regimens in otolaryngology. In 2013, a survey was published of Danish patients who underwent tonsillectomies and their number of days absent from work or school along with their pain score for the first 14 days postoperative time period.[18] A total of 549 patients returned the survey, with 30% dissatisfied with the information provided about postoperative complications and risks. The daily pain score was significantly higher in adults (>15 years) compared to children ($p < .0001$). Days missed were significantly higher in patients greater than 16 years (12 versus 9 days; $p < .0001$). Pain medications prescribed for the first week were a combination of paracetamol (APAP) and NSAIDs, according to age and weight. While the survey did find that most patients were satisfied with their outpatient tonsillectomy procedure, postoperative pain management warrants review. Unfortunately, no specifics on the dosing, frequency, and selection of NSAIDs were provided in the study.

A survey of parents of 324 children who underwent adenotonsillectomy was conducted to assess the opioid-sparing effects of postoperative ibuprofen use.[19] The pain regimen included the combination of APAP and ibuprofen or the combination hydrocodone/APAP and ibuprofen. Oral APAP was prescribed at 15–20 mg/kg every 6 h, ibuprofen was dosed at 7.5–10 mg/kg every 6 h, and hydrocodone/ APAP was dosed at 0.1 mg/kg of hydrocodone every 6 h. The two groups (opioid and nonopioid) were equally matched in gender, race/ethnicity, and insurance status. Most parents filling out the survey ranked their child's pain control as excellent or good/adequate, while only 9% without opioids ranked it as poor/inadequate and 5% with opioids. The authors concluded that nonopioid analgesic regimens following pediatric adenotonsillectomy did not result in worse parental satisfaction or poor/inadequately controlled pain in children.

Various studies have investigated whether adults could have their pain adequately managed without the use of opioids. In a randomized controlled study of adults undergoing thyroidectomy or parathyroidectomy surgery, 127 patients were randomized to either a narcotic arm ($n = 53$) or nonnarcotic arm ($n = 73$) for postoperative pain management.[20] The groups had some differences in baseline demographics with more patients in the nonnarcotic arm reporting alcohol use (10.9% versus 5% in narcotic arm; $p = .009$), while more patients in the nonnarcotic arm had an active illicit drug use (9.5% versus 0% in narcotic arm; $p = .03$). All patients received 1000 mg APAP alternating with 800 mg of ibuprofen every 4 h as needed for pain, along with ice packs on the incision (15 min on, 15 min off) and dyclonine throat lozenge to dissolve in the mouth every 2 h as needed for throat pain. Breakthrough pain while inpatient could be treated with 5 mg of oxycodone every 6 h as needed. Upon discharge, the nonnarcotic arm received 1000 mg APAP alternating with 800 mg of ibuprofen every 4 h as needed for pain, but no oxycodone for rescue. Upon discharge, the narcotic arm received the same APAP and ibuprofen instructions and prescriptions along with a prescription for 5 mg of oxycodone every 6 h as needed for breakthrough pain. Only 10 oxycodone tablets were prescribed in the narcotic arm. Patients were surveyed at postoperative days (POD) 0 and 5. When reviewing patients who received a narcotic after discharge from the PACU, either in the hospital or after discharge, there was no difference in age, sex, race, or history of chronic pain between the groups. The narcotic group had a larger percentage reporting alcohol consumption (15.1% vs. 2.8%; $p = .01$), active illicit drug use (9.6% vs. 1.4%; $p = .03$), previous opioid misuse (7.7% vs. 0%; $p = .02$), and smoking (41.5% vs. 15.1%; $p = .001$), while 98.6% in the narcotic-free group were opioid naïve and 86.8% ($p = .007$) in the narcotic group. Opioid naïve was defined as not having received narcotic within 3 months of surgery. The median pain score on POD 0 was 7 and 7.5 for narcotic versus nonnarcotic ($p = .1$), respectively. Each day until POD 5, the median pain score decreased by 1 and was evenly matched between the groups. On POD 5, it was 2.5 for the narcotic group and 2 for the nonnarcotic group ($p = .8$). The authors concluded that an opioid-sparing pain regimen provides effective analgesia for patients after a thyroidectomy or a parathyroidectomy. As a result of this study, the authors created a standardized approach to postoperative pain management after thyroidectomy and parathyroidectomy. The approach involves patient education regarding expectations for postoperative pain and where the pain is most likely to occur (incision site, throat, and neck, headache due to anesthesia, sometimes chest wall, and shoulder, jaw, and ear pain), no longer routinely prescribing narcotics at discharge, and the use of ice and dyclonine as adjuncts to APAP and ibuprofen. If the pain is uncontrolled with this regimen, three narcotic tablets are prescribed for rescue.

A study was conducted evaluating the effect of celecoxib added to the postoperative pain regimen. In a retrospective matched cohort study of patients undergoing head and neck cancer surgery with free tissue reconstruction, the amount of morphine equivalents per patient per day postoperative was measured in those who received celecoxib ($N = 51$) and the control group ($N = 51$).[21] The celecoxib group received 200 mg twice daily through a feeding tube for a minimum of 5 days starting on POD 1. Celecoxib use was associated with decreased use of opioids (30.9 mg mean morphine equivalents (MME) per day) compared to the control (44.9 mg MME/day; 14 mg of morphine equivalents per day difference (95% confidence interval: 2.6–25.4)). The reduction in MME is clinically significant, as the

Center for Disease Control has shown that 50 mg MME (equivalent to 33 mg of oxycodone) more than doubles the risk of overdose and other opioid-related complications. There were no statistically significant differences in complications between the two groups; flap dehiscence/surgical site infection (16% vs. 13% in control), hematomas (1.9% vs. 4.0% in control), free flap failure rate (4% in both groups), gastrointestinal complications (4% vs. 5.8% in control), cardiovascular complications (4% in both groups), and no difference in 30-day mortality (1.9% in both groups). The authors concluded that in head and neck cancer surgery patients that oral celecoxib helped to reduce morphine equivalent use in patients without increasing surgery and microvascular flap-related complications.

Common misconceptions

As discussed in the literature review earlier in this section, a significant increase in postoperative bleeding risk is not a clinically relevant concern in patients without risk factors like concomitant anticoagulation or antiplatelet therapy or significantly low hemoglobin, hematocrit, or platelet values. This should not be a concern when considering scheduled NSAID therapy, especially with the antiinflammatory properties of this drug class that often help with pain relief for patients.

In addition to the questions on bleeding risk, concern for immediate risk of perioperative acute kidney injury (AKI) due to NSAID use is also not a significant concern in patients without underlying kidney insufficiency, though ketorolac specifically can cause acute AKI even with short term use (can be seen within the first 7 days of use). Remembering to keep patients hydrated and regularly monitoring renal labs while inpatient is important to catch any developing AKI quickly and decrease unintended morbidity associated with this drug class.

In reviewing the role of IV ketorolac as part of a postoperative multimodal pain regimen, a common intervention that pharmacists make is the dose recommendation. There is evidence that there is a ceiling effect for ketorolac dosing that supports a lower dose of 15 mg (vs. 30 mg that is often ordered especially for younger patients with excellent renal function). In a randomized controlled trial ($N = 240$), patients were divided evenly into three groups where a single dose of IV ketorolac, either 10 mg, 15 mg, or 30 mg was given in the emergency department for acute pain.[22] The reduction in pain scores after 30 min between the three groups was similar and the differences were not statistically significant. Patients that had complete resolution of the pain also did so with ketorolac only and did not require an available rescue dose of IV morphine, which also shows the possibility of opioid-sparing effects in a multimodal pain regimen. This support for the lower dose of ketorolac in the setting of similar efficacy will also help more safely use this specific NSAID that can lead to AKI concerns more quickly as previously mentioned. Given this, the general recommendation is not to use scheduled ketorolac IV for more than five consecutive days—the approval studies did not study consecutive use for longer than this in human subjects, and there could be an increased risk of AKI development. That being said, if your patients cannot take medications orally after 5 days (and can be switched to an oral NSAID), risk versus benefit of extending therapy beyond 5 days should be considered, with a focus specifically on younger, healthy patients with no baseline or new renal insufficiency and no prior history of gastrointestinal (GI) ulcers or bleeding ulcers; daily checks of renal function and hemoglobin, hematocrit, and platelet counts are also recommended for safety monitoring.[15]

Another side effect often discussed for NSAIDs is GI ulcer development and whether stress ulcer prophylaxis with a proton pump inhibitor (PPI) is required for scheduled NSAID therapy for postoperative pain control. To answer this question, we really should look at the patient's risk factors for gastrointestinal toxicity with NSAID use. Joint guidelines from the American College of Cardiology, American College of Gastroenterology, and American Heart Association listed the following factors as high risk for GI toxicity and stress prophylaxis should be considered with NSAID use: history of ulcer disease or ulcer complication, patients on dual antiplatelet therapy, patients on anticoagulant therapy, and patients who meet two or three of the following criteria: age ≥ 60 years, glucocorticoid use, or dyspepsia or gastroesophageal reflux disease symptoms.[23] Patients meeting these criteria may warrant stress ulcer prophylaxis. In this scenario, PPIs are preferred for improved effectiveness regarding ulcer prevention over histamine H2 receptor antagonists, such as famotidine or ranitidine. Additionally, the ease of once-daily dosing with PPIs is helpful for improving patient adherence. Duration of NSAID use should also be considered as short durations of use (<1 week) are considered relatively low risk regardless of the presence of other risk factors. If stress ulcer prophylaxis is warranted, an important piece to remember is to ensure that the PPI is stopped when the scheduled NSAID therapy is stopped. This can often be overlooked leading to possible long-term polypharmacy with an unnecessary PPI increasing the risk for significant adverse events (*Clostridium difficile* infections, electrolyte/nutrient deficiencies, and osteoporosis-related bone fractures).

Another common misconception is that COX-2 selective inhibitors, such as celecoxib, are safer to use than nonspecific NSAIDs. While COX-2 selective inhibitors tend to carry a lower risk of gastroduodenal ulcer than nonspecific NSAIDs, the use of concomitant aspirin (including low-dose aspirin) negates this benefit. Additionally, COX-2 specific inhibitors have a similar to higher risk of myocardial infarction compared to other NSAIDs. This has led to the removal of rofecoxib and valdecoxib from the market. There is some data to suggest the risk of adverse cardiovascular events is dose dependent and can be mitigated by limiting celecoxib to a dose of no more than 200 mg per day. Alternatively, naproxen may carry some cardioprotective properties and therefore be the preferred agent in patients with risk factors for cardiovascular disease (prior history of cardiovascular event, diabetes, hypertension, hyperlipidemia, and obesity).[24] Based on this increased cardiovascular risk, a general higher cost (more than $4 per 100 mg tablet of celecoxib vs. less than $1 per 500 mg tablet of naproxen) and typically more difficulty with obtaining insurance coverage for COX-2 selective inhibitors, we suggest using naproxen as the NSAID of choice when patients have cardiovascular risk factors.[15]

Gabapentinoids

Overview

Gabapentinoids consist of a group of gamma aminobutyric acid (GABA) analogs, gabapentin and pregabalin. Although these agents have a close structural resemblance to GABA, they do not directly act on GABA receptors. However, they bind to voltage-gated calcium channels within the CNS to inhibit the release of excitatory neurotransmitters such as glutamate, norepinephrine, serotonin, and dopamine.[2,3] Both agents were originally designed to treat seizures but have become more commonly used for the treatment of neuropathic pain and potential synergistic effects when paired with other analgesics.[25]

Gabapentin has a dose-dependent nonlinear absorption, while pregabalin exhibits linear absorption.[2] Peak effects are reached within 1–2 h in a fasting state and 3–4 h when taken with food. Neither agent is hepatically metabolized and both are primarily eliminated unchanged through renal excretion. Half-life ranges from 4 to 8 h in the setting of normal renal function. See Table 8.1 for specific dosing recommendations.

Common adverse effects include the following: somnolence, dizziness, ataxia, headache, and tremor. Pregabalin is classified as a schedule V controlled substance due to increased reports of euphoria compared to placebo in clinical trials (4% vs. 1%, respectively).[2] While gabapentin does not carry a controlled designation, misuse and abuse have increased significantly over the past several years as regulations on opioids have become more stringent. There are minimal clinically significant drug–drug interactions.

Use in otolaryngology surgery

Gabapentinoids, including gabapentin and pregabalin, have been studied as part of a multimodal analgesia regimen as well as in randomized, placebo-controlled trials in otolaryngology surgeries including sinonasal, head and neck, tonsillectomy, and adenotonsillectomy. Studies including meta-analyses have conflicting conclusions on whether gabapentinoids dosed either perioperatively or postoperatively are efficacious for reduced postoperative pain control or decreased analgesic rescue. However, most studies reported less nausea and vomiting with gabapentinoids, but increased incidence of dizziness and somnolence.

A meta-analysis evaluated randomized controlled trials to determine the efficacy of perioperative gabapentinoids for the management of postoperative acute pain in adults.[26] Although 281 trials with over 24,000 patients were included, only 32 (10%) of trials with 2431 patients underwent ophthalmologic, maxillofacial, oral, and otolaryngologic surgeries. Gabapentinoids (including gabapentin and pregabalin) were administered as a single dose in 192 (68%) trials and multiple doses in 87 trials (31%). They were administered perioperatively, postoperatively, or both in 71%, 4%, and 25% of trials, respectively. For subgroup analysis, doses were considered high dose at 300 mg/day and above for pregabalin and at least 900 mg/day for gabapentin. Although there was slightly lower postoperative pain intensity at 6, 12, 24, and 48 h with gabapentinoids, this did not appear to be clinically significant. Gabapentinoids were associated with less postoperative nausea and vomiting but with more dizziness and visual disturbances. It was concluded that there was no clinically significant analgesic effect for perioperative gabapentinoids and use was not recommended.

Although the previous meta-analysis with a range of surgeries did not conclude benefit with gabapentin and pregabalin use, a systematic review of 15 randomized controlled trials with perioperative use of gabapentin in surgeries including tonsillectomy ($n = 4$), rhinologic surgery ($n = 3$), and thyroidectomy ($n = 3$) did show benefit.[27] Gabapentin doses ranged from 600 to 1200 mg for adults and 10–20 mg/kg for pediatric patients. Of the 15 trials, 13 used a single preoperative dose administered 1–2 h before anesthesia. The systematic review reported inconsistent results regarding gabapentin for perioperative pain control in tonsillectomies. Reductions in VASs were inconsistent. Of note, gabapentin was considered effective pain control for nasal surgery, with statistically significant reduction in VAS compared to control up to 24 h postoperatively ($p < .05$). This was not demonstrated in a retrospective comparison of sinonasal surgery patients receiving either gabapentin 600 mg 1 h preoperatively or no gabapentinoid.[28] Of note, approximately 6% of patients in the study were on chronic opioids. There was no significant difference in morphine equivalent doses or VAS scores between those that received gabapentin and those that did not. The authors concluded that perioperative gabapentin did not have an effect on postoperative pain or morphine equivalent doses. Lastly in a meta-analysis, four randomized, placebo-controlled trials reported reduced VAS pain scores with gabapentin administered perioperatively in thyroidectomies.[27] Studies also reported less nausea and vomiting, with a higher incidence of dizziness and somnolence.

In head and neck surgery, a randomized controlled trial and retrospective cohort review examined patients undergoing head and neck mucosal surgery and free flap reconstruction.[29,30] Ninety adult patients received either gabapentin 300 mg twice daily before surgery and up to 72 h after surgery ($n = 44$) or placebo ($n = 46$).[29] Oral morphine equivalents were similar between gabapentin and placebo groups. VAS scores were lower in the gabapentin group (after adjusting for differences in comorbidity and self-reported baseline pain levels). Patients reported higher satisfaction and less pain with gabapentin. There was less reported nausea in the gabapentin group, but again more dizziness. In the retrospective cohort study, patients received either gabapentin 600 mg before surgery ($n = 43$) or did not (control, $n = 43$).[30] Gabapentin was administered at 300 mg twice daily until postoperative day 5. APAP was also administered perioperatively and postoperatively. There was a statistically significant decrease in opioid consumption 5 days postoperatively and in daily pain scores. No adverse events occurred. The authors concluded that gabapentin is safe and effective.

A meta-analysis compared studies assessing preoperative gabapentinoids at a single dose from 300 to 1200 mg for postoperative pain after tonsillectomy.[31] A total of eight articles were included. Like previous meta-analyses, there was significant heterogeneity between trials. The meta-analysis included both adult and pediatric patients. Gabapentinoids resulted in statistically lower postoperative resting pain at four and 8 h, but not 12 and 24 h. The same trend was determined for swallowing pain, with differences at 2 and 8 h postoperative (compared to control) but not at 12 and 24 h. The time to analgesic administration and analgesic requirements were lower for gabapentinoids compared to controls during the first 24 h. While the incidence of postoperative nausea and vomiting were lower in the postoperative period (first 24 h) compared to control, there was no significant difference in dizziness or sedation.

Two trials compared APAP to gabapentinoids in adenotonsillectomy and ESS.[32,33] In a double-blind randomized study, children either received gabapentin 10 mg/kg orally or paracetamol (APAP) 20 mg/kg orally 2 h before anesthesia.[32] The gabapentin group had significantly lower pain scores (VAS scale) up to 8 h postoperatively, longer time to first analgesic, and less pethidine (meperidine) use compared to the APAP group. In the other randomized controlled trial, patients with nasal polyps received either pregabalin 50 mg three times daily or APAP 500 mg orally every 6 h for a total of 3 days.[33] The VAS score was significantly lower in the pregabalin group at 12–72 h postoperatively compared to the APAP group. Adverse events such as nausea, vomiting, headache, and bleeding were less in the pregabalin group as well. This lead to the conclusion that gabapentinoids may have advantages over oral APAP for pain control in otolaryngologic surgeries.

Lastly, a head-to-head randomized controlled trial was performed comparing gabapentin to APAP.[34] In a double-blind randomized control trial ($N = 60$), children 7–15 years old undergoing adenotonsillectomy were assigned to receive either gabapentin at 10 mg/kg ($n = 30$) or rectal APAP at 40 mg/kg (n-30) preoperatively. There was no difference between groups at any time point up to 24 h after surgery in regards to pain, and both had a statistically significant decrease in pain intensity ($p < .001$ for both groups). There was also no difference in the incidence of nausea and vomiting.

Common misconceptions

As seen in the literature review in this section, there are a few studies that showed no difference between gabapentin and placebo, but more studies indicated that the use of gabapentin in a multimodal pain regimen could reduce the use of opioids and may lead to improved subjective pain score reporting from patients. With this mixed literature on reduction in postoperative opioid use, there are multiple meta-analyses in various surgical specialties that have shown some clinically significant reduction in 24-h postoperative opioid consumption, though with varying doses of gabapentin and different opioids studied.

In clinical practice, the usual starting dose of gabapentin is 300 mg by mouth at bedtime, where dose and frequency titration (up to three times daily) should not occur more than every 3—4 days to allow the current dosing regimen to reach a steady state. This is important as gabapentinoids are known to cause somnolence and dizziness and should be dosed cautiously, especially in patients with renal impairment as well as older adults, where a lower starting dose of 100 mg by mouth at bedtime is common.[15]

To note, pregabalin is often used in preoperative pain regimens given its longer half-life compared to gabapentin to help with immediate 24-h postoperative opioid sparing. That being said, in clinical practice the general recommendation is to trial gabapentin first for postoperative scheduled regimens as part of a multimodal pain plan. It is much less costly than pregabalin, which often requires prior authorization and proven failure after trialing gabapentin before insurance companies will assist with drug cost coverage.

Multimodal analgesia

Many surgery centers are contemplating an opioid-free postoperative approach to pain management. A retrospective chart review was conducted of adult patients undergoing thyroid and parathyroid operations, before and after implementation of an opioid-free analgesia protocol.[35] The primary outcome was new postoperative opioid prescriptions, secondary outcomes were prescription characteristics (daily MME and days supply), as well as predictors of new opioid prescriptions. There were 240 patients in the preintervention group (May through October 2017) and 275 patients in the postintervention group (May through October 2018). The preintervention prescribing was traditionally hydrocodone/APAP (5/325 mg) 1—2 tablets every 6 h as needed for pain, for up to 10 days. This was at the discretion of the surgeon and practice differed among surgeons. In February 2018, the endocrine surgery group at the University of Kentucky implemented an opioid-sparing analgesia practice where patients would no longer receive opioid prescriptions postoperatively. Opioids were not discussed with or offered to patients and patients were instructed to take APAP 1000 mg every 6 h with ibuprofen up to 600 mg every 6 h. The time periods were selected to allow for an adequate 3-month washout period before and after the practice change. The opioid discharge prescriptions for the primary endpoint included buprenorphine, codeine, fentanyl, hydrocodone, hydromorphone, methadone, morphine, oxycodone, oxymorphone, tapentadol, or tramadol. The only statistically significant demographic between the two groups was preoperative opioid use, which was higher (12.5%) in the control (preimplementation) compared to the intervention (2.9%; $p < .001$). Patients were less likely to receive opioids postoperatively in the intervention group (12.0% vs. 59.6%; $p < .001$). Those patients that did receive a prescription postoperatively had lower doses and shorter durations, but it was not statistically significant. Hydrocodone/APAP accounted for 75.8% of all new prescriptions pre- and postimplementation. The patients in the intervention cohort were prescribed significantly fewer pills per prescription (21 vs. 64; $p < .001$). The authors concluded that a simple practice change of utilizing APAP and NSAIDs is effective for analgesia after thyroid or parathyroid operations. They also noted that the study adds to existing evidence that opioid-free surgeries may be possible even in environments with high baseline opioid utilization.

While the use of both NSAIDs and APAP could be considered in multimodal approaches, more investigation to refine multimodal pathways has been underway. A review of perioperative multimodal nonopioid alternatives for sinus and skull base surgery demonstrated that opioids should be reserved for breakthrough pain management.[36] Short-acting opioids are preferred over long-acting opioids for acute pain and the lowest reasonable dose to adequately control pain should be used to decrease misuse and overdose. Sinus surgery algorithms should begin with a preoperative assessment for medical and psychiatric comorbidities, medication review, history of chronic pain or substance abuse, postpostoperative pain plan, and checking the prescription drug monitoring program. Preoperative pain control should begin with anesthesia and the use of preoperative APAP, gabapentinoids, and α-2 agonists. Intraoperative pain control should involve tissue infiltration/nerve block with a local anesthetic. Postoperative pain control should include scheduled IV/PO APAP, scheduled IV/PO NSAIDs, a gabapentinoid, and oral opioids only for breakthrough pain. Discharge medication regimens should include scheduled APAP and NSAID, and if opioids are necessary the smallest dose and duration necessary should be used. Traditional NSAIDs utilized are ibuprofen, ketorolac, and celecoxib. Gabapentin is the most commonly used gabapentinoid.

An evidence-based review evaluated the studies behind specific multimodal agents and the benefit-harm assessment of their use in endoscopic sinus surgery.[37] The review utilized many elements of a Cochrane review. A total of 32 studies with 1812 patients were included in the review. APAP has a preponderance of benefit over harm and may adequately control postoperative pain and reduce the immediate need for opioid rescue. NSAIDs require consideration of benefit versus harm as many patients undergoing sinus surgery have asthma or nasal polyposis and are NSAID intolerant. They may also help reduce postoperative opioid consumption and manage mild-to-moderate pain. α-2 agonists, such as dexmedetomidine or clonidine, also require careful analysis of benefit versus harm as there is a possibility of hypotension, bradycardia, and dry mouth. Their use has been associated with reduced anesthetic requirements and can help with anxiolysis, sedation, and attenuation of sympathoadrenal response to laryngoscopy and intubation as well as postoperative analgesia. Regional sinonasal analgesia via a peripheral nerve block or local anesthetic-soaked sinus packs also have a preponderance of benefit over harm. They can reduce the need for any additional rescue analgesia, have a quick onset, and are simple to administer. Finally, gabapentin also has a preponderance of benefit over harm and also has a role in the treatment of chronic pain. In conclusion, the authors recommend scheduling agents rather than prescribing "as-needed" administration can increase efficacy, especially with medications such as APAP.

Conclusion

In light of the growing opioid epidemic in the United States, the need to find new ways to manage pain while minimizing opioid use and prescribing is greater than ever. Multimodal pain management strategies are one avenue for combating this problem. As demonstrated in this chapter, the use of nonopioid analgesic combinations has the potential to improve perioperative pain management and decrease opioid utilization. However, definitive conclusions on the optimal combination, dosing, and duration of medications cannot be made due to a paucity of high-quality data. There is a continued need for more large-scale, well-designed clinical studies to evaluate pain management using robust multimodal focused perioperative protocols to fill this gap in knowledge.

References

1. Gray ML, Fan CJ, Kappauf C, et al. Postoperative pain management after sinus surgery: a survey of the American Rhinologic Society. *Int Forum Allergy Rhinol.* 2018;8(10): 1199–1203.
2. Manufacturer's Official Product Labeling (Package Insert) and Other Product Labeling.
3. Brunton LL, Knollmann Bïrn C, Hilal-Dandan R, Goodman LS, Gilman AG. *Goodman & Gilman's the Pharmacological Basis of Therapeutics.* 13th ed. New York, NY: McGraw Hill Medical; 2018.
4. Thung AK, Elmaraghy CA, Barry N, et al. Double-blind randomized placebo-controlled trial of single-dose intravenous acetaminophen for pain associated with adenotonsillectomy in pediatric patients with sleep-disordered breathing. *J Pediatr Pharmacol Therapeut.* 2017;22(5):344–351.
5. Roberts CA, Shah-Becker S, O'Connell Ferster A, et al. Randomized prospective evaluation of intraoperative intravenous acetaminophen in pediatric adenotonsillectomy. *Otolaryngol Head Neck Surg.* 2018;158(2):368–374.
6. Chisholm AG, Sathyamoorthy M, Seals SR, et al. Does intravenous acetaminophen reduce perioperative opioid use in pediatric tonsillectomy? *Am J Otolaryngol.* 2019; 40(6):102294.
7. Tyler MA, Lam K, Ashoori F, et al. Analgesic effects of intravenous acetaminophen vs placebo for endoscopic sinus surgery and postoperative pain: a randomized clinical trial. *JAMA Otolaryngol Head Neck Surg.* 2017;143(8):788–794.
8. Kemppainen T, Kokki H, Tuomilehto H, et al. Acetaminophen is highly effective in pain treatment after endoscopic sinus surgery. *Laryngoscope.* 2006;116(12):2125–2128.
9. Koteswara CM DS. A study on pre-emptive analgesic effect of intravenous paracetamol in functional endoscopic sinus surgeries (FESSs): a randomized, double-blinded clinical study. *J Clin Diagn Res.* 2014;8(1):108–111.
10. Kemppainen TP, Tuomilehto H, Kokki H, et al. Pain treatment and recovery after endoscopic sinus surgery. *Laryngoscope.* 2007;117(8):1434–1438.
11. Moir MS, Bair E, Shinnick P, et al. Acetaminophen versus acetaminophen with codeine after pediatric tonsillectomy. *Laryngoscope.* 2000;110(11):1824–1827.

12. Laporta ML, O'Brien EK, Stokken JK, et al. Anesthesia management and postanesthetic recovery following endoscopic sinus surgery. *Laryngoscope*. 2021;131(3):E815–E820.

13. Campbell HT, Yuhan BT, Smith B, et al. Perioperative analgesia for patients undergoing otologic surgery: an evidence-based review. *Laryngoscope*. 2020;130(1):190–199.

14. U.S. Food and Drug Administration: Drug Safety Communications. Safety review update of codeine use in children: new boxed warning and contraindications on use after tonsillectomy and/or adenoidectomy. *FDA*; February 20, 2013:1–4. Accessed https://www.fda.gov/media/85072/download. Accessed April 22, 2021.

15. Lexicomp [internet database]. Hudson, OH: Wolters Kluwer. Updated periodically. Accessed April 11, 2021.

16. Liu C, Ulualp S. Outcomes of an alternating ibuprofen and acetaminophen regimen for pain relief after tonsillectomy in children. *Ann Otol Rhinol Laryngol*. 2015;124(10):777–781.

17. Merry AF, Gibbs RD, Edwards J, et al. Combined Acetaminophen and ibuprofen for pain relief after oral surgery in adults: a randomized controlled trial. *Br J Anaesth*. 2010;104(1):80–88.

18. Kamarauskas A, Dahl MR, Hlidarsdottir T, et al. Need for better analgesic treatment after tonsillectomy in ear, nose and throat practices. *Dan Med J*. 2013;60(5):A4639.

19. Adler AC, Mehta DK, Messner AH, et al. Parental assessment of pain control following pediatric adenotonsillectomy: do opioids make a difference? *Int J Pediatr Otorhinolaryngol*. 2020;134:110045.

20. Brady JT, Dreimiller A, Miller-Spalding S, et al. Are narcotic pain medications necessary after discharge following thyroidectomy and parathyroidectomy? *Surgery*. 2021;169(1):202–208.

21. Carpenter PS, Shepherd HM, McCrary H, et al. Association of celecoxib use with decreased opioid requirements after head and neck cancer surgery with free tissue reconstruction. *JAMA Otolaryngol Head Neck Surg*. 2018;144(11):988–994.

22. Motov S, Yasavolian M, Likourezos A, et al. Comparison of intravenous ketorolac at three single-dose regimens for treating acute pain in the emergency department: a randomized controlled trial. *Ann Emerg Med*. 2017;70(2):177–184.

23. Bhatt DL, Scheiman J, Abraham NS, et al. ACCF/ACG/AHA 2008 expert consensus document on reducing the gastrointestinal risks of antiplatelet therapy and NSAID use: a report of the American college of cardiology foundation task force on clinical expert consensus documents. *J Am Coll Cardiol*. 2008;52(18):1502–1517.

24. Lanza FL, Chan FK, Quigley EM. Guidelines for prevention of NSAID-related ulcer complications: practice parameters committee of the American College of Gastroenterology. *Am J Gastroenterol*. 2009;104(3):728. Epub 2009 Feb 24.

25. Radley DC, Finkelstein SN, Stafford RS. Off-label prescribing among office-based physicians. *Arch Intern Med*. 2006;166:1021–1026.

26. Verret M, Lauzier F, Zarychanski R, et al. Perioperative use of gabapentinoids for the management of postoperative acute pain: a systematic review and meta-analysis [published correction appears in Anesthesiology. 2020 Aug 21;:null] *Anesthesiology*. 2020;133(2):265–279.

27. Sanders JG, Dawes PJ. Gabapentin for perioperative analgesia in otorhinolaryngology-head and neck surgery: systematic review. *Otolaryngol Head Neck Surg*. 2016;155(6):893–903.

28. Gill KS, Chitguppi C, Haggerty M, et al. Assessment of narcotic use in management of post-op pain after functional endoscopic sinus surgery. *Laryngoscope Investig Otolaryngol.* 2021;6(1):42–48.

29. Townsend M, Liou T, Kallogjeri D, et al. Effect of perioperative gabapentin use on postsurgical pain in patients undergoing head and neck mucosal surgery: a randomized clinical trial. *JAMA Otolaryngol Head Neck Surg.* 2018;144(11):959–966.

30. Lee TS, Wang LL, Yi DI, et al. Opioid sparing multimodal analgesia treats pain after head and neck microvascular reconstruction. *Laryngoscope.* 2020;130(7):1686–1691.

31. Hwang SH, Park IJ, Cho YJ, et al. The efficacy of gabapentin/pregabalin in improving pain after tonsillectomy: a meta-analysis. *Laryngoscope.* 2016;126(2):357–366.

32. Amin SM, Amr YM. Comparison between preemptive gabapentin and paracetamol for pain control after adenotonsillectomy in children. *Anesth Essays Res.* 2011;5(2): 167–170.

33. Rezaeian A. Administering of pregabalin and APAP on management of postoperative pain in patients with nasal polyposis undergoing functional endoscopic sinus surgery. *Acta Otolaryngol.* 2017;137(12):1249–1252.

34. Haddadi S, Marzban S, Parvizi A, et al. Effects of gabapentin suspension and rectal APAP on postoperative pain of adenotonsillectomy in children. *Iran J Otorhinolaryngol.* 2020;32(111):197–205.

35. Oyler DR, Randle RW, Lee CY, et al. Implementation of opioid-free thyroid and parathyroid procedures: a single center experience. *J Surg Res.* 2020;252:169–173.

36. Nguyen BK, Svider PF, Hsueh WD, et al. Perioperative analgesia for sinus and skull-base surgery. *Otolaryngol Clin.* 2020;53(5):789–802.

37. Svider PF, Nguyen B, Yuhan B, et al. Perioperative analgesia for patients undergoing endoscopic sinus surgery: an evidence-based review. *Int Forum Allergy Rhinol.* 2018; 8(7):837–849.

Addiction management in the outpatient setting

9

Julia M. Shi, MD, FACP [1,2]**, Benjamin J. Slocum, DO** [3]**,**
Jeanette M. Tetrault, MD, FACP, FASAM [4]**, Ken Yanagisawa, MD, FACS** [5,6,7,8]

[1]*Medical Director, Primary Care Services, APT Foundation, New Haven, CT, United States;*
[2]*Associate Clinical Professor of Medicine, Yale University School of Medicine, New Haven, CT,*
United States; [3]*Family Medicine, Central Maine Healthcare, Gray, ME, United States;* [4]*Professor*
of Medicine and Public Health, Vice Chief for Education, Section of General Internal Medicine,
Program Director, Addiction Medicine Fellowship, Associate Director for Education and Training,
Program in Addiction Medicine, Yale University School of Medicine, New Haven, CT, United
States; [5]*Managing Partner, Southern New England Ear Nose Throat & Facial Plastic Surgery*
Group, LLP, New Haven, CT, United States; [6]*Section Chief of Otolaryngology, Yale New Haven*
Hospital, New Haven, CT, United States; [7]*Associate Clinical Professor of Surgery, Yale University*
School of Medicine, New Haven, CT, United States; [8]*Assistant Clinical Professor of Surgery, Frank*
H. Netter MD School of Medicine, Quinnipiac University, Hamden, CT, United States

Introduction

Since the 1990s, the increasing incidence of opioid use disorder (OUD) and overdose deaths involving opioids have reached epidemic proportions. Rising use has been associated with both medical and nonmedical opioid use. While opioids are an effective form of analgesia for acute and postoperative pain, the overprescribing of opioids, in part, has contributed to the escalation of opioid overdoses in the United States.

In 1996, the American Pain Society advocated for progressive evaluation of pain control with "the fifth vital sign" assessment. Although well intentioned and supported by physicians, patients, and professional societies, it promoted the aggressive treatment of both acute and chronic pain, often with opioids to improve subjective numeric pain scores at the point of care. During a similar time frame, opioid prescriptions rose dramatically, as did nonmedical opioid use. Individuals in the United States consumed more opioid medication than all other nations worldwide combined.[1]

In 2013, the economic cost of prescription opioid-related overdose and OUD exceeded $78.5 billion with a large portion spent on healthcare, substance use disorder treatment, and loss of work productivity.[2]

By 2017, opioid-related deaths continued to increase, and the United States government declared a public health emergency related to opioid use.[2]

According to the 2019 National Survey on Drug Use and Health, 9.7 million people reported nonmedical use of prescription pain medicine. In an evidence-based consensus report published in 2019, an estimated 2.1 million people suffered from

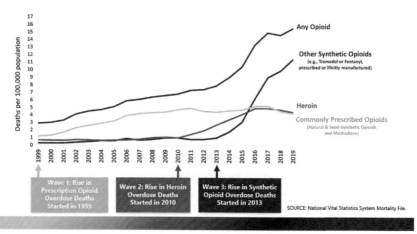

FIGURE 9.1

Three waves of the rise in opioid overdose deaths.

OUD, including 1.8 million with primary prescription opioid use and over 600,000 with primary heroin use.[3]

In 2019, more than 70,000 Americans died from a drug-involved overdose, including illicit drugs and prescription opioids. Synthetic opioids, primarily fentanyl, were the main driver of these drug overdose deaths with a nearly 14-fold increase from 2012 to 2019 resulting in more than 36,359 casualties.

The Centers for Disease Control and Prevention (CDC) summarizes the rise in opioid overdose deaths in three distinct waves in its publication, "Understanding the Epidemic" (Fig. 9.1).[4]

1. The first wave began with increased prescribing of opioids in the 1990s, with overdose deaths involving prescription opioids increasing since at least 1999.
2. The second wave began in 2010, with rapid increases in overdose deaths involving heroin.
3. The third wave began in 2013, with significant increases in overdose deaths involving synthetic opioids, particularly those involving illicitly manufactured fentanyl and its many analogs. Illicit fentanyl can be found in combination with heroin, counterfeit pills, and cocaine.

Many opioid-involved overdose deaths are associated with the use of multiple substances, including benzodiazepines, alcohol, cocaine, and methamphetamine.

There has been an ongoing public health crisis of infectious diseases driven by the opioid epidemic, including the transmission of the human immunodeficiency virus (HIV), hepatitis C, endocarditis, and infections of the skin, bones, and joints related to the rise of injection drug use. In addition to trauma and suicide risks, people with OUD have a 20-fold greater chance of early death.[5]

What is opioid use disorder?

OUD describes patients who have lost control and have a compulsion to use opioids. Physical dependence is the physical adaption to opioids characterized by symptoms

Table 9.1 Diagnostic criteria for opioid-use disorder.[a]

Use of an opioid in increased amounts or longer than intended
Persistent wish or unsuccessful effort to cut down or control opioid use
Excessive time spent in obtaining, using, or recovering from opioid use
Strong desire or urge to use an opioid
Interference of opioid use with important obligations
Continued opioid use despite resulting interpersonal problems, social problems (e.g., interference with work), or both
Elimination or reduction of important activities because of opioid use
Use of an opioid in physically hazardous situations (e.g., while driving)
Continued opioid use despite resulting physical problems, psychological problems, or both
Need for increased doses of an opioid for effects, diminished effect per dose, or both[b]
Withdrawal when dose of an opioid is decreased, use of drug to relieve withdrawal, or both[b]

[a] If two or three items cluster together in the same 12 months, the disorder is mild; if four or five items cluster, the disorder is moderate; and if six or more items cluster, the disorder is severe. Criteria are from the Diagnostic and Statistical Manual of Mental Disorders, fifth edition.
[b] If the opioid is taken only as prescribed, this item does not count toward a diagnosis of an opioid-use disorder.

of withdrawal when the drug is stopped and need to take more to get the desired effect. Physical dependence alone does not mean OUD. In fact, individuals who take opioids over a long enough period of time will develop physiologic dependence manifested by withdrawal and tolerance. The Diagnostic and Statistical Manual of Mental Disorders, Fifth Edition (DSM-5) criteria for OUD includes physical dependency, but differs as this is also characterized by the presence of cravings, compulsive use, and eventually loss of control, with continued use despite negative consequences from opioid use. Additionally, for patients prescribed opioids, physiologic dependence criteria should not be used in the diagnosis of OUD. The diagnostic criteria are summarized in Table 9.1.

Risk of developing opioid use disorder

OUD is considered a bio-psycho-social illness. Genetic factors, psychological factors, and social environments can place an individual at a higher risk of developing OUD. See Table 9.2. However, repeated opioid use alone can result in changes in neural structure and function and can change the brain's pleasure and reward pathways, leading to the development of OUD.

The likelihood of chronic opioid use after an opioid-naïve individual is prescribed an opioid medication has been shown to increase after as little as 3—5 days of opioid use.[9]

In a survey of individuals who use heroin, approximately 75% reported nonmedical use of a prescription opioid in the prior year, often obtained from a family members' prescription or from opioid diversion from another individual's prescription.[10]

Table 9.2 Risk factors for nonmedical opioid use.

Several reviews[6-8] have identified the most common risk factors for nonmedical opioid use:
- Young age
- Personal history of substance use disorder
- Use of other substances
- Family history of substance use disorder
- History of criminal activity or legal problems including DUI, incarceration
- Mental health disorder
- Frequent contact with high-risk people or high-risk environments
- Risk-taking or thrill-seeking behavior
- History of severe depression or anxiety
- Nonfunctional status due to pain
- Psychological stressors and/or traumas, in particular, preadolescent sexual abuse

A challenge that remains is the safe use of prescription opioids among surgical patients. More than 50 million Americans undergo inpatient surgery annually, and opioids remain a primary modality for postoperative acute pain management.[11]

Surgical patients routinely receive the most commonly prescribed opioids—oxycodone and hydrocodone—which are also the most commonly implicated in nonmedical use and drug overdose deaths.[5,12] Consequently, it is of the utmost importance that all medical providers who prescribe opioid medications adopt screening and safe prescribing practices.

The American Academy of Otolaryngology-Head and Neck Surgery Foundation's Clinical Practice Guideline on Opioid Prescribing for Analgesia After Common Otolaryngology Operations offers specialty-specific, evidence-based recommendations on the preoperative identification of OUD risk factors, and the postoperative management of pain, emphasizing prudent prescribing, storage, and disposal of opioids.[12]

Screening for opioid use disorder

Every clinical encounter is an opportunity to screen for substance use disorder, and this is especially important when considering prescribing opioid medication for acute or postoperative pain.

The screening, brief intervention, and referral to treatment (SBIRT) model is a useful technique to identify patients at risk of substance use disorders.[13] SBIRT is a comprehensive, integrated, public health approach to the delivery of early intervention for individuals with risky alcohol and drug use, as well as timely referral for treatment in those with substance use disorders. Primary care centers, hospital emergency rooms, trauma centers, and community health settings provide opportunities for early intervention before more consequences occur.

Screening

Ask every patient if they have any history of opioid use—prescribed or nonprescribed. A single question related to drug use (i.e., "How many times in the past year have you used an illegal drug or used a prescription medication for nonmedical reasons?") was found to be effective in detecting drug use among primary care patients. One or more times was considered a positive screen requiring further questioning.[14]

Brief Intervention

The goal of brief treatment is to raise awareness of the risky behavior, delegate responsibility to the patient for successful improvement, and advise on strategies for change. It is important to approach each individual with empathy and support and to encourage optimistic empowerment.

Referral to treatment

If there is a concern for OUD, then consider referring to an addiction medicine specialist or coordinating care with the patient's primary care provider.

A newer screening, treatment initiation, and referral (STIR) model (STIR for substance use treatment) also offers a clinically effective approach to the treatment of substance use in clinical care settings with initiation using medications.[15]

Training opportunities, resources, and treatment programs in addiction are available from the Substance Abuse and Mental Health Services Administration (SAMSHA).[16]

Safe prescribing practices

Pain following otolaryngological procedures can range from minimal to severe. Opioid prescriptions should be offered judiciously, with a high awareness for a preexisting OUD, and considerations for safe prescribing habits should be discussed to limit the potential for risk.

Patients who undergo otolaryngological procedures should be kept on limited opioids for postoperative pain control, or be treated with a nonopioid pain management modality if at all possible. Pain control and medication adherence should be assessed at appropriate postoperative follow-up.

Patients should be counseled on safe storage and disposal of opioid medications, as unused opioids can subsequently be diverted to nonmedical purposes by the patient, his or her family, or others who may have access to improperly stored medications. Studies have shown that the majority of patients kept their leftover pills in an unsecured location in their homes. Most patients were not given information on how to properly dispose of unused opioid medication.[9,12] CDC guidelines recommend disposing of unused opioids by dropping off medication at the community drug take-back program or your pharmacy mail-back program. Check with your local and state guidelines for any other options.[12,17]

Coprescribing naloxone with opioid medication is recommended to reduce the risk of opioid overdose. Naloxone comes in the following United States Food and Drug Administration (FDA)-approved forms: injectable, auto-injectable (Evzio), and prepackaged nasal spray. Instructions for administration should be reviewed with the patient and a household member, who may be assisting during the postoperative period.

Overview of opioid use disorder treatment

As with many chronic illnesses, treatment of OUD requires ongoing management and reduction of risks, rather than the attainment of a cure. Medication treatment of OUD is effective and enables people to counteract the disruptive effects on their brain and behavior and regain control of their lives.[18] Table 9.3 describes the goals of medication management.

An understanding of opioid clinical pharmacology, especially the affinity for specific receptors and anticipated analgesic effects, is necessary for the selection of the appropriate opioid and nonopioid medication for pain management.[19,20] Different opioid classes have different pharmacologic effects on intrinsic opioid receptor activity with increasing doses. These classes are as follows: full opioid agonists, partial opioid agonists, and opioid antagonists (Fig. 9.2).

- Full opioid agonists are substances that bind tightly to the opioid receptor and undergo a significant conformational change to produce a maximal effect. Examples of full opioid agonists include codeine, hydrocodone, oxycodone, morphine, methadone, fentanyl, and heroin.
- Partial opioid agonists are substances that cause less conformational change and receptor activation than full agonists. Examples of partial agonists include buprenorphine and pentazocine.

Table 9.3 Goals of medication for treatment of opioid use disorder.

- Alleviate physical withdrawal
- Opioid blockade
- Reducing opioid cravings
- Normalize altered brain changes and physiology
- In patients with concurrent pain, to stabilize pain
- Reduce return to use and risks of fatal overdose
- Restore functionality
- Improve quality of life
- Reintegrate into families and communities

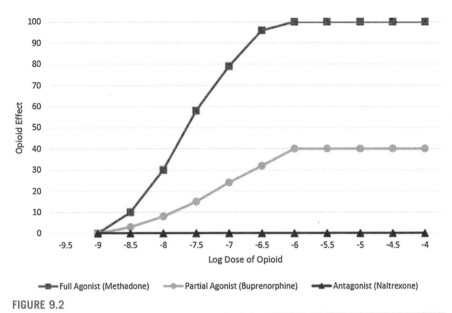

FIGURE 9.2

Pharmacological effects on intrinsic opioid receptor activity with different opioid classes.

- Opioid antagonists are substances that block the effects of opioids by competitive binding to the opioid receptor. Examples of opioid antagonists include naloxone and naltrexone.

In 2018, the National Institute on Drug Abuse and the SAMSHA commissioned the National Academies of Sciences, Engineering, and Medicine (the National Academies) with developing a Consensus Study Report to update the current knowledge on medication-based treatment for OUD and to highlight gaps for future research, policy, and service provision.[3]

A recent consensus report showed that medications are undeniably the most effective way to treat OUD, reducing the likelihood of overdose death by up to three-fold. Combining opioid agonist medications with behavioral health counseling may offer the best treatment outcomes of OUD.[3,5] Effective agonist medication used for an indefinite period of time is the safest option for treating OUD.

Opioid detoxification programs without continued pharmacotherapy have not been shown to have long-term efficacy for treating OUD due to low rates of retention in treatment, high rates of relapse posttreatment, and increased rates of overdose due to decreased tolerance after a period of abstinence.

Medications for opioid use disorder

Methadone, buprenorphine, and extended-release naltrexone are the three medications currently approved by the FDA for treating OUD. All three medications reduce opioid cravings and help to sever the ties between opioid use and established situational and emotional triggers. They all target the μ-receptor, though with distinct mechanisms of action and safety and efficacy profiles.[3,5,20] See Fig. 9.2.

Methadone

Methadone is a synthetic, long-acting, full μ-opioid receptor agonist, and as such, provides a sustained effect to reduce opioid cravings and withdrawal symptoms for more than 24 h. Methadone is 70%−80% bioavailable and metabolized by the CYP450 enzyme system. Methadone is a schedule II-controlled medication, and by law in the United States, outpatient methadone treatment can only be offered through state- or federally approved treatment centers. At initiating doses (20−30 mg orally), it alleviates all aspects of opioid withdrawal. The therapeutic dose may be achieved in 2 weeks or more, and at that dose (over 60 mg), it attenuates the euphoric "highs" of shorter-acting opioids, such as heroin and oxycodone. Patients enrolled in opioid treatment programs (OTPs) are required to have daily visits for supervised medication dispensing and regular counseling sessions with close monitoring. Eventually, stable patients may receive take-home doses if they meet certain criteria, such as stable periods without any illicit drug use.

Like all agonists, patients treated with methadone will have opioid tolerance and physical dependence, thus missing doses can cause opioid withdrawal. Methadone, even at a low dose, can be fatal to opioid-naïve individuals. Overdose risk is highest during the first 2 weeks of methadone induction, after which the risk of overdose death is significantly lower than for those with OUD and not in treatment. At the stabilization dose, the main effect of blocking or blunting the euphoria from other self-administered opioids usually deters from continued illicit opioid use. Recent high-potency fentanyl analogs have increased the risk of overdose in those with OUD, including patients taking methadone.[17] Use of other sedatives, including benzodiazepines, will increase the risks of an overdose in individuals taking methadone. The other potential side effects include sedation, which is worst at its peak serum concentration (2−4 h), though its effects are gradually blunted with tolerance; hypogonadism with low testosterone; and prolongation of the corrected QT (QTc) interval, which may potentially lead to Torsades de pointes. Risk of QTc prolongation increases by dose, combination with other medications that prolong the QTc interval, and acute medical conditions, such as hypokalemia. Drug interactions, especially those metabolized by the P450 system, have to be considered.

Despite the strong evidence supporting methadone treatment, patients taking methadone remain highly stigmatized.

Buprenorphine

Buprenorphine is a high-affinity partial μ-opioid receptor agonist and weak κ-opioid receptor antagonist. As a partial μ-opioid agonist, buprenorphine does not fully substitute for full opioid agonists, such as heroin, on the μ-receptors, and thus has limited euphoric effect. It is effective in alleviating opioid withdrawal symptoms and reducing cravings. As a partial agonist, it also acts as a competitive antagonist for full opioid agonists, thus blocking the effects of other opioids. Additionally, buprenorphine has a ceiling effect, thus limiting the respiratory depression effects and the risk of overdose. It is a schedule III-controlled medication.

Buprenorphine has poor oral bioavailability and has no oral formulation. Coadministration of other medications that use the CY450 pathway can affect the rate of buprenorphine metabolism, though it has fewer relevant drug interactions than methadone.

Formulations of buprenorphine are typically combined with the short-acting opioid antagonist, naloxone, in a 4:1 ratio, which serves to discourage nonmedical use of the medication. When this combination medication is taken properly in its sublingual (Suboxone, Zubsolv) or buccal (Bunavail) formulation, the naloxone component of the medication does not absorb to reach bioavailable levels in the body. If this combination medication were injected intravenously, then the user would experience the opioid antagonist properties of naloxone, counteracting the effects of buprenorphine. The dose range of the buprenorphine component in the sublingual product is between 8 and 16 mg. The maximum daily dose of buprenorphine is 24 mg, as dosages above this amount have shown no clinical advantage.

Buprenorphine is also available in extended-release monthly subcutaneous formulation (Sublocade)[21] and biannual subdermal implants (Probuphine), both necessitating administration by a medical provider, which makes them more difficult to divert and theoretically increases treatment adherence. A clinical trial of CAM2038, a weekly buprenorphine injection, is underway.[22]

In the United States, buprenorphine can be provided at an OTP but is commonly prescribed in an office-based setting, such as a primary care clinic or community health center. Patients are seen and evaluated by trained providers, frequently at first, and then with reduced frequency as the treatment progresses. The prescription can be dispensed at regular pharmacies, and patients self-administer the buprenorphine, similar to other medications of chronic diseases. Since FDA approval of buprenorphine in 2002, physicians, nurse practitioners, and physician assistants were required to undergo training and obtain a waiver from the Drug Enforcement Administration (DEA) to prescribe. As of 2021, medical providers treating 30 or fewer patients with buprenorphine-based treatment do not require a special DEA waiver.

Similar to methadone, patients are physically dependent on this medication, and discontinuation can lead to withdrawal, though buprenorphine's withdrawal syndrome may be less severe than that of methadone or other opioids. The most prominent risk of administering buprenorphine to a patient with OUD is the precipitation of nonlife-threatening opioid withdrawal at the first dose (induction). In general, induction of buprenorphine will require the patient to be in a mild-to-moderate withdrawal after opioid abstinence for 8−24 h, to minimize precipitated symptoms. Newer protocols such as buprenorphine-naloxone "microdosing" (Bernese method)[23,24] offer an alternative induction approach for the treatment of OUD in the wake of increasingly potent illicit drug marketing and sales. Patients have consistently reported that the induction process is well tolerated, with a reduction or elimination of cravings and avoidance of precipitated withdrawal.

With the initiation of buprenorphine treatment, the risks of opioid overdose-related death immediately decline. Hypogonadotropic effects are less with buprenorphine than with methadone. Buprenorphine is not associated with QTc prolongation or cardiac arrhythmia.

Extended-release naltrexone

Naltrexone is not an opioid, but rather a μ-opioid receptor full antagonist that blocks the euphoric and analgesic effects of opioids and helps maintain abstinence from opioids in highly motivated patients.

Naltrexone can be administered as an intramuscular injection for OUD (XR Naltrexone) or as an oral pill (FDA approved for alcohol use disorder). The intramuscular injection causes a transient peak blood concentration 2 h after injection and then another at 2—3 days after injection. After sustained use of extended-release (XR) Naltrexone, the patient's drug cravings decline. Treatment initiation of XR Naltrexone requires medically supervised withdrawal followed by at least 4—7 days without any opioids, including methadone or buprenorphine. This remains a key barrier to its popular use. The risk of overdose for patients being treated with the XR formulation may be reduced compared to treatment with a placebo, nonmedication-based treatments, and treatment with oral naltrexone. It is not uncommon for patients to try to use opioids while on extended-release naltrexone, but it is exceedingly rare that using any opioid can override the effect of naltrexone to yield any rewarding effects. Patients can experience an increased risk of overdose when they approach the end of the 28-day period of the XR formulation. The once-a-day 50 mg oral tablet was found to be no better than a placebo in retaining patients in treatment or eliminating opioid use, with a possible increased risk of opioid overdose compared to methadone if a user attempted an opioid challenge. This observation requires further validation.[25] Thus, the FDA only approved the injectable XR formulation (380 mg) for OUD treatment given on a monthly basis. No special training is required for medical providers to prescribe naltrexone. XR Naltrexone treatment is most effective when administered in combination with cognitive-behavioral therapy (Table 9.4).

Naloxone

The opioid antagonist naloxone is not a medication for OUD, but it is approved by the FDA to diagnose and treat the respiratory depressive symptoms of opioid use in a potentially fatal overdose. Naloxone is safe and effective, and it is the standard medication administered to reverse opioid overdose.

It is available in injectable and intranasal formulations. Guidance from the United States Department of Health and Human Services urges that all patients receiving medications for OUD be coprescribed naloxone.

Table 9.4 Comparison of medications for OUD.

Medication	Methadone	Buprenorphine	Naltrexone
Mechanism of action at μ-opioid receptor	Agonist	Partial agonist	Antagonist
Phase of treatment	Medically supervised withdrawal, maintenance therapy	Medically supervised withdrawal, maintenance therapy	Prevention of relapse following medically supervised withdrawal
Route of administration	Oral	Sublingual tablet/film, buccal film, subcutaneous extended-release injection, subdermal implant	Oral, intramuscular extended release
Possible adverse effects	Constipation, sedation, respiratory depression, sexual dysfunction, hypotension, QT prolongation, neonatal opioid withdrawal syndrome, nonmedical use potential	Constipation, fatigue, nausea, precipitated opioid withdrawal, respiratory depression (particularly if combined with benzodiazepines or other CNS depressants) neonatal opioid withdrawal syndrome, nonmedical use potential. Subcutaneous injection: injection site itching, pain, death from intravenous injection. Implant: nerve damage during insertion/removal, local migration or protrusion, accidental overdose or nonprescribed use if extruded.	Nausea, anxiety, depression, suicidality, insomnia, precipitated opioid withdrawal, dizziness/syncope, sedation, appetite changes, hepatotoxicity, vulnerability to opioid overdose. Intramuscular: Pain, swelling, induration (including some cases requiring surgical intervention).
Regulations and availability	Schedule II; only available at federally certified OTPs and the acute inpatient hospital setting for OUD treatment	Schedule III; requires waiver to prescribe outside OTPs (when treating more than 30 patients). Subcutaneous injection: healthcare setting and pharmacies must be certified in the sublocade risk evaluation and mitigation strategy (REMS) program and only dispense the medication directly to a provider to administration. Implant: prescribed must be certified in the probuphine REMS program. Providers who wish to insert/remove implants are required to obtain special training and certification in the REMS program.	Not a scheduled medication; not included in OTP regulations; requires prescription; office-based treatment or specialty substance use treatment programs including OTPs

Evidence on the effectiveness of FDA-approved medications in treatment for OUD[3]

Patients with OUD in long-term treatment with methadone or buprenorphine have a mortality reduction of approximately 50%, decreased risk of both all-cause and overdose-related mortality, reduced overdose deaths, lower rates of other opioid use, improved social functioning, decreased injection drug use, reduced HIV transmission risk behaviors, reduced risk of hepatitis C virus infection, and better quality of life compared to those not in OUD treatment. Methadone is also associated with reduced levels of criminality for individuals. In pregnant women with OUD, methadone maintenance is the standard of care, while buprenorphine treatment has been linked to improved maternal and fetal outcomes.

Considerations for special populations
Pregnancy in women with OUD[3,26]

Methadone and buprenorphine are widely used in the treatment of pregnant women with OUD to reduce opioid use and improve retention. Methadone is historically the standard of care for pregnancy. The use of buprenorphine (without naloxone) may be preferred to methadone, as it is associated with a shorter treatment duration and less medications needed to treat neonatal opiate withdrawal syndrome. Breastfeeding is encouraged while a patient is taking buprenorphine[26,27] or methadone,[28] as the exposure of infants to buprenorphine or methadone is minimal, and the benefits of breastfeeding outweigh the risks. Despite the standard of care, medication treatment is still underused for patients with OUD during pregnancy, which may be attributed to the stigmatization of OUD in pregnancy and childcare.

Psychiatric comorbidities

In 2018, National Survey on Drug Use and Health[29] reported that substance use was more common among both adolescent and adults who had a mental health issue than those who did not. 9.2 million adults (3.7% of all adults) had both acute mental illness and substance use disorder. Common comorbid psychiatric conditions for patients with OUD include major depression, anxiety disorders, posttraumatic stress disorder, antisocial personality disorder, borderline personality disorder, and other substance use disorders. A combination of the comorbidities is associated with poorer outcomes, though the treatment of these comorbid psychiatric conditions may improve treatment, psychosocial, and functional outcomes.[3]

People of color

The rate of overdose deaths among Black individuals in the United States has been rising.[30] There is a call to address the opioid epidemic within the Black/African

American communities.[31] There is significant historical mistrust of healthcare, social services, and criminal justice system in this population. It is critical to review the prevalence of opioid dependence in this population and to discuss the challenges to engage this population in their community for evidence-based prevention, treatment, and recovery.

Lesbian, gay, bisexual, transgender, and queer

There are limited studies examining opioid use disorders in the lesbian, gay, bisexual, transgender, and queer (LGBTQ+) population. This population appears to be at high risk for substance abuse, and work is underway to accurately identify opioid prevalence as well as effective means to engage and treat this population.[32,33]

Behavioral therapy in conjunction with medication treatment

At this time, evidence for behavioral interventions in conjunction with medication management for OUD is not conclusive. However, evidence-based behavioral interventions can be useful in engaging people with OUD in treatment and may improve retention, outcome, and quality of life.[3]

Postoperative management for individuals with history of opioid use disorder

Patients with a history of OUD may have pain that is more difficult to treat due to high opioid tolerance. Unfortunately, due to an ongoing stigma of addiction, these individuals are often labeled as "drug-seeking" when reporting acute or postoperative pain. As with the treatment of all postoperative pain, a multimodal approach to pain management should be provided, utilizing adjunctive medications, such as acetaminophen, nonsteroidal antiinflammatory drugs, neuropathic agents, topical analgesics, and regional anesthesia when appropriate. Opioid analgesic medications may be an appropriate option in the acute postoperative setting for an individual with OUD, whether or not they are currently being prescribed medications for OUD.

Pain management considerations for patients treated with medications for opioid use disorder

Acute pain management for patients on medications for OUD often requires coordination with addiction specialist or OTP, especially if opioids are required.[34,35]

Patients physically dependent on opioid agonists, including buprenorphine or methadone treatment, must be maintained on a daily equivalent opioid dose to avoid experiencing withdrawal. This maintenance requirement must be met before any analgesic effect for acute pain is observed with additional opioids.

Confirmation of the outpatient medication dosage with the patient's OTP provider or buprenorphine prescriber is the first step. If used for OUD, methadone is only provided by a federally qualified OTP. The dispensing of methadone is not accessible on the Prescription Drug Monitoring Program (PDMPs)—the electronic database that tracks controlled substance prescriptions. On the other hand, dispensing of buprenorphine is a class III drug and is included in the PDMPs with all the other controlled substances. States have implemented policies that require providers to check the state PDMPs before prescribing controlled substances. History of other controlled substance prescription or use, including benzodiazepines, opioids, and cannabis, may also affect the decision of pain management approach.

The management of peri-operative pain for any patient should involve a shared decision-making approach to make plans collaboratively and address individual concerns and expectations of the level of pain and care. A patient's OUD treatment provider can be a useful and critical resource during the preoperative and surgical risk evaluation, in particular, if opioid medications for acute pain are required.[36]

Any medication changes should be clearly communicated to the patient and outpatient provider at the time of postoperative discharge. Close surveillance and communication with the patient and providers are essential for successful postoperative pain control and optimal care management.

If prescribing an opioid for the treatment of pain, coprescription of naloxone is recommended.[37]

Patients taking methadone for treatment of opioid use disorder

The general approach to acute pain management in patients on methadone is similar to those patients on any other opioids on a chronic basis. The maintenance dose of methadone should be continued to meet the patient's opioid requirement. If the patient cannot take oral medication, parenteral methadone can be given (dose reduced to ½ the oral dosage). For mild acute pain, nonpharmacologic and nonopioid pharmacologic therapy should be maximized and is often adequate. If additional short-acting opioids are needed for breakthrough pain, then care should be taken to start low and go slow. Pain may be more difficult to control in patients who receive methadone because of the high affinity of methadone on the opioid receptor. These patients typically require higher doses of opioids (starting dose at oxycodone 10–20 mg) than opioid-naïve patients. For severe pain requiring intravenous opioids, close monitoring for respiratory depression and pain assessment is most important. In the outpatient setting, coadministration of methadone and short-acting opioid agonists poses an increased risk of overdose.

Methadone can prolong the QTc interval, and this should be taken into consideration if other agents with this effect are being administered in the peri-operative period, or if the patient has concerning cardiac conditions.

Patients taking buprenorphine for treatment of opioid use disorder

Buprenorphine is a partial agonist and has high affinity to the μ-receptor. Past recommendation of withholding buprenorphine for peri-operative analgesia was based on the concern that buprenorphine may block the effectiveness of additional opioids. With current reviews, there is no clear evidence that stopping buprenorphine or buprenorphine/naloxone during the peri-operative period is necessary or beneficial for the management of pain.[38–40]

One concern is that buprenorphine will counteract the effects of other opioid medications, however, despite buprenorphine's high affinity for the μ-opioid receptor, additional receptors remain available for a full opioid agonist to bind and provide effective pain relief if necessary.

Another concern is that coadministration of buprenorphine with full opioid agonists could induce precipitated withdrawal. This only occurs when buprenorphine is newly introduced to patients with already circulating opioids.

Temporarily discontinuing buprenorphine can introduce unnecessary complexity to a patient's treatment plan, placing the patient at risk of exacerbation of pain and opioid withdrawal, and predisposing the patient to return to use, relapse, or overdose if buprenorphine is not properly resumed.

In most cases, for patients with mild to moderate pain needs, the patient's total daily buprenorphine dose can be divided into three or four times per day dosing with possibly a dose increase to a maximum of 24 mg daily to provide the strongest analgesic effect. For patients with buprenorphine implants or receiving long-acting depot injections, the provider should proceed to full agonist opioids without any dose adjustment. Studies show that patients who continued buprenorphine experienced similar pain control, lengths of stay, and functional outcomes to controls with the addition of short-acting opioid medications; however, they may require higher doses of these medications to achieve adequate analgesia.[38]

For those with moderate pain, an advantage to continuing buprenorphine maintenance dose in the perioperative period is that this meets a patient's baseline opioid requirement while still allowing the use of additional short-acting opioid agonists as needed for pain. For these reasons, many institutions advise continuing buprenorphine at the same dose and adding short-acting opioid agonist medications like hydromorphone, oxycodone, or hydrocodone on an as-needed basis if indicated during the acute postoperative period, in conjunction with a defined plan to discontinue short-acting opioid agonists to avoid a return to use.

Some clinicians may hesitate to continue a buprenorphine prescription in the peri-operative period for fear they lack the necessary qualifications to prescribe buprenorphine in the inpatient setting. Clinicians do not necessarily require additional training or a special DEA waiver to administer buprenorphine to hospitalized patients. As of 2021, training requirements are limited to providers caring for more than 30 patients in the outpatient setting.

Ultimately, patient preference is extremely important in the management of both pain and OUD. After shared decision-making discussions, some patients may opt to hold buprenorphine in certain situations or consider alternative opioid treatment for pain. Creating such a mutually agreed upon pain control plan among the surgeon, OTP provider, and patient will bring about successful results.

Patients taking naltrexone for treatment of opioid use disorder

Acute pain management for patients who are taking extended-release injections of naltrexone can be challenging, as naltrexone occupies and blocks activation of μ-receptors, and thus blocks the effects of the opioid analgesic. The risks of side effects, especially respiratory depression, may be increased if opioid antagonism is overcome or is discontinued. Patients are at high risks of overdose with any opioid. Oral naltrexone may be discontinued 3 days before surgery, and XR formulation at least 1 month before surgery. If opioids are required while naltrexone is still in effect, close monitoring is necessary during opioid titration. Reinduction of naltrexone will require at least 7 days of opioid abstinence as active withdrawal may be activated.

Conclusion

Opioid overdose-related deaths continue to rise in the United States, posing serious public health risks. Prolonged opioid use alone can affect brain physiology and put one at risk of developing opioid use disorder. To reduce the incidence and consequences of an opioid use disorder, all medical providers, including otolaryngologists, should have the capacity to provide screening and referral to treatment. When opioid medications are being considered, it is important to adopt safe prescribing practices and discuss the risks of these medications.

For individuals with opioid use disorder, effective pharmacotherapy is available in the form of buprenorphine, methadone, and naltrexone-based treatment, often in combination with behavioral health counseling. Opioid agonist treatment alleviates symptoms of physical withdrawal, reduces cravings, normalizes altered brain physiology, provides opioid blockade, and reduces the risk of relapse and overdose.

Opioid medications may still be an appropriate option for the management of acute and postoperative pain, including for individuals with a known history of opioid use disorder or established in an OUD treatment program. A thoughtful approach to pain management, including shared decision making with the patient and collaboration with their addiction medicine specialist or outpatient provider, can optimize patient care.

References

1. Manjiani D, Paul DB, Kunnumpurath S, Kaye AD, Vadivelu N. Availability and utilization of opioids for pain management: global issues. *Ochsner J*. 2014;14(2):208−215.

2. Hedegaard H, Warner M, Miniño AM. *Drug Overdose Deaths in the United States, 1999−2016. NCHS Data Brief, No 294*. Hyattsville, MD: National Center for Health Statistics; 2017.

3. National Academies of Sciences, Engineering, and Medicine. *Medications for Opioid Use Disorder Saves Lives*. Washington, DC: The National Academies Press; 2019. https://doi.org/10.17226/25310.

4. CDC.gov. *Understanding the Epidemic*; 2021 [online] Available at: https://www.cdc.gov/drugoverdose/epidemic/index.html. Accessed April 15, 2021.

5. Schuckit M. Treatment of opioid-use disorders. *N Engl J Med*. 2016;375(4): 357−368.

6. Klimas J, Gorfinkel L, Fairbairn N, et al. Strategies to identify patient risks of prescription opioid addiction when initiating opioids for pain: a systematic review. *JAMA Netw Open*. 2019;2(5):e193365. https://doi.org/10.1001/jamanetworkopen.2019.3365.

7. Mayo Clinic. *Am I Vulnerable to Opioid Addiction?*; 2021 [online] Available at: https://www.mayoclinic.org/diseases-conditions/prescription-drug-abuse/in-depth/how-opioid-addiction-occurs/art-20360372. Accessed April 15, 2021.

8. Webster LR. MD risk factors for opioid-use disorder and overdose. *Anesth Analg*. 2017; 125(5):1741−1748. https://doi.org/10.1213/ANE.0000000000002496.

9. Shah A, Hayes C, Martin B. *Characteristics of Initial Prescription Episodes and Likelihood of Long-Term Opioid Use — United States, 2006−2015*. 2017.

10. Brummett CM, Waljee JF, Goesling J, et al. New persistent opioid use after minor and major surgical procedures in US adults. Published correction appears in JAMA Surg. 2019 March 1;154(3):272 *JAMA Surg*. 2017;152(6):e170504. https://doi.org/10.1001/jamasurg.2017.0504.

11. Hah JM, Bateman BT, Ratliff J, Curtin C, Sun E. Chronic opioid use after surgery: implications for perioperative management in the face of the opioid epidemic. *Anesth Analg*. 2017;125(5):1733−1740. https://doi.org/10.1213/ANE.0000000000002458.

12. Anne S, Mims J, Tunkel DE, et al. Clinical practice guideline: opioid prescribing for analgesia after common otolaryngology operations. *Suppl Otolaryngol-Head Neck Surg*. 2021;164(4):S1−S42. https://doi.org/10.1177/0194599821996297.

13. *Screening, Brief Intervention and Referral to Treatment (SBIRT) in Behavioral Healthcare. SAMHSA Report*; 2021. available at: https://www.samhsa.gov/sites/default/files/sbirtwhitepaper_0.pdf. Accessed April 15, 2021.

14. Smith PC, Schmidt SM, Allensworth-Davies D, Saitz R. A single-question screening test for drug use in primary care. *Arch Intern Med*. 2010;170(13):1155−1160. https://doi.org/10.1001/archinternmed.2010.140.

15. Bernstein SL, D'Onofrio G. Screening, treatment initiation, and referral for substance use disorders. *Addiction Sci Clin Pract*. 2017;12(1):18. https://doi.org/10.1186/s13722-017-0083-z. Published 2017 Aug 7.

16. Providers Clinical Support System. *An SBIRT Approach to Pain and Addiction - PCSS*; 2021 [online] Available at: https://pcssnow.org/event/an-sbirt-approach-to-pain-and-addiction/. Accessed April 15, 2021.

17. Cdc.gov; 2021 [online] Available at: https://www.cdc.gov/drugoverdose/pdf/aha-patient-opioid-factsheet-a.pdf. Accessed April 15, 2021.

18. National Institute on Drug Abuse. *Treatment and Recovery | National Institute on Drug Abuse*; 2021 [online] Available at: https://www.drugabuse.gov/publications/drugs-brains-behavior-science-addiction/treatment-recovery. Accessed April 15, 2021.

19. Painphysicianjournal.com; 2021 [online] Available at: https://www.painphysicianjournal.com/current/pdf?article=OTg3&journal=42. Accessed April 15, 2021.

20. Substance Abuse and Mental Health Services Administration. *Medications for Opioid Use Disorder. Treatment Improvement Protocol (TIP) Series 63, Executive Summary.* HHS Publication No. (SMA) 18-5063EXSUMM. Rockville, MD: Substance Abuse and Mental Health Services Administration; 2018.

21. NIDA. *Monthly Buprenorphine Injections Effective for Opioid Use Disorders.* National Institute on Drug Abuse; February 19, 2019. website https://www.drugabuse.gov/news-events/news-releases/2019/02/monthly-buprenorphine-injections-effective-for-opioid-use-disorders. Accessed April 15, 2021.

22. Clinicaltrials.gov. *Clinical Trial of CAM2038, Long-Acting Subcutaneous Buprenorphine Injections for Treatment of Patients with Opioid Dependence - Full Text View - ClinicalTrials.Gov*; 2021 [online] Available at: https://clinicaltrials.gov/ct2/show/NCT02651584. Accessed April 15, 2021.

23. Marwah R, Coons C, Myers J, Dumont Z. Buprenorphine-naloxone microdosing: tool for opioid agonist therapy induction. *Can Fam Physician.* 2020;66(12):891−894. https://doi.org/10.46747/cfp.6612891.

24. Randhawa PA, Brar R, Nolan S. Buprenorphine-naloxone "microdosing": an alternative induction approach for the treatment of opioid use disorder in the wake of North America's increasingly potent illicit drug market. *CMAJ (Can Med Assoc J).* 2020;192(3):E73. https://doi.org/10.1503/cmaj.74018.

25. Binswanger IA, Glanz JM. Potential risk window for opioid overdose related to treatment with extended-release injectable naltrexone. *Drug Saf.* 2018;41(10):979−980. https://doi.org/10.1007/s40264-018-0705-8.

26. Tran TH, Griffin BL, Stone RH, Vest KM, Todd TJ. Methadone, buprenorphine, and naltrexone for the treatment of opioid use disorder in pregnant women. *Pharmacotherapy.* 2017;37(7):824−839. https://doi.org/10.1002/phar.1958.

27. Jansson LM, Spencer N, McConnell K, et al. Maternal buprenorphine maintenance and lactation. *J Hum Lactation.* 2016;32(4):675−681. https://doi.org/10.1177/0890334416663198.

28. Glatstein MM, Garcia-Bournissen F, Finkelstein Y, Koren G. Methadone exposure during lactation. *Can Fam Physician.* 2008;54(12):1689−1690.

29. Substance Abuse and Mental Health Services Administration. *Key Substance Use and Mental Health Indicators in the United States: Results from the 2018 National Survey on Drug Use and Health.* HHS Publication No. PEP19-5068, NSDUH Series H-54. Rockville, MD: Center for Behavioral Health Statistics and Quality, Substance Abuse and Mental Health Services Administration; 2019. Retrieved from https://www.samhsa.gov/data/.

30. James K, Jordan A. The opioid crisis in Black communities. *J Law Med Ethics.* 2018;46(2):404−421. https://doi.org/10.1177/1073110518782949.

31. Substance Abuse and Mental Health Services Administration. *The Opioid Crisis and the Black/African American Population: An Urgent Issue. Publication No. PEP20-05-02-001. Office of Behavioral Health Equity.* Substance Abuse and Mental Health Services Administration; 2020.

32. Girouard MP, Goldhammer H, Keuroghlian AS. Understanding and treating opioid use disorders in lesbian, gay, bisexual, transgender, and queer populations. *Subst Abuse.* 2019;40(3):335−339. https://doi.org/10.1080/08897077.2018.1544963.

33. Moazen-Zadeh E, Karamouzian M, Kia H, Salway T, Ferlatte O, Knight R. A call for action on overdose among LGBTQ people in North America. *Lancet Psychiatry.* 2019;6(9):725−726. https://doi.org/10.1016/s2215-0366(19)30279-2.

34. Substance Abuse and Mental Health Services Administration. *Managing Chronic Pain in Adults with or in Recovery from Substance Use Disorders*. Advisory; 2021.

35. Quinlan J, Cox F. Acute pain management in patients with drug dependence syndrome. *Pain Rep*. 2017;2(4):e611. https://doi.org/10.1097/PR9.0000000000000611. Published 2017 July 27.

36. Veazie S, Mackey K, Bourne D, Peterson K. *Evidence Brief: Managing Acute Pain in Patients with Opioid Use Disorder on Medication-Assisted Treatment*. Washington (DC): Department of Veterans Affairs (US); August 2019.

37. Substance Abuse and Mental Health Services Administration. *SAMHSA Opioid Overdose Prevention Toolkit*. HHS Publication No. (SMA) 18-4742. Rockville, MD: Substance Abuse and Mental Health Services Administration; 2018.

38. Lembke A, Ottestad E, Schmiesing C. Patients maintained on buprenorphine for opioid use disorder should continue buprenorphine through the perioperative period. *Pain Med*. 2019;20(3):425−428. https://doi.org/10.1093/pm/pny019.

39. Mehta D, Thomas V, Johnson J, Scott B, Cortina S, Berger L. Continuation of buprenorphine to facilitate postoperative pain management for patients on buprenorphine opioid agonist therapy. *Pain Physician*. 2020;23(2):E163−E174.

40. Haber LA, DeFries T, Martin M. Things we do for No Reason™: discontinuing buprenorphine when treating acute pain. *J Hosp Med*. 2019;10:633−635. https://doi.org/10.12788/jhm.3265. Published online first August 21, 2019.

International perioperative pain management approaches

10

Catherine P.L. Chan, MRCSEd (ENT), MRes, MB ChB [1], **Jason Y.K. Chan, MBBS** [2]

[1]*Department of Ear, Nose and Throat, Prince of Wales Hospital, Shatin, Hong Kong SAR, China;*
[2]*Department of Otorhinolaryngology, Head and Neck Surgery, The Chinese University of Hong Kong, Shatin, Hong Kong SAR, China*

Introduction

Opioids were initially used for acute and cancer-related pain in the early 20th century. In a seminal campaign in 1996, the American Pain Society (APS) introduced "pain as the fifth vital sign" to address the issue of inadequate treatment of pain. Since then, opioid-class drugs were approved by the United States Food and Drug Administration (FDA) for pain management. Opioid therapy has hence been readily used internationally, not only for acute and cancer pain but also for chronic noncancer pain management.[2] Worldwide consumption of opioids for pain management surged by seven folds since the 1990s with an overprescription of opioids for pain management in the recent decades contributing to an opioid abuse epidemic in the United States.[3,4]

The Centers for Disease Control and Prevention estimated that there were approximately 450,000 death owing to opioid over-prescription, from 1999 to 2019.[5] In 2018 alone, there were close to 15,000 deaths due to opioid overprescription, comprising 32% of the 47,000 opioid-related deaths in total—equivalent to 41 deaths per day in 2018.[6]

A population-based statistical calculation of the total amount of opioid consumption per population of each country in 2019 illustrated that American and European countries, such as the United States and Germany, had an average consumption of narcotic drugs of 12,575—40,240 defined daily doses for statistical (S-DDD) purposes. This metric is defined as annual doses of opioids divided by 365 days, divided by the population of interest (in millions).[2,4] The consumption of opioids in Asian countries, in contrast, was low, ranging from 26 to 2409 S-DDD per million inhabitants per day.[4] According to the Central Registry of Drug Abuse in Hong Kong, the total number of reported drug abusers has declined by 4% in 2018. Nevertheless, there was an increasing number of young drug abusers (aged up to 35 years old), comprising 35% of all reported abusers. Tables 10.1A and B illustrate an overview of the prevalence of opioid use per country population, the average opioid consumption, and deaths related to opioid overdose and opioid use worldwide.[4,7]

Table 10.1A Overview on prevalence, opioid consumption and deaths related to opioid use in Asian countries[5,6].

Countries	Bangladesh	China	India	Japan	Philippines	Singapore	South Korea	Thailand	Vietnam
					Asia				
Prevalence (%) of opioid use in 2017 (relative changes between 1990 and 2017)	0.51% (+3%)	1.11% (−3%)	0.53% (+8%)	0.92% (+8%)	0.65% (−4%)	0.91% (+5)	0.91% (+9%)	0.85% (+13%)	0.69% (+13%)
Death from opioid overdose (number of deaths in 2017)	1,438,000	15,075,000	6,120,000	457,000	455,000	11,000	84,000	608,000	791,000
Direct death from opioid use disorder in 2017. Death per 100,000 individuals (relatives changes between 1990 and 2017)	2.55 (−10%)	1.28 (−57%)	0.93 (+29%)	0.33 (+237%)	0.68 (−49%)	0.25 (+126%)	0.22 (−23%)	0.93 (+92%)	1.21 (+50%)
Average consumption of narcotic drugs[a], in defined daily doses for statistical purposes (S-DDD) per million inhabitants per day (2015–17)	58	208	36	1413	26	577	2409	218	1883

[a] Drugs include buprenorphine, codeine, fentanyl, hydrocodone, hydromorphone, methadone, morphine, oxycodone and others.

Table 10.1B Overview on prevalence, opioid consumption and deaths related to opioid use in American, European and Oceanian countries[5,6].

Countries	America/Europe/Oceania					
	Australia	Brazil	Canada	Germany	United Kingdom	United States of America
Prevalence of opioid use in 2017 (%) and relative changes between 1990 and 2017	2.32% (+9%)	1.06% (+13%)	2.28% (+26)	0.88% (+15%)	1.66% (+13%)	3.45% (+46%)
Death from opioid overdose (number of deaths in 2017)	691,000	1,295,000	1,285,000	774,000	1,604,000	47,343,000
Direct death from opioid use disorder in 2017 death per 100,000 individuals (relative changes between 1990 and 2017)	4.05 (+83%)	0.98 (+116%)	4.95 (+258%)	2.06 (+27%)	4.23 (+191%)	18.75 (+802%)
Average consumption of narcotic drugs[a], in defined daily doses for statistical purposes (S-DDD) per million inhabitants per day (2015–17)	15,282	500	26,029	28,862	12,575	40,240

[a] Drugs include buprenorphine, codeine, fentanyl, hydrocodone, hydromorphone, methadone, morphine, oxycodone and others.

Motivation reviewing perioperative management in otolaryngology—head and neck surgery

Surgeons, after chronic pain physicians, were found to be the second most frequent prescribers of opioids. Almost every 4 out of 10 drug prescriptions for opioids were prescribed by surgeons.[8] Moreover, 10% of patients who were opioid naïve became long-term opioid users after being given opioids for short-stay low-risk surgeries.[9] Opioid naïve patients receiving postoperative opioid therapy were 44% more likely to become a long term opioid users in comparison to those who received nonopioid postoperative pain therapy.[9] A cross-sectional study at the University of Pennsylvania Medical Center showed a 6% prevalence rate of opioid prescription in otolaryngology-head and neck surgery (OHNS).[1] Inevitably, OHNS surgeons must take accountability for "opioid diversion," defined as nonmedical use of legally prescribed opioids, resulting in opioid misuse and overdose-related deaths.[10]

In this chapter, we will review international perioperative pain management approaches in OHNS. A preliminary search in MEDLINE was performed with combinations of the terms opioids and otorhinolaryngology to evaluate the relevant abstracts and establish the keywords in the main search. Relevant publications were identified through MEDLINE (1946 to April 2021), EMBASE (April 2021 via Ovid SP), and Google Scholar. The search used the following subject headings and keywords: opioid, otolaryngology, otorhinolaryngology, ear nose and throat, septoplasty, rhinoplasty, tonsillectomy, sinus surgery, ear surgery, adenoidectomy, perioperative pain, perioperative analgesia, enhanced recovery after surgery, and ERAS.

Overview of perioperative pain management globally

While surgery aims to remove pathological insults from the body, to repair and restore function, it creates another form of injury to the body requiring a subsequent healing process and rehabilitation. Surgical trauma has been shown to affect the immune response and thus hinder recovery, in addition to anesthetic effects, physical and psychological stress, and postoperative pain.[11] Beilin et al. highlighted the effects of postoperative pain optimization on attenuating surgery-associated immunosuppression in 2003.[12] Therefore, in the past two decades, activists worldwide proposed guidelines and protocols for perioperative pain management. In general, perioperative pain management is a structural pathway with both pharmacological and nonpharmacological treatments involving different healthcare parties including surgeons, nurses, anesthetists, pain specialists, or intensive care physicians before, during, and after the operative procedures. The APS and the American Society of Anesthesiologists compiled a guideline with evidence-based recommendations on perioperative pain management.[13] Similarly, the British and Australian counterparts published perioperative care guidelines such as the National Institute for Health and Care Excellence reviews for managing acute postoperative pain.[14,15] The principles of perioperative pain management include preoperative education, perioperative planning, application of different pharmacological and nonpharmacological modalities, organizational policies and procedures, and outpatient care planning.[13]

Preoperative counseling and education of patients and caregivers

It is recommended that patient-oriented, individually tailored education on options of postoperative pain therapy are provided to patients and their caregivers.[13] They should be counseled on the expectation of postoperative pain and reassured the pain would be monitored and optimally controlled with pain-relieving therapy. Active engagement of patients and caregivers for pain management reduces anxiety and corrects potential misconceptions about pain control therapy.[16] Safe use of opioids, proper storage, and proper disposal should be emphasized to avoid opioid diversion.[17]

Preoperative high-risk assessment

Preoperative evaluation should review medical comorbidities; current consumption of analgesics, opioids, psychiatric and anxiolytics drugs; social history including alcohol and substance abuse; and biopsychosocial assessment for pain. Any new prescriptions of opioids, benzodiazepines, sedative-hypnotics, anxiolytics, and central nervous systems depressants should be avoided before surgery.[18] It is particularly important in complex pain patients to avoid potential chronic opioid dependence after surgery.[19] If a high-risk case is anticipated, the patient should be referred to pain specialists for assessment.

Intraoperative preemptive analgesia

Studies have shown ongoing nociceptive stimuli increase the excitability of central nociceptive neurons, leading to central sensitization, lowering the activation threshold for pain.[20,21] Hence, the previously nonpainful low-intensity stimuli generates a painful sensation across the area of surgically injured tissue.[22] Preemptive analgesia hypothesizes that preoperative pain therapy before "preincision" stage may facilitate postoperative pain control when compared with the same analgesia given after the surgery.[23] The use of multimodal analgesia, for instance, paracetamol, NSAIDs such as celecoxib or ketorolac, gabapentin, or pregabalin—when given preoperatively—reduces postoperative pain scores.[13,15,17,19] While opioid-sparing perioperative therapy is suggested in opioid naïve patients, appropriate intraoperative opioid dosing should be administered in known chronic opioid-using patients to avoid acute withdrawal postoperatively.[18]

Postoperative pain assessment

Postoperative pain should be optimized before leaving the postoperative recovery bay to the ward or intensive care unit.[19] A validated pain assessment tool is recommended to monitor the response to pain management and to adjust the treatment plan accordingly.[13] Examples of validated pain intensity assessment scales include visual analog scales, numeric or verbal rating scales. In pediatric cases with nonverbal expression, the face, legs, arms, cry, and consolability five-item scale (each item scoring 0–2) is recommended for postoperative pain assessment during hospitalization.[24,25]

Postoperative multimodal analgesia and adverse effect monitoring

While single opioid use for analgesia could achieve postoperative pain relief, it has also been shown to have significant postoperative adverse reactions such as emesis and respiratory depression.[26] Systemic reviews recommend a multimodal analgesia regimen for postoperative pain control.[27] The European Society of Regional Anesthesia and Pain Therapy has proposed a procedure-specific postoperative pain management (PROSPECT) initiative with evidence-based recommendations for the treatment of pain across various types of operations.[28]

When postoperative pain control cannot be achieved by nonopioid analgesics such as paracetamol or NSAIDs, immediate-release and short-acting opioids should be offered to provide adequate pain relief.[13,19] Also, the oral route is preferred over intramuscular and intravenous routes for the administration of analgesics when the patients are able to tolerate oral intake.[13,14,17–19] If a parenteral route is needed, intravenous patient-controlled analgesia is recommended for systemic pain control. Nevertheless, routine basal infusion of opioids should be avoided in opioid-naïve adults.[13,14,18] When the patient receives opioid therapy, it is essential to monitor vital signs, level of consciousness, and respiratory status. Common side effects of opioids such as nausea and vomiting, and opioid-related constipation should not be overlooked. Additionally, the red flag warnings of opioid overdose—including excessive sedation, respiratory depression, and pinpoint sized pupils—should be recognized early and an opioid antagonist made promptly available.

Pain specialist consultation in high-risk cases

Some patients, in particular those who are opioid-tolerant, have substance abuse histories, or alcoholism, have a poor tolerance to postoperative pain despite the use of multimodal analgesia and opioids. It is recommended in these cases to refer or consult a pain specialist for interventional treatment.[13]

Transitioning to outpatient care

Recognizing the problem of illicit use of medical prescribed opioids, the Washington State Agency Medical Directors' Group (AMDG) provided a guideline of postoperative pain therapy on discharge depending on the extent of the surgery and expected progression of pain. AMDG recommended the use of multimodal analgesia with a plan for opioid tapering according to the length of expected recovery.[18] If minor surgery is performed and there is an expectation of minimal postoperative pain, it is suggested to discharge the patients with acetaminophen or NSAIDs only, or with a two to 3 day supply of short-acting opioids. Whether a patient is expected to have rapid recovery (Type 1), medium-term recovery (Type 2), or longer-term recovery (Type 3), acetaminophen and NSAIDs are still recommended as first-line therapy in postoperatively. In cases of severe pain, short-acting opioids should be prescribed with less than 3 day's quantity, 7 day's quantity, and 14 day's quantity respectively for type 1, type 2, and type 3 recoveries. For major surgeries, surgeons are responsible and are advised to taper the opioid use within 6 weeks.

Similarly, other guidelines have suggested opioid-sparing therapy or nonpharmacological therapy as first-line treatment and judicious use of opioid therapy for severe postoperative pain.[13,17,19] The emphasis of education on opioid dependence, the need of discontinuing opioid consumption after resolution of pain, prevention of opioid diversion, safe storage, and disposal of unused opioids are highlighted. Nursing consultation for patients and caregivers upon discharge, written instructions of recommended opioid dose, opioid supply and duration of use, and patient leaflets for opioid storage and disposal help to reinforce the cautious use of opioids after discharge.[13,23]

In pediatric cases, education to parents and caregivers on the appropriate use of analgesia is a large determinant of successful postoperative pain control in children. Parents' postoperative pain measure is recommended for parents to assess the severity of pain experienced by their children at home.[29]

Perioperative pain management in general otolaryngology—head and neck surgery procedures globally

Despite recommendations provided in the aforementioned guidelines describing the role of postoperative opioids, there is rarely clear guidance for perioperative pain management in procedures such as tonsillectomy, nasal surgery, and major head and neck surgery.

Tonsillectomy

Tonsillectomy is one of the most painful surgical procedures frequently performed by otolaryngologists.[30] The PROSPECT Initiative provides evidence-based recommendations for perioperative pain management after tonsillectomy.[31] There is strong evidence that NSAIDs should be administered preoperatively or intraoperatively and continued postoperatively. A single dose of intravenous dexamethasone given intraoperatively is highly recommended for postoperative analgesia and alleviation of postoperative nausea and vomiting. A Swedish group developed a national guideline for pediatric tonsillectomy-related pain management in 2012 and evaluated the effects in 2015.[32] Table 10.2 compares various global recommendations for perioperative pain management for tonsillectomies in both adult and pediatric groups.[31–34]

Table 10.2 Compares various analgesic protocols for tonsillectomy globally.

	Preoperative	Intraoperative	Postoperative	Discharge
PROSPECT[29]	• Combinations of paracetamol and NSAIDs at pre- or intraoperative period • A single intraoperative dose of IV dexamethasone		• Paracetamol (Grade D) • NSAIDs (Grade A) • Opioids for rescue (Grade D)	
Swedish guidelines[30]	• Paracetamol 40 mg/kg • Clonidine 2-3ug/kg • Betamethasone 0.2 mg/kg, max 8 mg	• Diclofenac 1 mg/kg IV/PR or • Ibuprofen 5–7 mg/ kg PR or • IV parecoxib 0.5 mg/ kg or • LA bupivacaine 5 mg/mL to wound 5 min	• IV paracetamol • Clonidine • Opioid titration • IV ondansetron 0.1 mg/kg, promethazine 0.1 mg/kg or droperidol 30ug/kg or • Regular panadol + NSAIDs/ celecoxib for 3 days	• Regular NSAIDs and paracetamol 5–8 days after tonsillectomy • Single dose clonidine, opioid (morphine/ oxycodone) PRN
French: SFORL[32]	-	• Dexamethasone (level 1 evidence) • Tramadol (1 mg/kg Q6H with vigilant use)	• Paracetamol (level 1 and 2 evidence) • Ibuprofen 5 mg/kg Q6H (level 1 and level 4 evidence)	• Paracetamol • Ibuprofen or tramadol
Australian: ANZCA[31]	• Gabapentin (10–20 mg/kg)	• Dexamethasone or • Peritonsillar infiltration of tramadol 2 mg/kg	• Paracetamol 15 mg/kg PO + diclofenac 1 mg/kg PO or • Paracetamol 15 mg/kg PO + Ibuprofen 4.5 mg/kg or • Paracetamol 30 mg/kg PO	
Hong Kong: Prince of Wales hospital	-	-	• Paracetamol 15–30 mg/kg PO Q4H • Ibuprofen 20 mg/kg/day PO TDS	

Other nonopioid agents were investigated for their analgesic benefits and side effect profiles. A systemic review of gabapentin for tonsillectomy did not find a statistically significant difference in postoperative pain in adult and pediatric populations at rest and during swallowing.[35]

Different research groups investigated the use of honey compared with peritonsillar injection of tramadol or as an adjunct with acetaminophen.[36–38] With honey, there was a reduction in pain in the first week of posttonsillectomy period when compared with the tramadol group; however, this did not reach statistical significance.[37,38] These findings may suggest that opioid analgesia does not provide a large incremental benefit.

Another study suggested the administration of low-dose ketamine intravenously with paracetamol just after adenotonsillectomy surgery in pediatric cases provides better pain control compared to paracetamol infusion alone. With low-dose ketamine there was better pain control at 0.5 and 6 h after the surgery, but no statistically significant improvement in pain control 12 h after the surgery when compared to acetaminophen infusion alone.[39] These studies also demonstrated the safety of ketamine analgesia, without a significant increase in common postoperative symptoms and signs such as nausea, vomiting, agitation, or sedation.[40]

Codeine, an opium alkaloid, is used for pain relief and as an antitussive agent. Codeine is converted into morphine via Cytochrome P450 2D6 enzyme. Although codeine was previously used for postoperative pain control after adenotonsillectomy, it was found that the use of codeine in pediatric patients could lead to rare but life-threatening adverse events or mortality in genetically susceptible children.[41] In 2013, the FDA issued a "Black Box Warning" and stated the use of codeine was contraindicated in all children below the age of 12 years. Hedenmalm et al. assessed the effectiveness of the codeine warning and observed a reduction in codeine prescriptions by 33%–84% to children younger than 12 years old in various European countries. In Germany, there was a continual decreasing trend in prescribing codeine after adenotonsillectomy from 0.4% to 0.6% in 2011 to 0.0% in 2015.[42]

Alternatively, Samba et al. compared opioids with nonopioid regimens for posttonsillectomy pain, showing a nonopioid regimen (acetaminophen and diclofenac) was at least as effective in pain control as the combined opioid drug regimens, without an increased risk in bleeding complications.[43] The treatment group with high-dose opioids and acetaminophen was found to be associated with poorer pain control and was almost five times more likely to seek emergency medical attention compared to the nonopioid regimen.[43]

Sinonasal surgeries

Sinonasal surgeries including rhinoplasty, septoplasty, endoscopic sinus surgery are common procedures performed by otolaryngologists. The intraoperative manipulation and bone work in addition to nasal packing postoperatively usually create postoperative pain, discomfort, and anxiety. However, there is no strong evidence for specific postoperative pain regimens adopted in sinonasal surgery, despite how common such procedures are. In one study otolaryngologists reported the number of opioid tablets prescribed, many stating the number dispensed was an arbitrary decision.[44] An average of 8.7 opioid tablets, only 36% of the total opioid prescription, were consumed by patients after rhinoplasty.[44] While otolaryngologists typically prescribed a standard regimen of 30 opioid tablets (5 mg of hydrocodone bitartrate and 325 mg of acetaminophen), studies showed 74%–89.5% of patients took fewer than 15 opioid tablets after sinonasal surgery.[44–47]

Raikundailia et al. reviewed the opioid consumption of patients after functional endoscopic sinus surgery (FESS), illustrating that 23% of patients required only nonopioid analgesics, and 45% of patients did not exceed usage of five opioid tablets within the first week of surgery.[48] The group also identified that patients who had bilateral FESS, received concurrent septoplasty and younger age tended to have increased opioid usage.[48]

Multimodal analgesia using NSAIDs, acetaminophen, preoperative use of pregabalin, and dexamethasone should be advocated to achieve satisfactory pain relief and reduce opioid consumption as well as postoperative nausea and vomiting.[15,49–51]

Otologic surgeries

In general, patients undergoing otologic surgeries such as external ear procedures, tympanoplasty, and middle ear surgery are categorized as having minor to intermediate procedures. With the improvement in camera systems and resultant resolution, endoscopic ear surgery offers a minimally invasive and low pain procedure. A study of the pain scores for microscopic and endoscopic ear surgeries showed the overall visual analog scale (VAS) pain score did not exceed four of 10. In fact, the highest pain score was reported after the retroauricular approach (3.17 of 10).[52] Most of the patients obtained satisfactory pain relief with paracetamol and NSAIDs and the average use of opioid tablets was taken 0–0.7 pills per patient.[52] Apart from pain, postoperative nausea and vomiting and vertigo increased patient fear and anxiety as well as the perception of pain. In pediatric patients undergoing myringotomies, intramuscular ketorolac was suggested to be an effective analgesic without significant postoperative emesis.[53] However, there was contradictory evidence suggesting the use of ketorolac showed no additional pain control over the use of paracetamol alone.[54,55]

While the extent of mastoid surgery and requirement of bone work is associated with higher pain intensity, regional anesthesia over the great auricular nerve distribution has been shown to have a comparable effect to intravenous morphine injection, and less postoperative nausea and vomiting events.[56]

Microlaryngology surgeries

Microscopic and endoscopic laryngeal surgeries are also common procedures performed by otolaryngologists. These short general anesthesia procedures usually generate minimal to mild pain with sore throat being the most frequent complaint.

These are often day surgeries or short stay procedures.[57] Taliercio et al. investigated the use of postoperative analgesics in direct microlaryngoscopy and found that 38% of patients did not require any form of pain medication and only around 13.6% required opioids for postoperative pain management.[58] Nevertheless, a cross-sectional survey revealed that 34% of otolaryngologists were still prescribing opioids for over two-thirds of the microlaryngoscopic procedures they performed.[46] As common laryngeal surgeries are considered to have minimal to mild pain postoperatively, multimodal and opioid-sparing analgesic regimens such as gabapentin preoperatively or acetaminophen and NSAIDs postoperatively are recommended.[46,59]

Major head and neck surgeries

Head and neck procedures including neck dissection, parotidectomy, thyroidectomy, major head and neck resection with or without reconstruction are associated with various degrees of pain and a wide range of opioid prescription practices for postoperative pain management.[60–63] It was observed that thyroid surgery had the lowest opioid use among otolaryngology—head and neck procedures.[64] Moreover, 69% of patients did not use the opioids prescribed at all.[61] The average pain scores found in thyroidectomy and parotidectomy peaked on postoperative day 1 with VAS 5.1/10 and 4.4/10, respectively, and trended downwards.[61] A study reported the pain mostly resolved in the fifth day of postthyroidectomy and less than 30 morphine milligram equivalents on average, that is, Four opioid tablets, were consumed by patients, while five times the average number of tablets used were prescribed.[65]

The opioid prescription pattern differs among various head and neck procedures. Higher opioid-based analgesics were given in major surgeries such as laryngectomy, neck dissection, and flap reconstruction.[63] Flap reconstructive surgery, for its large anatomical extent of surgery and complexity, increased the odds of prescribing opioids as postoperative pain therapy.[66]

Opioid use in perioperative pain management globally

Not only do the particular surgical procedures determine the opioid prescription patterns, but similar procedures performed in different global regions also show a serious variation in postoperative pain regimens. Li et al. evaluated the postoperative analgesic therapy of head and neck surgery patients between two academic institutions in Oregon, United States and in Hong Kong, China, illustrating a significantly lower rate of postoperative opioid prescription in the Hong Kong group (0.4%–1.6%) compared to that in the Oregon group (15.3%–86.8%) with comparable characteristics of diagnosis and head and neck procedures.[66] In addition, the nonopioid analgesic therapy prescribed between two groups was not statistically significantly different.

With more awareness on the opioid epidemic, opioid overprescription was described across various types of ear, nose, throat, and head and neck operations.

Among opioid naïve patients, there were 1.7—5 times overprescription of opioids compared to the actual quantity consumed, while there were 1.7—3.4 times overprescription in opioid exposed patients.[62] The unawareness of proper disposal and discontinuation of opioid medication has led to opioid misuse and diversion. The majority (72.2%) of patients kept the excess unused opioids in one study.[62] The overprescription of opioids might imply the surgeons' perception toward pain relief as an important cornerstone in shortening the recovery process. In view of this phenomenon, research groups advocate the adoption of multimodal opioid-sparing or opioid-reducing strategies for acute postoperative pain.[59] Kehlet et al. suggested that a mere provision of good analgesic effects after surgery had minimal effects on speed and quality of postoperative recovery[67]

As the ERAS Society was established in 2001, opioid-sparing multimodal analgesic regimen was incorporated in the development of the ERAS protocol in various surgeries. The ERAS principles underpinned the elements of a comprehensive multidisciplinary approach involving preoperative, intraoperative, and postoperative care to facilitate the recovery journey. With the complexity of head and neck oncologic surgeries, a consensus-based ERAS protocol concerning free flap reconstruction was assembled with the joint efforts of an international panel of expertise from Australia, Canada, Sweden, Switzerland, and the United States.[68]

One of the essential elements of providing a "fast-track" perioperative care is the implementation of a balanced multimodal analgesic therapy. This includes the use of nonopioid analgesics such as paracetamol, NSAIDs, gabapentin/pregabalin, and long-acting local and regional anesthesia.[15,69] This has been shown to reduce postoperative nausea and vomiting, facilitate the recovery journey, reduce postoperative comorbidities, and ensure adequate pain control with an opioid sparing regimen.[15,68,70] The benefit of opioid-sparing multimodal therapy does not only ascertain satisfactory pain control but also allows patients to achieve early enteral feeding, early mobilization, and improve ambulation to facilitate early discharge.[15,59]

Patient cultural backgrounds and perioperative opioid use

Li et al. presented the drastic difference in opioid prescribing patterns on similar head and neck procedures in the United States and in Hong Kong.[66] One of the contributing factors might be related to the pharmaceutical advertisement on underscoring the importance of pain relief with opioids but underemphasizing the addictive properties that worsened the opioid crisis. Also, the governments in eastern countries such as China and Japan historically feared the use of opium after World War II.[71] To date, despite the overall downward trend in substance abuse, the most common drugs abused in Hong Kong are still narcotics analgesics, mainly heroin. As opioid medication could only be obtained from the pharmacy of registered clinics or hospitals, the government emphasizes the harmful effects from opioids misuse and often publicizes the legal consequences through media and advertisement.[72]

The acceptance of pain intensity is also affected by culture and ethnicity. Japanese from the older generation believe in "gaman," a virtue meaning the enduring of unbearable suffering in silence. They are reluctant for opioid medication as pain intolerance requiring pain relief medication is considered "a very weak samurai (warrior)."[71] Another study reported African American children had higher postoperative pain scores after tonsillectomy, and thus required higher amounts of opioid medication compared to Caucasian children.[73]

Nonetheless, examples of postoperative pain therapy for major head and neck procedures by the Hong Kong group suggested the feasibility of rapid opioid discontinuation postoperatively and even complete nonopioid regimens to proactively reduce opioid utilization.[66]

Healthcare environments and perioperative opioid use

In consideration of the opioid epidemic, government policymakers and clinicians should adopt measures and education initiative committed to reducing opioid usage. A large national survey of the Medicare program was conducted and found 10% of Medicare beneficiaries became persistent opioid users, after previously being opioid naïve.[74] Surgeons are responsible for identifying high-risk patients and prescribe opioids with care. However, over 20% of otolaryngologists surveyed by the American Rhinologic Society reported to be "unsure if they were practicing evidence-based medicine" when it came to postoperative pain management.[75] Similarly, otolaryngology residents expressed their opioid prescribing patterns were mostly influenced by attending or senior preferences, while patient preference and fear of patient dissatisfaction were less influential.[76] This alarming result calls for standardized opioid prescribing education incorporated into otolaryngology residency training to establish a judicious use of opioids.

Conclusion

Pain is inevitable in the journey of life. The perception of pain could be influenced by physical, cognitive and emotional factors. Optimizing pain management after surgery reduces perioperative morbidities and surgical complications, shortens the length of stay, and also improves the efficiency and cost of care.[68] This chapter overviews the global approach of perioperative pain management in otolaryngology. In the opioid epidemic era, research support the use of multimodal and opioid-sparing analgesics to reduce potential opioid misuse. While otolaryngologists should ensure adequate pain control of our patients after operations, we should be vigilant of the adverse effects and consequences of opioid over-prescription. It is worth noting that appropriate perioperative pain management ideally would be a clearly outline algorithm with both pharmacological and nonpharmacological therapies and contributions from a multidisciplinary team. Patient education and the preparation for the surgical procedure, expectation of postoperative recovery pathways, and active involvement of patients and their love ones are paramount to responsible perioperative pain management in otolaryngology.

References

1. Jiang X, Orton M, Feng R, et al. Chronic opioid usage in surgical patients in a large academic center. *Ann Surg.* 2017;265(4):722−727.
2. Cheung CW, Chan T, Chen PP, et al. Opioid therapy for chronic non-cancer pain: guidelines for Hong Kong. *Hong Kong Med J.* 2016;22(5):496−505.
3. Cleary JF, Maurer MA. Pain and policy studies group: two decades of working to address regulatory barriers to improve opioid availability and accessibility around the World. *J Pain Symptom Manag.* 2018;55(2S):S121−S134.
4. *Board, I.n.c., Narcotic Drugs - Estimated World Requirements for 2019, Statstics for 2017.* United Nations Publication; 2019.
5. Center for Disease Control and Prevention, Drug Overdose Deaths.
6. Wilson N, Kariisa M, Seth P, Smith H, Davis NL. Drug and opioid-involved overdose deaths - United States, 2017-2018. *MMWR Morb Mortal Wkly Rep.* 2020;69(11): 290−297.
7. Roser M, Ritchie H. *Opioids, Cocaine, Cannabis and Illicit Drugs*; 2018. Available from: https://ourworldindata.org/illicit-drug-use.
8. Levy B, Paulozzi L, Mack KA, Jones CM. Trends in opioid analgesic-prescribing rates by specialty, U.S., 2007−2012. *Am J Prev Med.* 2015;49(3):409−413.
9. Alam A. Long-term analgesic use after low-risk surgery: a retrospective cohort study. *Arch Intern Med.* 2012;172(5):425−430.
10. Waljee JF, Li L, Brummett CM, Englesbe MJ. Iatrogenic opioid dependence in the United States: are surgeons the gatekeepers? *Ann Surg.* 2017;265(4):728−730.
11. Dabrowska AM, Slotwinski R. The immune response to surgery and infection. *Cent Eur J Immunol.* 2014;39(4):532−537.
12. Beilin B, Shavit Y, Trabekin E, et al. The effects of postoperative pain management on immune response to surgery. *Anesth Analg.* 2003;97(3):822−827.
13. Chou R, Gordon DB, De Leon-Casasola OA, et al. Management of postoperative pain: a clinical practice guideline from the American Pain Society, the American Society of Regional Anesthesia and Pain Medicine, and the American Society of Anesthesiologists' Committee on Regional Anesthesia, Executive Committee, and Administrative Council. *J Pain.* 2016;17(2):131−157.
14. Centre NG. *Perioperative Care in Adults [N1] Evidence Reviews for Managing Acute Postoperative Pain.* National Institute for Health and Care Excellence; 2020.
15. Schug SA, Scott DA, Alcock M, Halliwell R, Mott JF. *APM:SE Working Group of the Australian and New Zealand College of Anaesthetists and Faculty of Pain Medicine Acute Pain Management: Scientific Evidence.* 5th ed. Melbourne: ANZCA & FPM; 2020.
16. Relieving pain in America: a blueprint for transforming prevention, care, education, and research. *Mil Med.* 2016;181(5):397−399.
17. Commission, P.D.O.A. *Acute Care Opioid Treatment and Prescribing Recommendations: Summary of Selected Best Practices.* 2019.

18. Washington State Agency Medical Directors' Group (AMDG) in collaboration with an Expert Advisory Panel, A.P.P., Public Stakeholders, and Senior State Officials. *Interagency Guideline on Prescribing Opioids for Pain*. 2015.

19. Faculty of Pain Medicine of the Royal college of Anaesthetists. *Surgery and Opioids Best Practice Guidelines*. 2020.

20. Woolf CJ. What to call the amplification of nociceptive signals in the central nervous system that contribute to widespread pain? *Pain*. 2014;155(10):1911−1912.

21. Baron R, Hans G, Dickenson AH. Peripheral input and its importance for central sensitization. *Ann Neurol*. 2013;74(5):630−636.

22. Sandkühler J. Models and mechanisms of hyperalgesia and allodynia. *Physiol Rev*. 2009; 89(2):707−758.

23. Wall PD. The prevention of postoperative pain. *Pain*. 1988;33(3):289−290.

24. von Baeyer CL, Spagrud LJ. Systematic review of observational (behavioral) measures of pain for children and adolescents aged 3 to 18 years. *Pain*. 2007;127(1−2):140−150.

25. Voepel-Lewis T, Merkel S, Tait AR, Trzcinka A, Malviya S. The reliability and validity of the Face, Legs, Activity, Cry, Consolability observational tool as a measure of pain in children with cognitive impairment. *Anesth Analg*. 2002;95(5):1224−1229 (table of contents).

26. Van den Berg AA, Honjol NM, Prabhu NV, et al. Analgesics and ENT surgery. A clinical comparison of the intraoperative, recovery and postoperative effects of buprenorphine, diclofenac, fentanyl, morphine, nalbuphine, pethidine and placebo given intravenously with induction of anaesthesia. *Br J Clin Pharmacol*. 1994;38(6):533−543.

27. Curatolo M, Sveticic G. Drug combinations in pain treatment: a review of the published evidence and a method for finding the optimal combination. *Best Pract Res Clin Anaesthesiol*. 2002;16(4):507−519.

28. The European Society of Regional Anaesthesia and Pain Theraphy. *Better Postoperative Pain Management*; May 5, 2021. Available from: https://esraeurope.org/prospect/.

29. Chambers CT, Finley AG, McGrath PJ, Walsh TM. The parents' postoperative pain measure: replication and extension to 2-6-year-old children. *Pain*. 2003;105(3):437−443.

30. Gerbershagen HJ, Aduckathil S, van Wijck AJM, Peelen LM, Kalkman CJ, Meissner W. Pain intensity on the first day after surgery: a prospective cohort study comparing 179 surgical procedures. *Anesthesiology*. 2013;118(4):934−944.

31. Aldamluji N, Burgess A, Pogatzki-Zahn E, et al. *PROSPECT Guideline for Tonsillectomy: Systematic Review and Procedure-specific Postoperative Pain Management Recommendations. Anaesthesia*. 76. 2020.

32. Ericsson E, Brattwall M, Lundeberg S. Swedish guidelines for the treatment of pain in tonsil surgery in pediatric patients up to 18 years. *Int J Pediatr Otorhinolaryngol*. 2015;79(4):443−450.

33. *Acute Pain Management: Scientific Evidence*. 5th ed; 2019. Cited 25 May 2021; Available from: https://www.anzca.edu.au/news/top-news/acute-pain-management-scientific-evidence-5th-edit.

34. Constant I, Ayari Khalfallah S, Brunaud A, et al. How to replace codeine after tonsillectomy in children under 12 years of age? Guidelines of the French Oto-Rhino-Laryngology–Head and Neck Surgery Society (SFORL). *Eur Ann Otorhinolaryngol Head Neck Dis*. 2014;131(4):233−238.

35. Sanders JG, Dawes PJ. Gabapentin for perioperative analgesia in otorhinolaryngology-head and neck surgery: systematic review. *Otolaryngol Head Neck Surg*. 2016;155(6): 893−903.

36. Ozlugedik S, Genc S, Unal A, Elhan A, Tezer M, Titiz A. Can postoperative pains following tonsillectomy be relieved by honey? A prospective, randomized, placebo controlled preliminary study. *Int J Pediatr Otorhinolaryngol.* 2006;70(11): 1929−1934.

37. Hatami M, Mirjalili M, Ayatollahi V, Vaziribozorg S, Zand V. Comparing the efficacy of peritonsillar injection of tramadol with honey in controlling post-tonsillectomy pain in adults. *J Craniofac Surg.* 2018;29(4):e384−e387.

38. Boroumand P, Mahdi Zamani M, Saeedi M, Rouhbakhshfar O, Hosseini Motlagh S, Moghaddam F. Post tonsillectomy pain: can honey reduce the analgesic requirements? *Anesth Pain Med.* 2013;3(1):198−202.

39. Kimiaei Asadi H, Nikooseresht M, Noori L, Behnoud F. The effect of administration of ketamine and paracetamol versus paracetamol singly on postoperative pain, nausea and vomiting after pediatric adenotonsillectomy. *Anesth Pain Med.* 2016;6(1):e31210.

40. Erhan OL, Göksu H, Alpay C, Beştaş A. Ketamine in post-tonsillectomy pain. *Int J Pediatr Otorhinolaryngol.* 2007;71(5):735−739.

41. Kuehn BM. FDA: no codeine after tonsillectomy for children. *J Am Med Assoc.* 2013; 309(11), 1100-1100.

42. Hedenmalm K, Blake K, Donegan K, et al. A European multicentre drug utilisation study of the impact of regulatory measures on prescribing of codeine for pain in children. *Pharmacoepidemiol Drug Saf.* 2019;28(8):1086−1096.

43. Samba SRB, Noah S, Dworkin Valenti P. Adult post-tonsillectomy pain management: opioid versus non-opioid drug comparisons. *Arch Otolaryngol Rhinol.* 2020;6.

44. Patel S, Sturm A, Bobian M, Svider P, Zuliani G, Kridel R. Opioid use by patients after rhinoplasty. *JAMA Facial Plast Surg.* 2018;20(1):24−30.

45. Locketz GD, Brant JD, Adappa ND, et al. Postoperative opioid use in sinonasal surgery. *Otolaryngol Head Neck Surg.* 2019;160(3):402−408.

46. Huston MN, Kamizi R, Meyer TK, Merati AL, Giliberto JP. Current opioid prescribing patterns after microdirect laryngoscopy. *Ann Otol Rhinol Laryngol.* 2019;129(2): 142−148. https://doi.org/10.1177/0003489419877912.

47. Biskup M, Dzioba A, Sowerby LJ, Monteiro E, Strychowsky J. Opioid prescribing practices following elective surgery in Otolaryngology-Head & Neck Surgery. *J Otolaryngol Head Neck Surg.* 2019;48(1):29.

48. Raikundalia MD, Cheng TZ, Truong T, et al. Factors associated with opioid use after endoscopic sinus surgery. *Laryngoscope.* 2019;129(8):1751−1755.

49. Demirhan A, Tekelioglu UY, Akkaya A, et al. Effect of pregabalin and dexamethasone addition to multimodal analgesia on postoperative analgesia following rhinoplasty surgery. *Aesthetic Plast Surg.* 2013;37(6):1100−1106.

50. Rock AN, Akakpo K, Cheresnick C, et al. Postoperative prescriptions and corresponding opioid consumption after septoplasty or rhinoplasty. *Ear Nose Throat J.* 2019, 145561319866824.

51. Svider PF, Nguyen B, Yuhan B, Zuliani G, Eloy JA, Folbe AJ. Perioperative analgesia for patients undergoing endoscopic sinus surgery: an evidence-based review. *Int Forum Allergy Rhinol.* 2018;8(7):837−849.

52. Baazil AHA, Spronsen E, Ebbens FA, Dikkers FG, De Wolf MJ. Pain after ear surgery: a prospective evaluation of endoscopic and microscopic approaches. *Laryngoscope.* 2021; 131(5):1127−1131.

53. Pappas AL, Fluder EM, Creech S, Hotaling A, Park A. Postoperative analgesia in children undergoing myringotomy and placement equalization tubes in ambulatory surgery. *Anesth Analg.* 2003;96(6):1621−1624 (table of contents).

54. Rodríguez MC, Villamor P, Castillo T. Assessment and management of pain in pediatric otolaryngology. *Int J Pediatr Otorhinolaryngol.* 2016;90:138−149.

55. Rampersad S, Jimenez N, Bradford H, Seidel K, Lynn A. Two-agent analgesia versus acetaminophen in children having bilateral myringotomies and tubes surgery. *Paediatr Anaesth.* 2010;20(11):1028−1035.

56. Suresh S, Barcelona SL, Young NM, Seligman I, Heffner CL, Coté CJ. Postoperative pain relief in children undergoing tympanomastoid surgery: is a regional block better than opioids? *Anesth Analg.* 2002;94(4):859−862 (table of contents).

57. Okui A, Konomi U, Watanabe Y. Complaints and complications of microlaryngoscopic surgery. *J Voice.* 2020;34(6):949−955.

58. Taliercio S, Sanders B, Achlatis S, Fang Y, Branski R, Amin M. Factors associated with the use of postoperative analgesics in patients undergoing direct microlaryngoscopy. *Ann Otol Rhinol Laryngol.* 2017;126(5):375−381.

59. Cramer JD, Wisler B, Gouveia CJ. Opioid stewardship in otolaryngology: state of the art review. *Otolaryngol Head Neck Surg.* 2018;158(5):817−827.

60. Mom T, Bazin JE, Commun F, et al. Assessment of Postoperative Pain After Laryngeal Surgery for Cancer. *Arch Otolaryngol Head Neck Surg.* 1998;124(7):794−798. https://doi.org/10.1001/archotol.124.7.794.

61. Dang S, Duffy A, Li JC, et al. Postoperative opioid-prescribing practices in otolaryngology: a multiphasic study. *Laryngoscope.* 2020;130(3):659−665.

62. Pruitt LCC, Casazza GC, Newberry CI, et al. Opioid prescribing and use in ambulatory otolaryngology. *Laryngoscope.* 2020;130(8):1913−1921.

63. Bianchini C, Malago M, Crema L, et al. Post-operative pain management in head and neck cancer patients: predictive factors and efficacy of therapy. *Acta Otorhinolaryngol Ital.* 2016;36(2):91−96.

64. Kim M, Kacker A, Kutler DI, et al. Pain and opioid analgesic use after otorhinolaryngologic surgery. *Otolaryngol Head Neck Surg.* 2020;163(6):1178−1185.

65. Tharakan T, Jiang S, Fastenberg J, et al. Postoperative pain control and opioid usage patterns among patients undergoing thyroidectomy and parathyroidectomy. *Otolaryngol Head Neck Surg.* 2019;160(3):394−401.

66. Li RJ, Loyo Li M, Leon E, et al. Comparison of opioid utilization patterns after major head and neck procedures between Hong Kong and the United States. *JAMA Otolaryngol Head Neck Surg.* 2018;144(11):1060−1065.

67. Kehlet H. Multimodal approach to control postoperative pathophysiology and rehabilitation. *Br J Anaesth.* 1997;78(5):606−617.

68. Dort JC, Farwell DG, Findlay M, et al. Optimal perioperative care in major head and neck cancer surgery with free flap reconstruction: a consensus review and recommendations from the enhanced recovery after surgery society. *JAMA Otolaryngol Head Neck Surg.* 2017;143(3):292−303.

69. Kehlet H, Wilmore DW. Evidence-based surgical care and the evolution of fast-track surgery. *Ann Surg.* 2008;248(2):189−198.

70. Practice guidelines for acute pain management in the perioperative setting: an updated report by the American Society of Anesthesiologists Task Force on Acute Pain Management. *Anesthesiology.* 2012;116(2):248−273.

71. Times, T.N.Y. *Japanese Slowly Shedding Their Misgivings About the Use of Painkilling Drugs.*[September 10, 2007 May 09, 2021]; Available from: https://www.nytimes.com/2007/09/10/health/10painside.html.

72. Narcotics Division, S.B., Hong Kong S.A.R. *Government, Understanding Drug Abuse Problem.*

73. Sadhasivam S, Chidambaran V, Ngamprasertwong P, et al. Race and unequal burden of perioperative pain and opioid related adverse effects in children. *Pediatrics.* 2012; 129(5):832−838.

74. Santosa KB, Hu HM, Brummett CM, et al. New persistent opioid use among older patients following surgery: a Medicare claims analysis. *Surgery.* 2020;167(4):732−742.

75. Gray ML, Fan CJ, Kappauf C, et al. Postoperative pain management after sinus surgery: a survey of the American Rhinologic Society. *Int Forum Allergy Rhinol.* 2018;8(10): 1199−1203.

76. Klimczak J, Badhey A, Wong A, Colley P, Teng M. Pain management and prescribing practices in otolaryngology residency programs. *Am J Otolaryngol.* 2020;41(1):102265.

A systems approach to perioperative pain management

11

Jay K. Ferrell, MD [1], **Maisie L. Shindo, MD** [2]

[1]*Division of Head and Neck Surgery, Department of Otolaryngology-Head and Neck Surgery, UT Health San Antonio Long School of Medicine, San Antonio, TX, United States;* [2]*Head & Neck Endocrine Surgery, Thyroid and Parathyroid Center, Department of Otolaryngology-Head and Neck Surgery, Oregon Health and Science University, Portland, OR, United States*

Introduction

As a result of the ongoing public health crisis of opioid addiction in the United States, increased focus and scrutiny have been placed on physicians' pain management practices. Moreover, postoperative opioid prescribing practices after routine surgical procedures are often not standardized and can vary widely.[1] While the current epidemic of opioid addiction is multifactorial and cannot solely be ascribed to surgeons' prescribing practices, the impact of conscientious and evidence-based perioperative pain management has certainly become clearer and more evident. However, reducing opioid prescribing is only one piece of a larger puzzle. Effective perioperative pain management is multifaceted, and, as with many other aspects of surgical practice, it is most successful when implemented systematically. To that end, this chapter will discuss several key components of a systems-based approach for perioperative pain management in otolaryngology including preoperative pain management assessment and education, current best evidence for perioperative pain management strategies, and incorporating pain management into successful enhanced surgical recovery (ERAS) processes.

Why a systems-based approach to perioperative pain management?

A *systematic* or *systems-based* approach to healthcare is an evolving concept that has gained popularity and traction in recent years. However, the idea that solutions to complex problems are multifaceted and interconnected is far from novel. In fact, it can be traced as far back as the philosopher Aristotle who famously remarked that *the whole is greater than the sum of its parts*. This simple yet insightful observation is especially pertinent to surgical practice where fostering a strong team dynamic is foundational. However, translating this abstract concept into more defined,

Opioid Use, Overuse, and Abuse in Otolaryngology. https://doi.org/10.1016/B978-0-323-79016-1.00010-6

systems-based approaches is challenging. While a full discussion of the theory and nuances of systems-based healthcare delivery is beyond the scope of this chapter, it is important for clinicians to have a general understanding of how this concept relates to the ongoing conversations on how to improve current perioperative pain management practices.

Proponents of a systematic approach to healthcare delivery cite similarities between medicine and other "high-risk" industries such as commercial aviation and petroleum engineering.[2] While these are admittedly imperfect analogies to surgical practice, there is a common theme—namely mitigating and managing potential risks and continuously pursuing higher-level goals of safety and quality. In response to reports published by the Institute of Medicine detailing disparities in quality and patient safety, the President's Council of Advisors on Science and Technology (PCAST) recommended that a systems [based] approach be promoted at all levels of the American healthcare system.[3] The PCAST report went on to recommend employing key principles of systems engineering—i.e., integrating pertinent disciplines, understanding the operational environment, and utilizing available metrics to evaluate quality and performance—to improve the quality and efficiency of healthcare delivery.[3] Although germaine in theory, applying these principles to actual clinical practice has proven challenging. Critics of systems-based healthcare argue that such approaches lead to overreliance on standardized, formulaic care, reduce clinician autonomy, and shift responsibility and accountability for errors away from individuals and onto a faceless "system." While these concerns are certainly valid, as Dekker and Levenson observe, such reservations often result from a misunderstanding of what is meant by a systems-based approach.[4] Far from simply creating standardized checklists, the goals of systems-based healthcare are to recognize the inherent linkages within a given healthcare environment and to design evidence-based frameworks that promote synergy, collaboration, and accountability. Successful real-world examples of systems-based approaches to healthcare delivery include the Surviving Sepsis Campaign to promote early identification and directed therapy for sepsis in critical care patients, employing information technology resources to track and support evidence-based care in chronic health conditions, and navigation programs to improve access and coordination of complex, multidisciplinary care for cancer patients.

The consequences of the historically fragmented and disparate approaches to postoperative pain management have been rendered even more salient by the ongoing opioid addiction crisis. As with other surgical specialties, significant variations in pain management and opioid-prescribing practices have been repeatedly demonstrated among otolaryngologists—head and neck surgeons performing common procedures. A retrospective review of five common outpatient surgical procedures demonstrated significant variations in the total amounts of opioids prescribed with the widest variance seen in patients undergoing thyroidectomy.[5] Similarly, a recent survey study demonstrated divergent pain management practices among a cohort of endocrine-focused head and neck surgeons and a heavy reliance on postoperative opioids following outpatient thyroid and parathyroid surgery.[6] These studies are just a few examples among many with similar results that speak to the scope and scale of the problem.

The reasons for such varying perioperative pain management practices are myriad and include a historical lack of evidence-based recommendations, practice variations as a result of training and location, disparate expectations between providers and patients, and shifting societal knowledge and priorities. Moreover, this problem goes beyond simply overprescribing and overreliance on opioids. A complex problem like this requires innovative solutions, and we need a systematic review and revamping of how we approach and manage perioperative pain. Therefore, shifting focus from simply trying to alter individual clinicians' behavior to pursuing systems-based approaches has so much potential benefit. As Dekker and Leveson aptly observe[4]:

> It is unrealistic to believe that [physician] behavior is not affected by the context in which it occurs ... The goal of a systems approach is ... to design a system in which individual responsibility and competence can effectively create desired outcomes.

With this rationale in mind, surgeons are well advised to work within their respective institutions and healthcare systems to construct clinical care pathways that promote and support perioperative pain management. In the following sections, we will discuss the rationale and available evidence for the primary components of a systematic approach to perioperative pain management including preoperative patient-specific pain assessment, surgeon-performed pain management counseling and education, multimodality pain regimens, and enhanced recovery protocols as a comprehensive, systematic approach to perioperative pain management.

Preoperative pain assessment and counseling

A systematic, comprehensive approach to perioperative pain management spans the continuum of the surgical encounter and begins at the initial preoperative consultation. To promote successful postoperative outcomes, surgeons are well accustomed to assessing patients' underlying medical risk factors and providing educative counseling regarding surgical complications and expectations. Similarly, evaluating patient-specific risk factors for perioperative pain and delivering focused counseling on pain management risks and expectations are important elements of the preoperative consultation. Just as failing to recognize an underlying cardiac or hematologic disorder increases the risk of serious surgical complications, failing to appreciate patients' unique pain management requirements and indiscriminate prescribing of opioid medications can have significant, negative consequences. As evidence, it has been reported that up to 20% of people suffering from opioid addiction were initially exposed to opiates via legitimately obtained prescriptions.[7] Even more alarming, a recent large-scale study of opioid-naïve patients found that those prescribed opioids for even short-term management of acute postoperative pain experience a 44% relative risk of long-term opioid use, and as many as 10% of those patients may still be taking an opioid medication at 12 months or beyond after surgery.[8] Thus, the potential positive or detrimental impacts of perioperative pain management practices cannot be overstated.

Preoperative pain risk assessment

In 1978, The International Association for the Study of Pain (IASP) provided one of the first consensus definitions of pain as a negative experience associated with actual or potential tissue damage.[9] However, to better articulate the complex, multifaceted nature of pain, the IASP recently revised its decades-old definition. The updated definition describes pain as, "an unpleasant sensory and emotional experience associated with, *or resembling that associated with*, actual or potential tissue damage.[10]" In essence, this updated definition recognizes that pain is a *personal* experience that is impacted by multiple variables (i.e., biological, sociologic, psychologic, etc.) beyond the apparent nociceptive stimuli. Surgeons should recognize there is no uniform perioperative pain experience for patients and, as a result, there is not a one-size-fits-all approach to perioperative pain management. Patients' postoperative pain management outcomes are impacted by several patient specific-variables, and the astute clinician should be proactive in assessing for and gaining a clear understanding of these factors well before the patient ever enters the operating room.

Several patient-specific factors have been identified that can portend an increased risk of higher postoperative pain levels and potentially higher opioid consumption. These include chronic or preexisting pain conditions, preoperative opioid use, prior postoperative painful experiences, inappropriate expectations or anxiety regarding proposed surgery, concomitant psychological issues (e.g., generalized anxiety disorder, major depressive disorder, etc.), and preexisting functional pain conditions (e.g., fibromyalgia).[11] Within the otolaryngology literature, independent factors that have clearly been identified in patients undergoing outpatient head and neck surgery are age less than 45 years and prior use of opioid medications.[12] Other factors that have been suggested include socioeconomic status, chronic medical conditions, history of tobacco or alcohol abuse, and even preoperative use of common nonopioid prescription medications—for example, benzodiazepines, selective serotonin reuptake inhibitors, and angiotensive converting enzyme inhibitors.[8,13] As part of the preoperative assessment, surgeons should proactively screen for patient-specific factors and counsel patients on postoperative pain expectations and developing a pain management plan.

Patient-centered perioperative pain management counseling

Physician—patient communication is a crucial component of effective healthcare delivery. While patient-centered health management education is well-established in other clinical conditions (e.g., diabetes), its value and utility in supporting efforts to reduce opioid consumption and improve perioperative pain outcomes are relatively novel and emerging concepts. However, the rationale and theoretical benefits of patient education certainly make intuitive sense as part of a systematic approach to perioperative pain management.

Sugai et al.[14] provided one of the earliest studies objectively evaluating the impact of surgeon-performed pain education on postoperative pain outcomes. In their study, 90% of the experimental cohort—which received oral and written educational materials emphasizing the benefits, risks, and rationale of multimodality nonopioid versus opioid postoperative pain management—subsequently declined a postoperative opioid prescription following outpatient cosmetic procedures. Similarly, a recent single-institution study of orthopedic trauma patients found that those patients who were specifically counseled preoperatively regarding expected pain levels and duration of postoperative opiate use were significantly more likely to have stopped taking opioid medications by postoperative week 6 versus those receiving no such counseling.[15] Incorporating pain expectation and management counseling has been demonstrated to have similarly positive results in head and neck surgery. Shindo and colleagues[16] demonstrated that clinician-performed counseling focused on pain expectations and multimodality pain management strategies is a key component in programmatic efforts to reduce unnecessary postoperative opioid use while maximizing postoperative pain outcomes.

Selecting an appropriate setting can be an equally important component of effective pain management counseling. From the patient's perspective, the preoperative office visit is an ideal setting for a conversation given its privacy and personalized context. While preoperative pain education and counseling can be composed of different topics, in general it is recommended that it at least focus on assessing past experiences with medical procedures and pain control, understanding past usage and issues with analgesics, and ascertaining patients' impressions and prior experiences with opioid medications. Once an understanding of the patient's unique situation and pain management expectations has been established, the surgeon can better outline the anticipated perioperative pain management approach. It is important to recognize the understandable consternation that can result from the anticipation of postoperative pain. To that end, effective preoperative education should also provide patients with a clear understanding that some measure of mild, manageable pain is expected and is part of the normal, uncomplicated postoperative healing process. Additionally, surgeons should highlight the proven efficacy of alternative pain management interventions (e.g., nonopioid medications, cool compresses, throat lozenges, etc.) while also clearly communicating that the proposed regimen can be appropriately tailored based on the patient's specific postoperative pain experience. To promote consistency and efficacy clinicians should consider integrating into their preoperative assessment of factors that may influence postoperative pain management, which can be in the form of a checklist, and counseling regarding expectations and plans for managing postoperative pain. An example of a pain assessment and counseling reference tool is provided in Fig. 11.1.

In summary, a successful systems-based approach to perioperative pain management begins at the initial preoperative encounter with both an assessment of patient-

1. How satisfied have you been with your pain management experiences after prior medical, surgical, or dental procedures (such as tooth extractions, root canal, etc.)?
   - ☐ Very satisfied
   - ☐ Somewhat satisfied
   - ☐ Somewhat dissatisfied
   - ☐ Very dissatisfied
   - ☐ I have never had any prior medical, surgical, or dental procedures

2. Which of the following best describes any current conditions you are experiencing that require daily use of pain medication(s)? (May select more than one answer)
   - ☐ Back/spinal pain
   - ☐ Osteoarthritis
   - ☐ Rheumatoid arthritis
   - ☐ Chronic headaches
   - ☐ Multiple sclerosis
   - ☐ Fibromyalgia
   - ☐ Nerve damage (neuropathy)
   - ☐ Other (Please specify) _____
   - ☐ I do not have any current pain condition

3. If you have any of the above pain conditions, what type(s) of prescription or over-the-counter medication(s) do you take? (May select more than one answer)
   - ☐ Opioids (hydrocodone, oxycodone, tramadol, Tylenol with codeine)
   - ☐ Tylenol (Acetaminophen)
   - ☐ NSAIDs (Advil, Aleve, Celebrex, ibuprofen, aspirin)
   - ☐ Nerve pain medication (Neurontin, Lyrica, gabapentin)
   - ☐ Other (Please specify) _____

4. Have you ever had any side effects or other bad reactions to any of the following types of pain medications?
   - ☐ Opioids (hydrocodone, oxycodone, tramadol, Tylenol with codeine)
   - ☐ Tylenol (Acetaminophen)
   - ☐ NSAIDs (Advil, Aleve, Celebrex, ibuprofen, aspirin)
   - ☐ Nerve pain medication (Neurontin, Lyrica, gabapentin)
   - ☐ Other (Please specify) _____
   - ☐ I have never had any side effects or bad reactions to a pain medication

5. If you have had any bad reaction(s) to a pain medication, which of the following best describes the reaction(s)? (May select more than one answer)
   - ☐ Nausea/vomiting
   - ☐ Constipation
   - ☐ Stomach pain
   - ☐ Drowsiness/decreased energy/mental cloudiness
   - ☐ Difficulty breathing
   - ☐ Rash/swelling
   - ☐ Other (Please specify) _____

6. Do you take any of the following medications? (Select all that apply)
   - ☐ Benzodiazepines (Xanax, Valium, Ativan, Klonopin)
   - ☐ SSRIs (Prozac, Lexapro, Zoloft, Celexa, Paxil)
   - ☐ ACE inhibitors (Lisinopril, enalapril, benazepril)

7. Have you ever experienced issues with addiction to alcohol or medications (prescription or non-prescription)?
   - ☐ Yes
   - ☐ No

8. The patient and I have discussed postoperative pain expectations and our pain management plan.
   - ☐ Yes
   - ☐ No

FIGURE 11.1

Example clinical reference tool for preoperative pain risk and expectation assessment.

specific pain risk factors and a clinician-lead discussion of pain management expectations. These exercises can truly set the tone and tenor of patients' subsequent postoperative pain experience. While clinicians can certainly modify the preoperative educational discussion to suit the needs of their patients and practice patterns, it should at minimum include the following topics: (1) accurate description of typical, expected postoperative discomfort; (2) reassurance that some pain is normal in the postoperative recovery period; (3) explaining the benefits and merits of nonopioid multimodality pain management; (4) discussing the risks of opioids and rationale of limiting their use in the postoperative period; and (5) describing processes to respond to patients' concerns about postoperative pain and to adjust their pain management as needed. The fundamental goals of this important physician–patient communication are to set realistic, up-front expectations regarding postoperative pain and its management, to promote patients' confidence in and acceptance of non-opioid, multimodality pain regimens, and to enable patients to feel more empowered and involved in their perioperative pain management experiences.

Perioperative multimodality pain management

As with many other surgical specialties, opioids have traditionally been a corner-stone of perioperative pain management in otolaryngology. As evidenced by several recent survey studies, there has been an overreliance on opioid medications across the spectrum of otolaryngologic procedures including endoscopic sinus surgery,[17] facial plastic surgery,[18] pediatric otolaryngology, and head and neck surgery.[6] Several reasons may underscore this including the potent efficacy of opioids in managing acute pain, surgeons' relative familiarity and experience with their use, and conventional hesitancy to using alternative medications (e.g., NSAIDs) due to potential perioperative complications such as postoperative hemorrhage. However, in light of contemporaneous evidence demonstrating both excessive amounts of pre-scribed opioids[5] and the risk of secondary opioid addiction following even short-term postoperative use,[19] increased interest and academic focus have been placed on the feasibility and utility of multimodality pain regimens that employ synergistic combinations of nonopioid analgesics and adjunctive interventions. The dual goals of this shifting paradigm are to effectively manage perioperative pain while reducing (or in some cases eliminating) the need for opioid medications.

Preoperative pain management

Effective multimodality pain management begins in the preoperative phase of care before the patient has experienced any nociceptive stimuli. Beneficial outcomes have been described with single-agent as well as combinatory use of several nonop-ioid medications—namely acetaminophen, gabapentinoids, and nonsteroidal antiin-flammatory drugs (NSAIDs). Otolaryngologists should be familiar with the primary medications available for preoperative administration as well as their associated risks and benefits.

Acetaminophen (APAP)—also known as *N*-acetyl para-aminophenol or paracetamol—is a well-established and widely available analgesic with numerous applications. Although the primary mechanism of action remains unclear, its anal-gesic properties are thought to be the result of inhibition of the cyclooxygenase

(COX) pathway within the central nervous system.[20] However, as it does not directly bind to either COX-1 or COX-2, APAP does not exhibit antiplatelet activity which makes it particularly attractive for preoperative use. Additionally, APAP can be administered either orally or intravenously. The intravenous form of APAP is relatively newer—as the FDA only approved it for use in 2010. The potential benefits of preoperative IV APAP include lower reported postoperative pain levels and decreased opioid requirements,[21,22] reduced incidence of postoperative nausea/vomiting (PONV),[23] and shorter postoperative hospital stay.[22,23] Considering these benefits, it is nonetheless important to note that IV APAP is considerably more expensive than oral formulation. The efficacy versus cost-effectiveness of preoperative IV versus PO APAP has been studied in a recent randomized control trial that demonstrated no significant differences in postoperative pain control or PONV with IV APAP.[24] While many patients can be adequately managed with PO APAP, the IV formulation may have specific benefits in select circumstances such as patients unable to tolerate oral medications, those with hepatic insufficiency, or those with gastrointestinal issues that would compromise parenteral medication uptake. A single preoperative dose of 1000 mg of APAP is reasonable and efficacious for a majority of otolaryngologic procedures.

NSAIDs have also shown promise in the preoperative setting. The primary mechanism of action of this class of analgesics is direct inhibition of COX-mediated inflammatory pathways. While this makes them efficacious in the management of acute postoperative pain, their use in the preoperative setting has historically been limited due to concerns regarding their antiplatelet activity. As a result, data on the safety and efficacy of preoperative NSAIDs for head and neck procedures are somewhat limited and heterogeneous compared to APAP. With respect to postoperative pain and opioid requirements, preoperative dosing of intravenous ibuprofen was shown to be superior to APAP in patients undergoing odontogenic procedures.[25] Preoperative use of NSAIDs in pediatric tonsillectomy has been shown to be effective but, based on a recently published meta-analysis, the data on the risk of secondary posttonsillectomy hemorrhage is equivocal due to lack of robust, prospective randomized studies.[26] Regarding concerns of intraoperative and postoperative bleeding, a recent report on the use of preoperative ketorolac in endoscopic sinus surgery showed no increase in intraoperative or postoperative bleeding compared to placebo.[27] Alternatively, selective COX-2 inhibitors (coxibs) have been advocated for postoperative pain due to their reduced effects on normal coagulation. Preoperative administration of both classes of NSAIDs has been shown to have benefits both in reducing postoperative pain levels and decreasing patients' opioid requirements in the first 24 h after surgery.[28–30]

Lastly, gabapentinoid agents such as gabapentin and pregabalin have gained popularity as adjunctive analgesics. Gabapentinoids are derivatives of the inhibitory neurotransmitter γ-aminobutyric acid and are primarily used in the prevention of epileptic seizures and the management of anxiety disorders. As analgesics, these medications have shown benefits in the treatment of pain from diabetic neuropathy and postherpetic neuralgia. As they also have a low overall abuse potential, their use has expanded to off-label applications such as acute perioperative pain. Recent studies have suggested positive albeit contradictory results in the preoperative use of gabapentin and pregabalin.[31,32] In addition, suggested dosages can vary widely from 150 to 1200 mg and untoward sequela such as blurred vision, somnolence, dizziness, and mood disturbances have been reported.[33,34] Specifically, regarding head and neck applications, a meta-analysis performed by Arumugam and colleagues[35] suggested that preoperative gabapentin may reduce cumulative postoperative opioid requirements following thyroidectomy. Lastly, clinicians should be aware of recent FDA warnings regarding potential respiratory and neurologic depression and should also counsel patients about the off-label use of gabapentinoids for perioperative pain.

Based on currently available evidence in the otolaryngology literature, multimodality regimens appear to be superior to single-agent therapy for preoperative analgesia. Oltman et al.[36] described a standardized regimen of meloxicam, acetaminophen, and gabapentin in patients undergoing outpatient thyroid, parathyroid, and parotid surgery. The authors demonstrated low resting and peak pain scores, and 60% of patients completely avoided postoperative opioids. Moreover, there were no treatment-specific complications and 90% of patients reported high-to-very-high levels of satisfaction with their perioperative pain management experience. A summary of commonly used preoperative analgesic agents, their typical dosing, and potential contraindications is provided in Table 11.1.

Table 11.1 Commonly used medications for preoperative analgesia.

Medication	Suggested dosage	Contraindications
Acetaminophen	1000 mg PO/IV	■ Hepatic insufficiency or cirrhosis ■ Heavy daily alcohol consumption (>3 drinks/day)
Ibuprofen	400–800 mg PO	■ Renal insufficiency (CrCl <30) ■ Peptic ulcer disease or history of gastrointestinal bleeding ■ History of coronary artery disease or prior CABG ■ Hypersensitivity to aspirin or NSAIDs
Celecoxib	200–400 mg PO	■ Hypersensitivity to aspirin or NSAIDs ■ History of CABG
Gabapentin	Age <65, CrCl >60: 900 mg PO Age >65 or CrCl <60: 600 mg PO	■ Renal insufficiency (CrCl <30) ■ Hypersensitivity to gabapentin or pregabalin

CABG, *coronary artery bypass graft surgery*; CrCl, *creatine clearance (mL/minute)*; NSAIDs, *nonsteroidal antiinflammatory drugs.*

Intraoperative pain management

Excellent discussions on intraoperative pain management from an anesthesiology perspective are provided elsewhere in this text. It suffices to say that surgeons should be cognizant that well-intentioned pain management efforts can be compromised by overutilization of opioid medications intraoperatively. Aside from good surgical technique and careful tissue handling, additional adjunctive options that can be employed by the surgical team to preemptively reduce postoperative pain include local and regional anesthetics.

Local anesthesia consists of subcutaneous or submucosal injection of lidocaine or one of its derivatives (e.g., bupivacaine or ropivacaine). Among otolaryngology procedures, the safety and efficacy of peri-incisional anesthetic infiltration have been most thoroughly studied in pediatric tonsillectomy, thyroidectomy, and neck dissection. A recent systematic review of over 1300 patients across 18 randomized trials synthesized the evidence for bupivacaine injections for pain prophylaxis in thyroidectomy. The authors concluded that there was strong evidence for the routine use of peri-incisional bupivacaine as it significantly reduced both acute postoperative pain levels and the need for "rescue" analgesia with IV opioids. Based on the available evidence, the authors recommended local injection of 20–75 mg of bupivacaine (i.e., approximately 10–30 mL of 0.25% bupivacaine) either before or immediately following skin closure.

For open neck procedures (e.g., thyroidectomy or neck dissection), regional anesthesia consisting of superficial (SCB) or deep cervical plexus blocks (DCB) can also be used. These interventions can be performed in the preoperative area or intraoperatively after induction. Based on available evidence, SCB is more commonly used for neck procedures as it can be performed easily and safely using palpable external landmarks. Injection in the midpoint of the posterior border of sternocleidomastoid muscle targets the sensory roots of C2-4 resulting in sensory blockade of the anterolateral neck extending from the lower external ear superiorly to the acromioclavicular joint inferiorly.[37] This renders SCB particularly useful for thyroid and parathyroid surgeries as well as lateral neck dissections. However, the published evidence on the efficacy of routine SCB is mixed. A double-blind randomized study published in 2010 comparing bilateral SCB to placebo for thyroidectomy demonstrated significantly lower visual analog scale (VAS) scores with SCB.[38] Interestingly, the authors did not observe either lower overall use of on-demand analgesics or reduced length of hospital stay compared to placebo. In contrast, a randomized controlled study by Eti et al. comparing the effects of local wound infiltration with bupivacaine versus SCB in patients undergoing thyroidectomy found no significant difference in either VAS scores or postoperative opioid requirements.[39] However, it should be noted that all patients in this study received meperidine patient-controlled analgesia starting immediately postoperatively. In the setting of current efforts to reduce perioperative opioid consumption, the benefits of local and regional nerve blocks are being reevaluated in the context of multimodal pain management.[40] Lastly, while DCB has also been described for use in head and neck procedures, it is less commonly utilized as it requires more time-intensive ultrasound guidance, a higher level of technical expertise and also carries the serious albeit rare risks of intravascular injection or inadvertent paresis of adjacent nerves such as the cervical sympathetic (Horner's syndrome), phrenic (diaphragmatic paralysis), vagus or recurrent laryngeal (dysphonia or acute airway compromise).[41] Additionally, a recent comparative study by Suh et al. has failed to demonstrate any additive analgesic benefit with deep cervical blocks.[42]

Postoperative pain management

A successful systematic pain management approach continues seamlessly through the transition to the postoperative recovery setting and eventual discharge. Efforts to avoid the overuse of opioids can be inadvertently compromised in the postanesthesia care unit (PACU) if nursing and ancillary staff are not educated and familiar with the desired pain management goals. In addition to reducing the risk of secondary dependence, limiting opioids in the postoperative period carries several additional benefits such as preventing constipation, delirium, nausea/emesis, and sedentary behavior that can increase the secondary risks of postoperative atelectasis or deep vein thrombosis.

Multimodality strategies that can be employed in the PACU setting include the following: early initiation of scheduled, alternating dosing of acetaminophen and ibuprofen; application of cold compresses to external surgical sites and incisions upon arrival in PACU; and the liberal use of anesthetic oral lozenges to reduce throat pain associated with endotracheal intubation or instrumentation of the oral cavity, oropharynx, or hypopharynx. Additionally, PACU nursing staff should be encouraged to assess pain based on patients' functional status—that is, ability to sit up comfortably, neck range of motion, ease of oral intake—instead of relying solely on numerical pain measures such as a 1–10 visual analog scale. Before discharge, it is recommended that a member of the surgical team reassess the adequacy of patients' pain management. A subset of patients may require limited amounts of prescribed opioids at discharge, but this determination should be made by the surgical team on an individualized basis. If deemed necessary, it is strongly recommended that low-potency opiates are utilized for the shortest possible duration. This recommendation is based on a preponderance of evidence from multiple, contemporary studies demonstrating that the majority of opioid-naïve patients who require opiates for breakthrough pain after outpatient, otolaryngologic procedures can be successfully managed with total dosages of <75 morphine milligram equivalents (MME)—which equates to <15 tablets of hydrocodone 5 mg or <10 tablets of oxycodone 5 mg based on the standard conversions illustrated in Table 11.2.

In our experience, the use of a comprehensive multimodality pain strategy can often reduce the total opioid dosage requirements for opioid-naïve patients undergoing outpatient thyroid and parathyroid procedures to <20 MME. Moreover, it is important to recognize that a sizable proportion of those patients can be successfully managed without opioids. Lastly, the transition from postoperative recovery to discharge and home recovery is a crucial opportunity. PACU nursing staff are an invaluable link between patients and surgical team at this phase care. As part of

Table 11.2 Opioid morphine milligram equivalents (MME).

Type of opioid (strength units)	MME conversion factor
Tramadol (mg)	0.1
Codeine (mg)	0.15
Hydrocodone (mg)	1
Oxycodone (mg)	1.5

Adapted from National Center for Injury Prevention and Control. CDC compilation of benzodiazepines, muscle relaxants, stimulants, Zolpidem, and opioid analgesics with oral morphine milligram equivalent conversion factors, 2016 version. https://www.cdc.gov/drugoverdose/media/.

the discharge process, they can support comprehensive pain management efforts by reinforcing the goals and expectations for at-home pain management, ensure patients' understanding and comfort with the major elements of a nonopioid pain control regimen (e.g., cold compresses, scheduled administrations of NSAIDs/acetaminophen, etc.), providing education on safe opioid use and storage, and escalating pain management concerns to the surgical team. Furthermore, surgeons' clinical office staff can maintain these lines of communication in the days following discharge and should be educated and well versed in appropriately responding to and escalating patients' pain management concerns. Requests for new or additional opioid medications during the acute postoperative period should be documented in the electronic health record and addressed directly by a member of the surgical team. This practice ensures accountability and responsiveness to patients' concerns, promotes conscientious opioid prescribing, and can allow for early identification of postoperative complications that may be heralded by an unexpected increase in pain (e.g., surgical site infection or hematoma/seroma).

In summary, effective multimodality pain management is built on the synergistic use of preoperative, intraoperative, and postoperative interventions. To ensure sustainability and reduce variability in execution, close collaboration between the perioperative nursing staff, anesthesia and surgical teams, and PACU staff is essential. Lastly, the transition at discharge is a crucial window of opportunity to ensure patients are able to successfully continue with multimodality pain management at home. To support patients during the acute postoperative period, surgeons should ensure that all members of the clinical care team—including and especially PACU, trainees, and outpatient office staff—are familiar with the goals of multimodality pain management and how to recognize patient-reported pain concerns that deviate from expected parameters.

Enhanced recovery after surgery: a model for systems-based perioperative pain management

Formed in Europe in 2010, The ERAS society is a multidisciplinary working group of anesthesiology and surgical specialists that aims to optimize perioperative care.

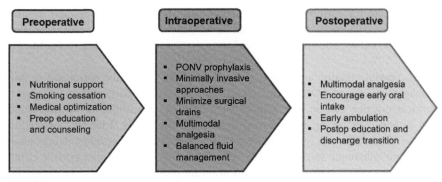

FIGURE 11.2

Schematic example of a standard ERAS workflow.

Although the group initially focused on evidence-based approaches to decrease the length of stay after major thoracic and abdominal procedures, ERAS protocols have since expanded to include multiple surgical specialties and procedures—including head and neck surgery. ERAS encompasses several facets and interventions spanning the major phases of the perioperative encounter. As would be expected, optimized pain management is one of its key provisions as it promotes early postoperative recovery while avoiding the detrimental effects of opioid overutilization (see Fig. 11.2).

Based on these foundational elements of ERAS, enhanced recovery protocols (ERPs) are quickly gaining popularity and supportive evidence in the published literature. Several recent reports have demonstrated the efficacy of implementing systematic ERAS pain management practices in short-stay head and neck surgery. Yip et al. recently described their pain management experience for thyroid and parathyroid surgery before and after ERP implementation.[43] Their protocol emphasizes preoperative diet modifications with high-protein and carbohydrate intake the week before surgery; prophylactic analgesia with APAP (1000 mg PO) and gabapentin (300–600 mg PO); preventing PONV via the use of total intravenous anesthesia and avoidance of intraoperative opioids; routine use of field neural blockage with bupivacaine; and multimodality postoperative pain management with PRN APAP or APAP with codeine for breakthrough pain. Comparing the ERP cohort to their historical pre-ERP control group, the authors demonstrated a 72% reduction in the total amounts of prescribed opioids, a significant percentage of patients receiving no perioperative opioids (21%), and reduced need for ondansetron or scopolamine for PONV. Lide et al. reported similar beneficial effects of a systems-based ERAS pain protocol.[40] Unique elements of their protocol include the use of ibuprofen in addition to APAP and gabapentin for preoperative prophylaxis, routine use of ketamine and dexamethasone during general anesthesia, and regional nerve block performed preoperatively by an anesthesia provider. Following initiation of a consistent ERAS pain protocol, the authors observed a reduction in prescribed opioids with overall improved patient-reported pain outcomes. Successful use of the

ERAS model for perioperative pain management has also been reported in other areas of otolaryngology-head and neck surgery including pediatric adenotonsillectomy, transoral robotic surgery, otologic surgery, and head and neck reconstructive surgery.[44–47]

Successful creation and integration of an ERAS model for perioperative pain management are not without their challenges. Effecting broad, systemic change in surgical practice can be met with barriers such as an initial lack of stakeholder buy-in and overcoming institutional inertia. In their study, Lide and colleagues discuss steps they took to overcome initial implementation barriers and encourage consistent adherence to their established ERAS protocol. These supportive efforts included providing evidence-based education for providers and patients, improving visibility and access to protocol medications in pre- and postoperative care sites, creating a dedicated order set in the electronic health record system, and sending automatic electronical protocol reminders to the primary anesthesia and surgical team members 24 h before surgery. With these efforts, the authors observed adherence to the ERAS protocol in over 75% of surgical cases by the end of the study period.[40] Likewise in their recent report on the feasibility of an ERAS protocol for major head and neck surgery, Low et al. identified several strategies to promote successful ERAS implementation.[48] They specifically highlighted the value and importance of early, multidisciplinary collaboration, identifying and building upon successful ERAS protocols within the institution, creation of standardized electronic order sets, and utilization of validated patient-reported outcomes measures for protocol assessment and improvement.

Although the data on their use in otolaryngology are relatively nascent, ERAS protocols represent a progressive shift toward a comprehensive, systems-based approach to perioperative pain management. This transition has several potential benefits such as promoting evidenced-based pain management, encouraging greater collaboration among members of the surgical team, avoiding unnecessary variability in perioperative pain management, and improving patients' clinical care experience. However, it is also important to recognize that the principles of ERAS are a general framework, and perioperative care teams can and should tailor ERPs to best fit the unique needs and resources of their respective institutions. This is an area ripe for further investigation, and larger, prospective studies are clearly needed to provide high-quality evidence and guidance on utilizing ERPs to promote more effective, comprehensive perioperative pain management.

Summary

Effective pain management is a cornerstone of good perioperative care and can significantly impact postoperative outcomes. Successful pain management spans the continuum of the perioperative encounter and is built upon good surgeon–patient communication, multimodal analgesia, and dynamic collaboration among all members of the perioperative care team. The opioid addiction crisis has made it clear that our historically fragmented and capricious approaches to perioperative pain management must be redressed and improved. To that end, systems-based care—as exemplified by the emerging concept of ERAS—synergizes several key elements to support comprehensive and sustainable pain management practices.

References

1. Hill MV, Mcmahon ML, Stucke RS, Barth RJ. Wide variation and excessive dosage of opioid prescriptions for common general surgical procedures. *Ann Surg.* 2017;265(4): 709–714. https://doi.org/10.1097/SLA.0000000000001993.
2. Hudson P. Applying the lessons of high risk industries to health care. *Qual Saf Health Care.* 2003;12(Suppl. 1):i7. https://doi.org/10.1136/qhc.12.suppl_1.i7.
3. Cassel CK, Saunders RS. Engineering a better health care system: a report from the president's council of advisors on science and technology. *J Am Med Assoc.* 2014;312(8): 787–788. https://doi.org/10.1001/jama.2014.8906.
4. Dekker SWA, Leveson NG. The systems approach to medicine: controversy and misconceptions. *BMJ Qual Saf.* 2015;24(1):7–9. https://doi.org/10.1136/bmjqs-2014-003106.
5. Nooromid MJ, Blay E, Holl JL, et al. Discharge prescription patterns of opioid and non-opioid analgesics after common surgical procedures. *PAIN Rep.* 2018;3(1):e637. https://doi.org/10.1097/PR9.0000000000000637.
6. Ferrell JK, Singer MC, Farwell DG, Stack BC, Shindo M. Evaluating contemporary pain management practices in thyroid and parathyroid surgery: a national survey of head and neck endocrine surgeons. *Head Neck.* 2019;41(7). https://doi.org/10.1002/hed.25694.
7. Lipari RN, Hedden SL, Hughes A. Substance use and mental health estimates from the 2013 national survey on drug use and health: overview of findings. In: *The CBHSQ Report.* Substance Abuse and Mental Health Services Administration (US); 2013:1–10.
8. Clarke H, Soneji N, Ko DT, Yun L, Wijeysundera DN. Rates and risk factors for prolonged opioid use after major surgery: population based cohort study. *BMJ.* 2014;348: g1251. https://doi.org/10.1136/bmj.g1251.
9. Pain terms: a list with definitions and notes on usage. Recommended by the IASP Subcommittee on Taxonomy. *Pain.* 1979;6(3):249.
10. Raja SN, Carr DB, Cohen M, et al. The revised International Association for the Study of Pain definition of pain: concepts, challenges, and compromises. *Pain.* 2020;161(9): 1976–1982. https://doi.org/10.1097/j.pain.0000000000001939.
11. Chou R, Gordon DB, De Leon-Casasola OA, et al. Management of postoperative pain: a clinical practice guideline from the American pain society, the American society of regional anesthesia and pain medicine, and the American society of anesthesiologists' committee on regional anesthesia, executive committee, and administrative council. *J Pain.* 2016;17(2):131–157. https://doi.org/10.1016/j.jpain.2015.12.008.
12. Lou I, Chennell TB, Schaefer SC, et al. Optimizing outpatient pain management after thyroid and parathyroid surgery: a two-institution experience. *Ann Surg Oncol.* 2017; 24(7):1951–1957. https://doi.org/10.1245/s10434-017-5781-y.
13. Cramer JD, Wisler B, Gouveia CJ. Opioid stewardship in otolaryngology: state of the art review. *Otolaryngol Head Neck Surg.* 2018;158(5):817–827. https://doi.org/10.1177/0194599818757999.

14. Sugai DY, Deptula PL, Parsa AA, Don Parsa F. The importance of communication in the management of postoperative pain. *Hawaii J Med Public Heal.* 2013;72(6):180–184. https://www.ncbi.nlm.nih.gov/pmc/articles/PMC3689499/pdf/hjmph7206_0180.pdf.

15. Holman JE, Stoddard GJ, Horwitz DS, Higgins TF. The effect of preoperative counseling on duration of postoperative opiate use in orthopaedic trauma surgery. *J Orthop Trauma.* 2014;28(9):502–506. https://doi.org/10.1097/BOT.0000000000000085.

16. Shindo M, Lim J, Leon E, Moneta L, Li R, Quintinalla-Diek L. Opioid prescribing practice and needs in thyroid and parathyroid surgery. *JAMA Otolaryngol Head Neck Surg.* 2018. https://doi.org/10.1001/jamaoto.2018.2427.

17. Gray ML, Fan CJ, Kappauf C, et al. Postoperative pain management a er sinus surgery: a survey of the. *Am Rhinol Soc How Cite Article.* 2018;8(10):1199–1203. https://doi.org/10.1002/alr.22181.

18. Sethi RKV, Lee LN, Quatela OE, Richburg KG, Shaye DA. Opioid prescription patterns after rhinoplasty. *JAMA Facial Plast Surg.* 2019;21(1):76–77. https://doi.org/10.1001/jamafacial.2018.0999.

19. Brummett CM, Waljee JF, Goesling J, et al. New persistent opioid use after minor and major surgical procedures in us adults. *JAMA Surg.* 2017;152(6). https://doi.org/10.1001/jamasurg.2017.0504.

20. Smith HS. Potential analgesic mechanisms of acetaminophen. *Pain Physician.* 2009;(4):269–280.

21. Tyler MA, Lam K, Ashoori F, et al. Analgesic effects of intravenous acetaminophen vs placebo for endoscopic sinus surgery and postoperative pain: a randomized clinical trial. *JAMA Otolaryngol Head Neck Surg.* 2017;143(8):788–794. https://doi.org/10.1001/jamaoto.2017.0238.

22. Shaffer E, Pham A, Woldman R, Spiegelman A, Strassels SA, Wan GJ, Zimmerman EL. *Estimating the Effect of Intravenous Acetaminophen for Postoperative Pain Management on Length of Stay and Inpatient Hospital Costs.* 2016. https://doi.org/10.1007/s12325-016-0438-y.

23. Hansen RN, Pham AT, Böing EA, et al. Hospitalization costs and resource allocation in cholecystectomy with use of intravenous versus oral acetaminophen. *Curr Med Res Opin.* 2018;34(9):1549–1555. https://doi.org/10.1080/03007995.2017.1412301.

24. Pelzer D, Burgess E, Cox J, Baker R. Preoperative intravenous versus oral acetaminophen in outpatient surgery: a double-blinded, randomized control trial. *J PeriAnesthesia Nurs.* 2020. https://doi.org/10.1016/j.jopan.2020.07.010.

25. Viswanath A, Oreadi D, Finkelman M, Klein G, Papageorge M. Does pre-emptive administration of intravenous ibuprofen (caldolor) or intravenous acetaminophen (ofirmev) reduce postoperative pain and subsequent narcotic consumption after third molar surgery? *J Oral Maxillofac Surg.* 2019;77(2):262–270. https://doi.org/10.1016/j.joms.2018.09.010.

26. Stokes W, Swanson RT, Schubart J, Carr MM. Postoperative bleeding associated with ibuprofen use after tonsillectomy: a meta-analysis. *Otolaryngol Head Neck Surg.* 2019;161(5):734–741. https://doi.org/10.1177/0194599819852328.

27. Moeller C, Pawlowski J, Pappas AL, Fargo K, Welch K. The safety and efficacy of intravenous ketorolac in patients undergoing primary endoscopic sinus surgery: a randomized, double-blinded clinical trial. *Int Forum Allergy Rhinol.* 2012;2(4):342–347. https://doi.org/10.1002/alr.21028.

28. Smirnov G, Terävä M, Tuomilehto H, Hujala K, Seppänen M, Kokki H. Etoricoxib for pain management during thyroid surgery–a prospective, placebo-controlled study.

Otolaryngol Head Neck Surg. 2008;138(1):92−97. https://doi.org/10.1016/j.otohns. 2007.10.022.

29. Schopf S, Ahnen M, Ahnen T, Neugebauer EAM, Schardey H. Effect of local anesthesia and COX-2 inhibitors after thyroid resection on postoperative pain. Results of two consecutive randomized controlled monocenter studies. *J Pain Manag.* 2012;5:279−287.

30. Karamanlioğlu B, Arar C, Alagöl A, Colak A, Gemlik I, Süt N. Preoperative oral cele-coxib versus preoperative oral rofecoxib for pain relief after thyroid surgery. *Eur J Anaesthesiol.* 2003;20(6):490−495. https://doi.org/10.1017/s0265021503000796.

31. Brogly N, Wattier JM, Andrieu G, et al. Gabapentin attenuates late but not early postop-erative pain after thyroidectomy with superficial cervical plexus block. *Anesth Analg.* 2008;107(5):1720−1725. https://doi.org/10.1213/ane.0b013e318185cf73.

32. Kim SY, Jeong JJ, Chung WY, Kim HJ, Nam KH, Shim YH. Perioperative administration of pregabalin for pain after robot-assisted endoscopic thyroidectomy: a randomized clin-ical trial. *Surg Endosc.* 2010;24(11):2776−2781. https://doi.org/10.1007/s00464-010-1045-7.

33. Hema VR, Ramadas KT, Biji KP, Indu S, Arun A. A prospective, observational study to evaluate the role of gabapentin as preventive analgesic in thyroidectomy under general anesthesia. *Anesth Essays Res.* 2017;11(3):718−723. https://doi.org/10.4103/aer. AER_250_16.

34. Nguyen BK, Stathakios J, Quan D, et al. Perioperative analgesia for patients undergoing thyroidectomy and parathyroidectomy: an evidence-based review. *Ann Otol Rhinol Lar-yngol.* 2020. https://doi.org/10.1177/0003489420919134, 3489420919134.

35. Arumugam S, Lau CS, Chamberlain RS. Use of preoperative gabapentin significantly re-duces postoperative opioid consumption: a meta-analysis. *J Pain Res.* 2016;9:631−640. https://doi.org/10.2147/jpr.S112626.

36. Oltman J, Militsakh O, D'Agostino M, et al. Multimodal analgesia in outpatient head and neck surgery: a feasibility and safety study. *JAMA Otolaryngol Head Neck Surg.* 2017; 143(12):1207−1212. https://doi.org/10.1001/jamaoto.2017.1773.

37. Hipskind JE, Ahmed AA. *Cervical Plexus Block.* StatPearls Publishing; 2021. http://www.ncbi.nlm.nih.gov/pubmed/32491314. Accessed April 26, 2021.

38. Steffen T, Warschkow R, Brändie M, Tarantino I, Clerici T. Randomized controlled trial of bilateral superficial cervical plexus block versus placebo in thyroid surgery. *Br J Surg.* 2010;97(7):1000−1006. https://doi.org/10.1002/bjs.7077.

39. Eti Z, Irmak P, Gulluoglu BM, Manukyan MN, Gogus FY. Does bilateral superficial cer-vical plexus block decrease analgesic requirement after thyroid surgery? *Anesth Analg.* 2006;102(4):1174−1176. https://doi.org/10.1213/01.ane.0000202383.51830.c4.

40. Lide RC, Creighton EW, Yeh J, et al. Opioid reduction in ambulatory thyroid and para-thyroid surgery after implementing enhanced recovery after surgery protocol. *Head Neck.* 2021;(January):1−8. https://doi.org/10.1002/hed.26617.

41. Kim JS, Ko JS, Bang S, Kim H, Lee SY. Cervical plexus block. *Korean J Anesthesiol.* 2018;71(4):274−288. https://doi.org/10.4097/kja.d.18.00143.

42. Suh YJ, Kim YS, In JH, Joo JD, Jeon YS, Kim HK. Comparison of analgesic efficacy between bilateral superficial and combined (superficial and deep) cervical plexus block administered before thyroid surgery. *Eur J Anaesthesiol.* 2009;26(12):1043−1047. https://doi.org/10.1097/EJA.0b013e32832d6913.

43. Yip L, Carty SE, Holder-Murray JM, et al. A specific enhanced recovery protocol de-creases opioid use after thyroid and parathyroid surgery. *Surgery.* 2021;169(1): 197−201. https://doi.org/10.1016/j.surg.2020.04.065.

44. Ganti A, Eggerstedt M, Grudzinski K, et al. Enhanced recovery protocol for transoral robotic surgery demonstrates improved analgesia and narcotic use reduction. *Am J Otolaryngol Head Neck Med Surg.* 2020;41(6):102649. https://doi.org/10.1016/j.amjoto.2020.102649.

45. Zhang Y, Liu D, Chen X, Ma J, Song X. An enhanced recovery programme improves the comfort and outcomes in children with obstructive sleep apnoea undergoing adenotonsillectomy: a retrospective historical control study. *Clin Otolaryngol.* 2021;46(1):249—255. https://doi.org/10.1111/coa.13655.

46. Tan JQ, Chen YB, Wang WH, Zhou SL, Zhou QL, Li P. Application of enhanced recovery after surgery in perioperative period of tympanoplasty and mastoidectomy. *Ear Nose Throat J.* 2020. https://doi.org/10.1177/0145561320928222.

47. Clark BS, Swanson M, Widjaja W, et al. ERAS for head and neck tissue transfer reduces opioid usage, peak pain scores, and blood utilization. *Laryngoscope.* 2021;131(3):E792—E799. https://doi.org/10.1002/lary.28768.

48. Low GMI, Kiong KL, Amaku R, et al. Feasibility of an Enhanced Recovery After Surgery (ERAS) pathway for major head and neck oncologic surgery. *Am J Otolaryngol Head Neck Med Surg.* 2020;41(6):102679. https://doi.org/10.1016/j.amjoto.2020.102679.

Index

225

Printed and bound by CPI Group (UK) Ltd, Croydon, CR0 4YY

03/10/2024

01040300-0001